THE COTA EXAMINATION REVIEW GUIDE

Caryn Johnson, MS, OTR/L, FAOTA
Fieldwork Coordinator
Department of Occupational Therapy
Thomas Jefferson University
Philadelphia, Pennsylvania

formerly
Fieldwork Coordinator
Occupational Therapy Assistant Program
Harcum College
Bryn Mawr, Pennsylvania

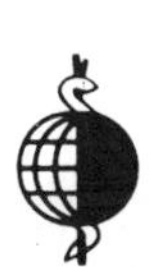

F.A. DAVIS COMPANY • Philadelphia

F.A. Davis Company
1915 Arch Street
Philadelphia, PA 19103
http://www.fadavis.com

Printed in the United States of America

Last digit indicates print number: 10 9 8 7 6 5 4 3 2

Publisher: Jean-François Vilain
Senior Editor: Lynn Borders Caldwell
Cover Designer: Louis J. Forgione

PREFACE

The purpose of this workbook is to give occupational therapy assistant students a general review of the profession and study tools to use while preparing to take the certification examination. It will also serve as an excellent review for occupational therapy assistants reentering the field or changing areas of practice.

The questions in this book are designed to facilitate study for the examination. While some have been written to simulate the exam, others have been written to maximize review of important content areas. The textbooks cited as references for most answers are those most commonly required for purchase by students in occupational therapy assistant programs across the United States. Because original sources may not be available to all students, we chose to cite books and journals to which most students have easy access. In this way, the COTA Examination Review Guide complements occupational therapy assistant curricula. In some cases we cite less well-known references because they provide the best rationales. Students can access these books through their own occupational therapy libraries or libraries of other occupational therapy or occupational therapy assistant programs. In addition, many of the books cited are available from the Wilma West Library at AOTA headquarters.

This workbook's format will encourage users to synthesize knowledge and become comfortable with the format of the National Board for Certification in Occupational Therapy (NBCOT) certification examination.

Please keep in mind that this workbook will not:

- be a comprehensive guide to practicing as an occupational therapy assistant,
- replicate the examination or any of the questions on the examination, or
- offer the student a guarantee of passing the examination.

This work book will:

- provide a general review of practice as an occupational therapy assistant,
- help readers identify the strengths and weaknesses in their knowledge of occupational therapy,
- acquaint the student with the format of questions used on the examination,
- help the student organize and set priorities for study time, and
- provide the student with a reference list from which further study may be pursued.

CONTRIBUTORS

Caryn Johnson, MS, OTR/L, FAOTA, served as Fieldwork Coordinator for the Occupational Therapy Assistant Program at Harcum College in Bryn Mawr, Pennsylvania, at the time this book was undertaken. She is currently Fieldwork Coordinator for the Occupational Therapy Program at Thomas Jefferson University in Philadelphia, where she has taught since 1983. Caryn received her Bachelor's Degree in Occupational Therapy from Tufts University in 1978 and an advanced Masters Degree in Occupational Therapy from Thomas Jefferson University in 1991. In addition, she is on the Board of Directors of the Pennsylvania Occupational Therapy Association and is president of Occupational Therapy Associates, a private practice specializing in aquatic rehabilitation.

Kerstin Potter, MA, OTR/L, has had a longstanding interest in the fields of teaching and pediatrics. She received her Bachelor's Degree in elementary education from Freiburg Teachers College in Germany in 1971 and a Masters Degree in Occupational Therapy from Boston University in 1977. As a clinician, she has enjoyed working with children in a wide range of settings. In 1984, she began teaching at Dominican College in NY, a program specifically designed for COTAs working to become OTRs. Kerstin is currently the Program Director at Harcum College in Bryn Mawr, Pennsylvania, where she continues to combine her interests in human development, occupational therapy, and COTA education. Kerstin also plays music and dances with a Renaissance performance group and develops and performs puppet shows emphasizing folk traditions and cultural awareness.

Debra N. Anderson, OTR, is the Administrative Director of Occupational Therapy at Frye Regional Medical Center in Hickory, North Carolina. She is the primary author of *The Occupational Therapy Examination Review Guide*.

Florence Hannes, OTR/L, is an Associate Professor at Orange Conty Community College in Middletown, New York, where she has been an OTA educator for the past 20 years. She is a senior member of the AOTA Accreditation Council for Occupational Therapy Education, representing technical level education, and a member of the Board of Directors of the Mental Health Association in Orange County. She is involved in promoting community-based occupational therapy programs. Flo maintains her own mental health as a stand-up comedienne. Her one-woman evening of comedy, "Conversations with a Jewish Mother," has received national acclaim.

Jolene Marie Jacobson, OTR, is a staff occupational therapist at the HealthSouth—Northern Kentucky Rehabilitation Hospital in Edgewood, Kentucky, where she is actively involved in COTA supervision. She received a Bachelor's Degree in Occupational Therapy from the University of Kansas in 1986 and is NDT certified.

Mary Kathryn Cowan, MA, OTR, FAOTA, is an Associate Professor of Occupational Therapy at the University of Texas—Pan American, a new program connected with the University of Texas—San Antonio Health Sciences Center. Mary earned her undergraduate degree in occupational therapy at the University of Minnesota and later completed a Master of Arts program in Educational Psychology at the same institution. She has worked clinically with children with all types of handicaps in public school and rehabilitation centers in Minnesota, Denmark, New Mexico, and Kentucky. She is certified in the Bobath Approach for the treatment of children with cerebral palsy and the administration and interpretation of the Southern California Sensory Integration and Praxis Tests. Mary's teaching experience includes the University of Illinois, University of Minnesota, the College of St. Catherine (in St. Paul, Minnesota), and Eastern Kentucky University. She has been recognized as a Fellow of the American Occupational Therapy Association.

Jean Steffan Smith, MS, OTR, was an Associate Professor in the Department of Occupational Therapy at Eastern Kentucky University.

ACKNOWLEDGMENTS

The input and enthusiasm of many individuals has made this book possible. I especially want to thank Lynn Borders Caldwell for her guidance and support and Debra Anderson for collaborating with me on the adaptation of her original book. I also want to express my sincere appreciation to Kerstin Potter for her organizational, collegial, and professional support and to Flo Hannes for her perserverence. My thanks also to the OTA students at Harcum College, for their input, and to Monifa Ferguson of FA Davis, for her significant contribution. My deepest thanks to my friends and family, for tolerating me while I lost myself to this project for the last year.

Finally, the following educators from Occupational Therapy Assistant educational programs across the country reviewed every question to make sure they are accurate and appropriate for the OTA student. Their work is greatly appreciated.

Roselyn Armstrong, MA, OTR
Department Chair
Occupational Therapy Assistant Program
Pitt Community College
Greenville, North Carolina

Deena Baenen, MA, LSW, OTA
Preceptor
Occupational Therapy Assistant Program
Cuyahoga Community College
Cleveland, Ohio

Rebecca R. Bahnke, OTR
Program Director
Occupational Therapy Assistant Program
Parkland College
Champaign, Illinois

Linda M. Barnes, MSEd, OTR
Associate Professor
Occupational Therapy Assistant Program
Pennsylvania College of Technology
Williamsport, Pennsylvania

Marilyn L. Blaisdell, MA, OTR
Assistant Professor/Fieldwork coordinator
Occupational Therapy Assistant Program
Becker College
Worcester, Massachusetts

Carol Davis, OTR
Program Director
Occupational Therapy Assistant Program
Riverland Community College
Austin, Minnesota

Edith Carter Fenton, MS, OTR
Program Coordinator and Associate Professor
Occupational Therapy Assistant Program
Becker College
Worcester, Massachusetts

Lynn Gitlow, MEd, OTR
Assistant Professor
Occupational Therapy Program
Lewiston–Auburn College
Lewiston, Maine

Liane Hewitt, MPH, OTR
Program Director
Occupational Therapy Assistant Program
Loma Linda University
Loma Linda, California

Patricia M. Holz, OTR
Instructor/Coordinator
Occupational Therapy Assistant Program
Fox Valley Technical College
Appleton, Wisconsin

Helen Nodzak, MOT, OTR
Director
Occupational Therapy Assistant Program
Soutwestern Community College
Sylva, North Carolina

Yvonne Parde, MS, OTR
Program Director
Occupational Therapy
Clarkson College
Omaha, Nebraska

Pat Pegels, MS, OTR
Professor
Erie Community College-North
Buffalo, New York

Helen M. Quarles, MS, OTR
Director
Occupational Therapy Assistant Program
Montana State University College of
Technology - Great Falls
Great Falls, Montana

Diane Sauter-Davis, OTR
Program Director
COTA Program
Kennebec Valley Technical College
Fairfield, Maine

CONTENTS

PREPARING FOR THE EXAMINATION

WHAT IS THE NBCOT EXAMINATION?

Successful completion of the certification examination is required for anyone who wants to practice as an occupational therapy assistant. Passing the National Board for Certification in Occupational Therapy (NBCOT) examination is the culmination of academic and fieldwork study. The examination tests the student's depth of knowledge. The questions require that the individual apply knowledge of occupational therapy or synthesize bits of knowledge to select the correct answer. The purpose of the examination is to identify those candidates who demonstrate entry-level competence for practicing as an occupational therapy assistant. Once candidates have successfully completed the examination, they are certified as occupational therapy assistants. The examination is given on the third Saturdays in March and September each year. Examinations are given for both certified occupational therapy assistant (COTA) and registered occupational therapist (OTR) candidates.

WHO CAN TAKE THE CERTIFICATION EXAMINATION?

The NBCOT oversees the certification examination and eligibility of candidates. Candidates must have graduated from an accredited occupational therapy assistant education program and successfully completed the required fieldwork by the day before the examination is to be given. Candidates are required to submit official transcripts from their occupational therapy assistant programs. After completing fieldwork and graduating from an accredited program, the candidate should take the exam the first or second time it is offered. Failure to do so means the forfeiture of one of the three opportunities to take the examination each candidate is allowed.

In cases where graduation is not scheduled until after the examination date, students must be cleared for graduation (both academically and financially) by the institution's registrar prior to the examination date. If complete official transcripts cannot be submitted, the student must have the "NBCOT Academic Credential Verification Form" completed by the registrar and submitted to the NBCOT. An official transcript must be submitted *no later* than 6 months after the date of the examination. Failure to do so may result in loss of certification.

Anyone seeking to take the examination who is not a recent graduate of an accredited US program must contact NBCOT for additional information. Internationally educated candidates must be screened by NBCOT to get approval to take the examination. Graduates who did not take the examination at the first opportunity and those who are taking the examination for a second or third time must meet additional requirements.

ABOUT THE NBCOT CANDIDATE HANDBOOK

Detailed and critical information is included in the NBCOT Candidate Handbook, which the candidate should read from cover to cover before completing the application form. Most schools provide students with a postcard to mail to NBCOT requesting the handbook and application to take the examination. If your school does not provide postcards, you can request the handbook and application by writing to NBCOT at: NBCOT Candidate Handbook, c/o Capital Fulfillment, PO Box 70, Waldorf, MD 20604-0070. You should include a self-addressed, pressure-sensitive label with your letter.

The handbook includes an application for the examination, a few examples of study questions, and general information regarding the examination. It also includes information on eligibility criteria, time tables, and information about test administration and scoring. Read this handbook thoroughly and save it until after you have received your test scores.

HOW TO APPLY FOR THE EXAMINATION

The fee for taking the examination is approximately $250. (Additional fees may be incurred by requesting a special test site, reports of scores to state regulatory agencies, or processing of a late application.) To avoid late fees, applications for the examination must be postmarked no later than December 15 for the March examination and June 15th for the September examination.

Candidates who do not receive the handbook may contact the NBCOT at (301) 990-7979. Upon receiving the application, NBCOT mails confirmation to the candidate. Candidates can send the application by certified mail to receive a "returned receipt" from the Post Office. Individuals from outside the United States must meet certain criteria and must be pre-screened by the NBCOT. Foreign candidates are required to successfully complete three English proficiency tests before taking the NBCOT examination.

There are more than 50 testing sites within the United States and approximately eight other sites in foreign countries, including Canada, China, England, India, and Israel.

WHAT IS THE FORMAT OF THE EXAMINATION?

The certification examination is composed of 200 multiple-choice questions that use the four-option format. No combination or "K" questions are used. Candidates have 4 hours to complete the examination. The questions for the examination are developed by the Certification Examination Development Committee. The group consists of content experts, both occupational therapists and occupational therapy assistants, from a variety of treatment settings accross the United States. A content outline for the certification examination was developed from the "National Study of the Profession of Occupational Therapy," a study published by the American Occupational Therapy Certification Board (now the NBCOT) in 1995. This approach provides a comprehensive overview of the service areas and issues pertaining to the practice of occupational therapy.

Every time the examination is given, a new set of questions is drawn from a "pool" or "item bank." The item banks for the OTR and COTA examinations are separate. The questions on each examination correspond to the content outline for either OTR or COTA candidates. The content outline specifies how many items should be asked for each major practice area. Each item has the same weight in scoring, and every question on the examination will have only one correct answer. There is not a penalty for guessing, so you should *never* leave a question unanswered. The raw scores of correct answers are statistically converted to a "scaled socre," which may range from 300 to 600 points. A scaled socre of 450 or more is required to pass the examination. The score does not actually reflect how many questions the candidate got right or wrong.

THE DAY OF THE EXAMINATION

Do you have the right date? The examination is offered the third Saturday in March and the third Saturday in September.

Bring your admission ticket.

Bring two forms of identification, including one photo ID.

Be on time. Registration starts at 8:00 am. You will not be admitted after 8:30.

Bring 3 sharpened No. 2 pencils and erasers. No other supplies or food are permitted.

Bring a watch to help you stay on schedule during the 4-hour test.

WHAT HAPPENS AFTER THE EXAMINATION?

Test results are mailed approximately 5 weeks after the certification examination. The percentage of students who pass the examination is usually 94% or higher. As previously stated, a score of 450 or higher is required to pass the certification examination. A grievance process is outlined in the NBCOT Handbook. The NBCOT tells program directors how many of their students have passed, but does not given them individual names. You may choose to tell your program director what your results are.

Candidates can request that results be sent to the licensing agency of the state(s) in which they will choose to practice. There is a $10 fee for each report you request—no reports are sent free of charge. Almost all states require a copy of the report. It is recommended that the candidate complete an application for state licensure before taking the examination. Often, these applications require a notarized copy of transcripts from an accredited occupational therapy assistant program, letters of reference, a picture identification, and so forth. Depending on the state licensure laws and facility requirements, COTAs may or may not be able to work with a temporary permit until examination results are received. Candidates should contact the licensing agency as soon as they know in which state they will be practicing. Candidates should learn as early as possible what information will be necessary for licensure and when applications should be submitted.

Candidates who fail the examination must retake the entire examination. Candidates may take the examination twice more, if necessary, provided they do so, each time, at the next possible opportunity. Each time the examination is offered, the score is counted in the attempt total, whether the candidate actually takes the examination or not. If, for example, you take the examination for the first time in March and fail, you only have two more chances to take the exam—the following September and then the following March. If you miss one of these, you cannot make it up.

HOW TO USE THIS WORKBOOK

This workbook has five complete sample tests of 200 questions that simulate the actual examination by asking questions in a four-option multiple-choice format. In addition, there is a section of test-taking tips. The "tips" help the reader identify his or her strengths and weaknesses and organize and set priorities for study time. The test-taking tips are followed by the five practice examinations. In the first four examinations, questions are grouped by practice areas, for example pediatrics, physical disabilities, psychosocial dysfunction, and service management and professional practice. Within the first three topic areas (pediatrics, physical disabilities, and psychosocial dysfunctions) the questions are divided among the following item areas:

14% Data Collection
17% Treatment Planning
20% Treatment Implementation
12% Evaluate the Treatment Plan
10% Discharge Planning.

The Service Management and Professional Practice topic areas are divided into two item areas:

13% Support Service Management
14% Promote Professional Practice

These areas are the same as those used by the NBCOT in the "content outline." The content outline, which specifies the percentage of questions to be asked for each major area of practice, is printed in the Candidate Handbook. Dividing each of the first four simulation examinations into these item areas enables the reader to focus on one area at a time. The final examination, Simulation Examination 5, mixes the topic areas, as does the actual examination. This arrangement is a bit more difficult in that it requires the reader to change topic and item areas frequently. This final examination enables the reader to evaluate how well he or she has retained and been able to implement the techniques recommended in this book. The mix of questions in each test covers the range of occupational therapy interventions, from referral through to discharge, thus providing a general review of the profession. A complete set of answers follows each examination. In order to help the student as much as possible, the workbook provides rationales for each answer, which explain why wrong answers are wrong and why the right answers are right. In addition, each answer provides the reader with a reference from which further information may be obtained on the subject matter. A complete bibliography including primary textbooks that the reader is likely to own is located after the final chapter.

WHERE TO BEGIN

Viewed as one task, preparing to take the examination can seem overwhelming. Breaking the process into smaller parts makes it easier to manage. The first step is to identify your areas of strength and weakness. The personal study plan chart shown in Tables 1 and 2 can help you through this process. Once you have completed this step, the second step is to complete your study plan. The final step is to pull all of the information together to take the practice examinations. It may be helpful to review the test-taking tips occasionally.

TEST-TAKING TIPS

Test-Taking Tip 1

Create a personal study plan. The question most frequently asked by occupational therapy assistant students preparing for the examination is "How do I start?" This guide will help you put all your educational preparation together and organize your study time. It will also make you comfortable with multiple-choice questions. All students preparing for the examination should have their course work at their fingertips, including books, notes, handouts, et cetera. Once you have assembled the stacks of information accumulated over the years, the question arises: "Where do I start?"

Complete Table 2 by defining you strengths and weaknesses. To do this, choose a main practice area and then go through all the component parts of that area. Classify the areas in which you are weakest as "A," and those in which you are strongest as "D." Assign "B" or "C," with "B" being weaker than "C," to the remaining practice areas. Within each letter grouping, identify the weakest subject with a number 1 and sequentially number through to the strongest subject.

Once this has been completed, your individualized studying needs have been organized and priorities set for accomplishment. The lower the number, the higher your study priority.

Now that you have set your priorities for studying, set target dates for completing your review of each area or subject. For instance, you may choose to work on the area of pediatrics during the month of March. Another individual may choose to review pediatric assessments the first week of March, developmental stages the second week of March, and so forth. Design your study plan to meet your needs. Set target dates that are realistic and attainable.

Now that the planning is complete, it is time for the study to begin. Start with the area listed as "A1" (high priority and need) and work your way through to the last "A." Once this is finished, continue with the "B" and "C" and "D" items. When all areas have been reviewed you may choose to begin again at A1 or to reset priorities for your studying needs. The easiest part of this task will be defining the time frame in which to study specific topics. The toughest challenge will be implementing the examination review plan!

Test-Taking Tip 2

Be prepared. The more prepared that you are to take the examination, the more comfortable you will feel during the examination. Preparation includes studying the knowledge base of occupational therapy, getting a good night's sleep, and bringing pencils to the examination. Once your studying is done, most of the preparation is complete. However, when asked to identify the single most important thing in preparing for the examination, a graduating class of students all agreed that the answer was getting a good night's sleep. Plan to arrive at the test site 20 to 30 minutes before the examination. Doing so will give you time to register and to get used to the environment. And remember, make sure you have three to four sharpened No. 2 pencils and an eraser.

Test-Taking Tip 3

Prepare your body as well as your mind! Eating a well-balanced breakfast can actually help your performance on the examination. A breakfast high in carbohydrates and low in fat will increase your energy and not produce a sluggish feeling. Avoid caffeine, because its ultimate effect will be to leave you tired and drowsy in the middle of the examination. Finally, wear comfortable clothes in layers to allow you to adjust as necessary to the temperature of the room.

Test-Taking Tip 4

Review the test packet briefly before starting the test. As you review the test booklet to verify that all of the test materials needed are provided, you will get a basic idea of the length of the test. If something is missing from the booklet, the error may be quickly corrected at the beginning of the examination and need not break your concentration.

Test-Taking Tip 5

Pace yourself. The test is to be completed within 4 hours. Within this time frame, you have to answer 200 multiple-choice questions. One technique for pacing the examination is to divide the test booklet into four equivalent sections mark each section by bending down the upper right corner of the first page in each section. You should aim to complete each of the four sections within 50 minutes to 1 hour. Understanding the format of the test and budgeting your time will help you work through the questions more efficiently and in the allotted time. Another pacing technique is to use a watch. This may be done one of two ways. The first method is to synchronize your watch with the clock being used by the individual administering the examination. At the end of every few pages of questions, briefly glance at your watch to keep an eye on your pace. If questions remain incomplete within the last 10 minutes of the examination, select one letter and fill in all of the remaining questions with that letter. *Remember, there is no penalty for guessing—only for leaving questions unanswered!* The second option is to wear a watch that can be set to signal on the hour. When the examination begins, set the watch for 12:00. Then you will know that at 4:00, the allotted time for taking the examination is up. Between 12:00 and 4:00, the watch will signal each hour, so that you can check your pace without having to "watch the clock." The goal is to complete at least 25% of the examination, or 50 questions, within each hour. Avoid wasting time by looking frequently at your watch.

Test-Taking Tip 6

Write as needed in the test booklet. It is permissible and often times helpful to write in the test booklet, crossing off answers as they are eliminated or circling logical answers. The key here is to mark the correct answer on the answer sheet after completing each question. Those who attempt to save time by writing the answers in the book and later transferring them to the answer sheet run the risk of making errors. These errors ultimately affect their score or their constructive use of time. For instance, a candidate may mark the correct answer, but in the wrong number on the answer sheet, resulting in a wrong answer. One way to avoid this is to avoid skipping any questions and answers in the test booklet or on the answer sheet. If you are uncertain of an answer, make the best logical guess and fill it in on the answer sheet. In general, you will be able to eliminate one or two of the incorrect answers. As an answer is eliminated, cross off the letter of the answer in the booklet. Again, there is no penalty for guessing, only for leaving questions unanswered!

Test-Taking Tip 7

When you use the same letter for more than three answers in a row, double check the questions to verify each answer. Test writers usually break up strings of four or more of the same letter or answer. The multiple-choice format is generally set so that three consecutive answers of the same letter is the maximum. If there are four or more of the same letters consecutively, it may be beneficial to recheck the answers. *Save this task for the end of the examination!*

Test-Taking Tip 8

Mark your answers clearly on the score sheet. Stray marks may invalidate answers. If the mark is too light, it may not be scanned appropriately by the scoring machine. If the mark is too big, it may be interpreted incorrectly as one of the adjacent letters. If you anticipate problems in this area, you can arrange to have the answer sheet scored by hand. There is an extra charge for this service, but it may make the difference between passing and failing the examination. Look at the following examples of correct and incorrect marking of answers.

22. Ⓐ Ⓑ Ⓒ ● Overmarking an answer.
23. Ⓐ ● Ⓒ Ⓓ Stray mark on answer sheet.
24. ● Ⓑ Ⓒ Ⓓ Incomplete marking of an answer.
25. Ⓐ Ⓑ ● Ⓓ Correct marking of an answer.

Test-Taking Tip 9

Use key techniques to help select the correct answer.

1. ***Follow your instincts when answering questions.*** The first answer chosen is usually the correct one. Change an answer only if you later realize that it is absolutely correct.
2. ***Ask, "What is this question about?"*** Try to decipher what the question is testing by selecting the key terms in the questions and not being distracted by peripheral information. By sorting through the information provided to identify what the question is testing, you may be more likely to select the correct answer.
3. **Anticipate the answer.** Many times you may anticipate an answer while reading a question. If so, look for the anticipated answer among the options. However, it is important to read and consider all of the options to verify that the anticipated answer is the correct answer.
4. ***Use logical reasoning.*** A commonly used technique is the process of deduction—eliminating answers that are incorrect. Doing this allows you to concentrate on the options that remain. (You are allowed to cross off answers in the test booklet as you eliminate them.)

Table 1. EXAMPLE OF COMPLETED CERTIFICATION EXAMINATION STUDY PLAN

	PEDIATRICS	PHYSICAL DISABILITIES	PSYCHOSOCIAL DYSFUNCTION
Data Collection			
Obtain/review background information	D/18	D/4	D/5
Interview techniques	D/19	D/5	D/6
Observation of performance	A/15	D/6	D/7
Knowledge and administration of nonstandardized tests with supervision	B/3	C/5	A/4
Knowledge and administration of standardized tests with supervision	B/4	C/6	A/5
Report data collected to OTR	C/13	C/7	C/17
Document using appropriate terminology	A/11	A/7	A/6
Uniform terminology	D/17	D/1	C/18
Using activities for assessment	D/16	D/3	C/19
Medical terminology	D/15	D/2	D/8
Treatment Planning			
Developing short-term goals	D/14	D/7	D/1
Developing long-term goals	A/14	D/8	D/2
Activity analysis	D/13	D/9	D/9
Familiarity with media and methods	C/14	D/10	D/4
Activity selection to address goals	C/15	C/8	C/16
Grading treatment activities	C/16	C/9	C/15
Adapting process, tools, and environment	D/12	C/10	C/14
Documentation	B/9	A/5	A/3
Components of a treatment plan	D/20	B/6	B/11
Normal/abnormal development	D/11	A/6	A/7
Team members	C/10	C/4	C/13

Table 1. *(continued)*

	PEDIATRICS	PHYSICAL DISABILITIES	PSYCHOSOCIAL DYSFUNCTION
Treatment Implementation			
Use of low- and high-tech activity	C/11	C/11	C/1
Physical management and positioning	A/13	B/7	C/2
Functional mobility training	B/10	B/8	C/3
Assistive devices and adaptive equipment	B/11	B/9	C/12
ADL training	D/10	D/11	D/3
Splinting	A/6	A/4	A/8
Precautions and contraindications	C/12	C/3	B/1
Compensatory techniques (work simplification and energy conservation)	B/12	B/10	B/9
Group formats and group development	A/7	A/8	A/9
Group activities and group process	B/8	B/5	A/10
Instructional methods	B/14	B/4	B/10
Sensory activities	B/13	C/13	C/7
Motor activities	B/9	C/14	C/8
Perceptual activities	C/17	C/15	C/9
Cognitive activities	C/18	C/16	C/10
Psychosocial activities	C/19	C/17	C/11
Verbal and nonverbal communication techniques	C/20	C/12	C/4
Evaluation of Treatment			
Recognizing and responding to individuals' responses to treatment	C/8	C/18	C/6
Knowledge of expected outcomes of various treatments	C/9	C/2	C/5
Modifying the treatment plan	B/15	B/3	B/8

Table 1. *(continued)*

	PEDIATRICS	PHYSICAL DISABILITIES	PSYCHOSOCIAL DYSFUNCTION
Documenting change	A/9	A/2	A/2
SOAP notes and other documentation formats	A/8	A/1	A/1
Discharge Planning			
Community resources	B/1	B/11	B/5
Identifying post-discharge needs	B/2	B/12	B/2
Discharge documentation	D/6	A/3	B/3
Discharge planning process	B/7	B/1	B/4
Developing home programs	C/7	C/1	B/7
Patient/family/caregiver training	C/6	B/2	B/6

	PROFESSIONAL PRACTICE AND SERVICE MANAGEMENT
Referral process	D/4
Policies and procedures	D/3
Quality assurance and program evaluation	C/4
Emergency and safety procedures and infection control	C/5
Supervision	D/5
Insurance, billing, and reimbursement	A/5
Use of aides and volunteers	C/3
Code of Ethics	B/6
Standards of practice	A/10
State regulation of OT practice	A/3
Liability and malpractice issues	A/4

	PROFESSIONAL PRACTICE AND SERVICE MANAGEMENT
Changes and trends in OT practice	A/3
Professional behavior	C/2
Fieldwork and student supervision	C/1
Service competency	B/5
COTA/OTR role delineation	D/7
OT history	D/1
Legislative actions affecting OT	A/2
Roles of AOTA and NBCOT	A/1
Maintaining supplies and equipment	D/8

Table 2. CERTIFICATION EXAMINATION STUDY PLAN

	PEDIATRICS	PHYSICAL DISABILITIES	PSYCHOSOCIAL DYSFUNCTION
Data Collection			
Obtain/review background information			
Interview techniques			
Observation of performance			
Knowledge and administration of nonstandardized tests with supervision			
Knowledge and administration of standardized tests with supervision			
Report data collected to OTR			
Document using appropriate terminology			
Uniform terminology			
Using activities for assessment			
Medical terminology			
Treatment Planning			
Developing short-term goals			
Developing long-term goals			
Activity analysis			
Familiarity with media and methods			
Activity selection to address goals			
Grading treatment activities			
Adapting process, tools, and environment			
Documentation			
Components of a treatment plan			
Normal/abnormal development			
Team members			

Table 2. *(continued)*

	PEDIATRICS	PHYSICAL DISABILITIES	PSYCHOSOCIAL DYSFUNCTION
Treatment Implementation			
Use of low- and high-tech activity			
Physical management and positioning			
Functional mobility training			
Assistive devices and adaptive equipment			
ADL training			
Splinting			
Precautions and contraindications			
Compensatory techniques (work simplification and energy conservation)			
Group formats and group development			
Group activities and group process			
Instructional methods			
Sensory activities			
Motor activities			
Perceptual activities			
Cognitive activities			
Psychosocial activities			
Verbal and nonverbal communication techniques			
Evaluation of Treatment			
Recognizing and responding to individuals' responses to treatment			
Knowledge of expected outcomes of various treatments			
Modifying the treatment plan			

Table 2. *(continued)*

	PEDIATRICS	PHYSICAL DISABILITIES	PSYCHOSOCIAL DYSFUNCTION
Documenting change			
SOAP notes and other documentation formats			
Discharge Planning			
Community resources			
Identifying post-discharge needs			
Discharge documentation			
Discharge planning process			
Developing home programs			
Patient/family/caregiver training			

	PROFESSIONAL PRACTICE AND SERVICE MANAGEMENT
Referral process	
Policies and procedures	
Quality assurance and program evaluation	
Emergency and safety procedures and infection control	
Supervision	
Insurance, billing, and reimbursement	
Use of aides and volunteers	
Code of Ethics	
Standards of practice	
State regulation of OT practice	
Liability and malpractice issues	

	PROFESSIONAL PRACTICE AND SERVICE MANAGEMENT
Changes and trends in OT practice	
Professional behavior	
Fieldwork and student supervision	
Service competency	
COTA/OTR role delineation	
OT history	
Legislative actions affecting OT	
Roles of AOTA and NBCOT	
Maintaining supplies and equipment	

As you complete the questions in the book, remember these techniques and practice using them when you have difficulty answering a question.

Test-Taking Tip 10

Read the questions before reading a case history. Reading the questions first will prepare your mind to seek out the answers while reading the selection. A small percentage of questions on the examination are grouped with case histories. Try your skills with this in the following case history and three questions.

Case History

Mrs. P is a 49-year-old white female who was referred to occupational therapy for evaluation. In the initial assessment, Mrs. P's right upper extremity was flaccid, passive range of motion was within normal limits for the elbow and hand, but the shoulder was limited to 90 degrees of pain-free shoulder flexion. A subluxation of one-and-a-half fingers width was noted. Mrs. P. had absent sensation for hot and cold, light touch, and sharp and dull. She required moderate assistance to stand at a table.

Based on this information, answer the following questions:

1. **What performance components were assessed in the above scenario?**
   A. Visual perceptual.
   B. Cognition
   C. Pyschosocial.
   D. Sensorimotor.

2. **The best way for the COTA to position Mrs. P's right arm is:**
   A. with a sling.
   B. on a lap tray
   C. on the armrest of the wheelchair
   D. resting in her lap.

3. **During meal-preparation activities, Mrs. P:**
   A. should protect her right upper extremity from injury.
   B. may use the right upper extremity for a functional assist.
   C. will tend to ignore items on her right side.
   D. will experience enhanced role performance.

The answers are as follows:

1. (D) Sensorimotor. Because both active and passive movement were assessed as well as sensation, the correct answer is sensorimotor. Based on the information given, areas involving memory, problem solving, concentration, visual tracking, visual discrimination, and figure ground were not assessed. Thus answers A and C are incorrect. Answer B is also incorrect because information regarding the individual's living situation, roles, and interests were not documented, as would be seen in a psychosocial assessment. See reference: AOTA: Uniform terminology.

2. (B) on a lap tray. A lap tray provides the safest position for the flaccid upper extremity. It supports the arm in a position that can prevent the force of gravity from causing subluxation and that prevents the arm from falling off the wheelchair during wheelchair mobility. Slings (answer A) place the arm in a position that may increase tone and discourage use. A flaccid arm placed on the armrest of a wheelchair (answer C) is likely to fall off and be bruised. An unsupported flaccid arm resting in the lap (Answer D) can lead to increased pain, subluxation, and deformity. See reference: Pedretti (ed): Davis, JZ: Neurodevelopmental treatment of the adult hemiplegia: The Bobath approach.

3. (A) should protect her right upper extremity from injury. A flaccid, insensate upper extremity is prone to injury and should be protected from sharp tools and hot surfaces during meal-preparation activities. With no tone or functional movement, Mrs. P would not be able to use her RUE as a functional assist (answer B). Nothing in the note indicated that Mrs. P had a right side neglect (answer C) or that the role of cook (answer D) was one of her previous roles. See reference: Pedretti (ed): Foti, D, and Pedretti, L. W., and Lille, S: Activities of daily living.

Answers to questions provide the student with an explanation for the correct selection. In addition, references are listed so that students may obtain further information for study. References are listed by author of the book, followed by the chapter author(s), and chapter title of the work referenced. To find the book title, simply cross-reference the book author with the bibliography at the end of this book.

The tips provided here are not an exhaustive list of what individuals have found to be useful in preparing examinations. You may have developed some of your own techniques that have proven successful. Select only the tips that feel comfortable to you, and practice using these techniques as you work through this book.

BIBLIOGRAPHY

National Board for Certification in Occupational Therapy, Inc: NBCOT 1997 Candidate Handbook. The National Board for Certification in Occupational Therapy, Gaithersburg, MD, 1997.

AOTCB Information Exchange. The American Occupational Therapy Certification Board (now NBCOT), Gaithersburg, Maryland, Winter 1994.

Gronlund, N: How to Construct Achievement Tests. Prentice-Hall, Englewood Cliffs, NJ, 1987.

Martinson, T: SuperCourse for the GMAT, ed 3, Prentice-Hall, New York, 1991.

Millman, J and Pauk, P: How to Take Tests. McGraw-Hill, New York, 1969.

Robinson, A and Katzman, J: The Princeton Review: Cracking the GRE 1997. Villard Books, New York, 1997.

McFadden S. and Woodbridge, E: Certification. OT Week's Today's Student. The American Occupational Therapy Association, Bethesda, MD, Spring 1995.

SIMULATION EXAMINATION 1

Directions: Circle the correct answer to the following questions. When you have completed this examination, check your answers against the answer key that follows. As you will see, an explanation is given for each answer along with a reference for further study: the book author is listed as well as the chapter author. See the bibliography for complete references. Study the areas in which your comprehension was low, then test yourself again by taking Simulation Examination 2.

PEDIATRIC QUESTIONS

Data Collection

1. The purpose of screening a child who has been referred to occupational therapy is to:
A. obtain necessary information for an occupational therapy consultation with teachers/parents.
B. test a wide variety of developmental behaviors.
C. establish an information base for the occupational therapy treatment plan.
D. determine the need for further occupational therapy evaluation.

2. A COTA is working with an infant and observes the presence of the first stage of voluntary grasp. This would be noted as:
A. radial palmar.
B. pincer.
C. ulnar palmar.
D. palmar.

3. The BEST method to find out more about deficits in performance areas in a 3-year-old with cerebral palsy is a:
A. standardized test of motor development.
B. review of the medical record.
C. developmental screening test.
D. home visit and interview with the parents.

4. When observing a child with spastic diplegia, the COTA would anticipate involvement in the following areas:
A. both upper extremities
B. both lower extremities.
C. lower extremities, trunk, and mild upper extremities.
D. both upper extremities and both lower extremities

5. When interviewing the parents of a 1-year-old client, the COTA obtains information by asking a certain number of prepared questions, which she adheres to closely. This type of interview is called:
A. semistructured.
B. structured.
C. criterion-referenced.
D. open-ended.

6. When collecting data through skilled observation of a 4-year-old with autism, the COTA should focus attention on:
A. gross and fine motor development.
B. muscle tone.
C. perceptual skills.
D. ability to relate to others.

7. The COTA administers an Interest Checklist to a newly referred 13-year-old with a diagnosis of conduct disorder. The checklist consists of 30 questions assembled by the OTR to reflect current interests of local teenagers. This type of assessment is classified as:
A. normative.
B. structured.
C. unstructured.
D. projective.

8. The COTA observes the dressing skills of a 5-year-old girl. She is able to put on a jacket, zip the zipper, and tie a knot in the draw string but needs verbal cuing to tie a bow. The COTA determines that the child's dressing skills are:
A. age appropriate.
B. delayed.
C. advanced.
D. limited.

9. When reporting the results of a dressing assessment of an 8-year-old with developmental dyspraxia, the COTA should focus on the following information:

A. social skills, frustration tolerance, motivation.
B. ability to follow verbal directions, attention span.
C. age appropriateness, functionality of skills, family priorities.
D. need for adaptations such as zipper pulls and Velcro closures.

10. The COTA greets her 6-year-old client with autism: "Good morning, Daniel!" The little boy responds: "Morning, Daniel!" The correct term for this behavior is:
A. rigidity.
B. echolalia.
C. learned helplessness.
D. nystagmus.

Treatment Planning

11. Occupational therapy practitioners can contribute their assessment and planning information to an "Individual Educational Plan" or IEP. The setting in which an IEP is used as the central plan for a child is a(n):
A. rehabilitation center.
B. public school system.
C. outpatient care center.
D. home health agency.

12. The MOST important items to include in the goals and objectives for a child's occupational therapy program are:
A. the child's priorities.
B. the priorities of the parents or caregivers.
C. solution to the problems identified in the occupational therapy evaluation.
D. child, caregiver, and therapist priorities.

13. An ultralight wheelchair would be appropriate for a child with the following functional needs:
A. sliding transfers.
B. desk work.
C. wheeling efficiency.
D. work surface height adjustment.

14. The early intervention team discusses with the family an IFSP for a 4-month-old child with multiple congenital malformations. "IFSP" stands for:
A. infant and family social program.
B. individual family service plan.
C. initial facilitation and schooling program.
D. intervention for families of special populations.

15. A COTA is working with a 7-year-old child with mild spastic cerebral palsy. The evaluation has shown the therapist that the child has poor in-hand manipulation skills. What type of activity would BEST develop this ability?
A. Grasping blocks to build a building.
B. Placing pegs from one pegboard to another.
C. Carrying a bag of Lego blocks with a handle.
D. Removing a nut from a bolt.

16. The IEP for a child in a special needs preschool lists development of kindergarten readiness skills as a primary goal. The MAIN focus of the COTA will therefore be on facilitating:
A. a dynamic tripod grasp.
B. mature use of scissors.
C. an adequate attention span.
D. independent shoe tying.

17. A 12-year-old girl with behavior problems has difficulty with peer interactions. The MOST important factor to incorporate into her treatment plan is:
A. provide activities in an authoritarian environment.
B. allow her the opportunity to develop basic social skills on her own.
C. provide enjoyable activities in a safe and accepting environment.
D. establish rules for group play.

18. The long-term goal for a 7-year-old with fine motor delay has been formulated as follows: "Linda will exhibit a mature pencil grasp using wrist and finger movement to control writing." A relevant short-term goal would be: "Within 2 weeks, Linda will demonstrate improved:
A. eye-hand coordination, by maintaining visual focus on the pencil for 30 seconds."
B. shape recognition skills, by matching five out of five shapes with 100% accuracy."
C. elbow and wrist stability, by wheelbarrow-walking ten steps while being held at the knees."
D. hand-to-mouth patterns, by spoon feeding herself apple sauce without spilling."

19. Juan has poor postural stability because of reduced muscle tone. A good activity to promote beginning antigravity control is:
A. pull-to-sit, leaning back against therapy ball.
B. prone scooter obstacle course.
C. hippity-hop races.
D. batting a balloon while Juan is suspended in net.

20. Angela has poor visual attention, which affects her school work. To increase her visual attention, the COTA recommends the following:
A. increase competing sensory input— work with lively background music.
B. increase competing visual input—work against a patterned background.
C. reduce competing sensory input—use headphones during work.
D. reduce visual input—use dim lighting.

21. For a group of preadolescents with behavior management problems, an effective way of promoting adherence to rules and a sense of self-management is to:

A. use aversive consequences (take away privileges) for breaking rules.
B. ignore transgressions consistently.
C. enlist the help of families to enforce rules.
D. involve the children in the rule-making process.

22. The COTA is working with a 19-year-old man receiving a wheelchair for the first time. The MOST important habit for the COTA to work with him on developing is:
A. performing regular weight shifts.
B. using wheelchair gloves.
C. keeping wheelchair speed moderate.
D. avoiding sandy surfaces.

Treatment Implementation

23. The COTA sets up an unstructured obstacle course for a child. Which type of play does this exemplify?
A. Exploratory.
B. Symbolic.
C. Creative.
D. Recreational.

24. When teaching children with moderate mental retardation to feed, groom, and dress themselves, the following method is the MOST effective:
A. forward and backward chaining.
B. practice and repetition.
C. demonstration.
D. role-modeling.

25. A COTA is using an adaptive device to support a child during functional mobility in creeping. This is helpful for the developmental and mobility experience. A disadvantage to using it, however, is that:
A. transitional movements to sitting are restricted.
B. leg movements are restricted.
C. arm movements are restricted.
D. weight bearing is restricted.

26. The COTA is demonstrating to a parent how to bathe a child with hypertonicity. Which of the following approaches should be employed?
A. Avoid using adaptive equipment.
B. Provide few explanations of procedure.
C. Handle the child slowly and gently.
D. Stand and lean over the tub to support and wash the child.

27. A first grader has difficulty with handwriting skills, resulting from poor finger isolation. The MOST appropriate activity for the COTA to recommend is:
A. crayon drawing on sandpaper.
B. copying shapes from the blackboard.
C. rolling out Play Doh with a rolling pin.
D. picking up raisins with a pair of tweezers.

28. A 10-year-old child with multiple handicaps who is functioning at a low cognitive level needs to work on self-feeding skills. Of the following approaches, which would provide the MOST support for learning this skill?
A. Physical guidance.
B. Verbal cues.
C. Visual cues.
D. Forward chaining.

29. Joey is a 3-year-old with spastic diplegia. Of the following, which mobility device is MOST appropriate for assisting Joey with exploration in space?
A. A prone scooter.
B. An airplane mobility device.
C. A tricycle.
D. A power wheelchair.

30. Leroy has difficulty self-feeding, as a result of abnormal muscle tone. When discussing mealtime with his parents the COTA should address which issue first?
A. The type of chair he should sit in.
B. The foods he should be served.
C. The utensils he should use.
D. The place where his meals should be served.

31. Joanne has difficulty controlling food in her mouth when swallowing. Which foods should the COTA recommend to the parents when helping plan snacks?
A. Chicken noodle soup.
B. Peanut butter.
C. Carrot sticks.
D. Applesauce.

32. Mikey is in second grade. His hydrocephalus is treated with a ventricular-peritoneal shunt to relieve cerebrospinal fluid pressure. On School Sports Day, which relay race should he be advised NOT to participate in?
A. Three-legged race (partner race with one leg tied to partner).
B. Egg walk (balancing a raw egg on a spoon while walking).
C. Wheelbarrow race (walking on hands, held at knees by teacher).
D. Dribbling race (dribble basketball to goal and back).

33. Jamie is in fourth grade and has a diagnosis of attention deficit disorder (ADD) as well as perceptual deficits. The activity that would MOST successfully train for visual attention is:
A. playing a game of "Memory" in which images are matched from memory.
B. assembling a 200-piece puzzle.

C. finding "Waldo" against a complex visual background.
D. blowing cotton balls into a target.

34. Connie is 13-years old and has a diagnosis of athetoid cerebral palsy. She would like to be able to dress herself independently. The COTA recommends looking for the following features when Connie selects clothing:
A. Mini Tees made of elasticized fabric.
B. dresses with side zippers and zipper pulls.
C. oversized tee shirts and elastic-top pants.
D. shirts with front closures, such as snaps or large buttons.

35. A 12-year-old girl with juvenile rheumatoid arthritis demonstrates hand weakness. Which of the following pieces of adaptive equipment would be MOST effective in preventing hand fatigue?
A. Reacher.
B. Jar opener.
C. Pencil gripper.
D. Plate guard.

Evaluation of the Treatment Plan

36. Although her lower extremities are correctly positioned, Kim, a child with cerebral palsy, tends to flex forward while riding her adapted tricycle. The adaptation that would BEST enable her to maintain a more upright position is:
A. raising the seat height.
B. raising the handlebars.
C. lowering the seat height.
D. lowering the handlebars.

37. After many months of therapy, a 3-year-old child with Down syndrome has begun to demonstrate protective reactions when falling to either side. What type of arm movements have been facilitated?
A. Flexion.
B. Extension.
C. Internal rotation.
D. External rotation.

38. Ida is 4 years old and is attending a special needs preschool. Her teacher reports that Ida is very motivated to use the scissors but cannot cut on a line yet. The COTA recommends that she practice:
A. cutting out a circle first.
B. cutting thinner paper.
C. snipping the edge of a paper ("making fringes").
D. cutting with her other hand.

39. Michelle is a 5-year-old with developmental delay. She is working on bilateral hand skills and has just learned to bring her hands to midline for clapping. The COTA decides to promote Michelle's great love of music as well as her bilateral development by recommending playing the following instrument as the next step:
A. bells on wrist straps worn on both hands.
B. a drum held in one hand with the drumstick in the other.
C. a set of cymbals.
D. a toy piano played with both hands.

40. Sebastian is 4 years old and is just beginning to develop independent play skills. He had come to the preschool afraid to touch any toys or get involved with the other children. The COTA observes Sebastian as he tries to place a triangular block in the square hole of a puzzle box by pressing harder to make it fit. To further promote the development of his play skills, she:
A. hands him the correct block to promote a successful experience.
B. acknowledges his efforts and encourages his active experimentation.
C. verbally explains his difficulties to him to promote problem analysis.
D. provides him with an easier toy to avoid his getting frustrated.

41. Chuck is 12 years old and has a history of traumatic brain injury. He is relearning to prepare simple foods but has been having difficulties with sequencing. Using a chart, he has just learned to prepare his favorite sandwich without "losing his place" in the process. He does, however, continue to need occasional verbal reminders to look at the chart for the next step and to ensure safety. The COTA documents his MOST recent level of independence as:
A. independent.
B. independent with setup.
C. supervision.
D. minimal assist.

42. Ricardo is 12 years old and has a diagnosis of spastic cerebral palsy. He has responded with great enthusiasm to the introduction of computer-assisted learning. Although he is making significant progress in written communication, he complains of general fatigue, body aches, and eye strain. Based on this information, which of the following areas would the COTA reassess FIRST?
A. The time he spends at the computer.
B. The size of the computer screen.
C. The challenge level of the learning program.
D. His control of the keyboard.

43. The COTA is monitoring use of a static wrist splint for a 12-year-old girl with juvenile rheumatoid arthritis. The PRIMARY purpose of the splint is to:
A. inhibit hypertonus.
B. increase range of motion.

C. prevent deformity.
D. correct deformity.

Discharge Planning

Questions 44 and 45 pertain to this case study:

Matthew, 5 years old, is diagnosed with autism and is being discharged to a school program for children with severe emotional impairments.

44. A preparatory vestibular activity should be used in the classroom to decrease his level of arousal so that he will be able to concentrate on simple activities. The MOST appropriate activity would be:
A. bouncing while sitting on a large therapy ball.
B. manual rocking while in prone on a therapy ball.
C. spinning in supine while on a hammock swing.
D. rolling down a large wedge.

45. Which of the following is MOST important to include in Matthew's discharge summary?
A. Matthew should participate in preparatory vestibular activities to enable him to concentrate on simple activities.
B. Matthew will demonstrate the ability to concentrate on simple activities for 5 minutes, three out of five attempts.
C. Matthew states he enjoys parachute activities.
D. Matthew's parents indicate he has difficulty concentrating on simple activities.

46. Ross is a 9-year old with a diagnosis of mental retardation. He has been receiving occupational therapy to become independent in dressing and feeding and is now being discharged. The BEST advice for the COTA to give his parents in order to maintain Ross's independence in dressing at home is:
A. give assistance to Ross when he asks for it to provide a success experience.
B. give praise for completed dressing; do not help him get dressed.
C. give him oversize clothing with Velcro closures and large snaps.
D. give him verbal prompts when needed and help with closures only.

47. The COTA is providing information to the OTR concerning readiness for discharge of a 5-year-old preschooler with mild developmental delay. The MOST important information for the COTA to focus on is:
A. independence in dressing.
B. improved socialization and impulse control.
C. attainment of kindergarten readiness skills.
D. independence in toileting.

48. A COTA and OTR are planning for the discharge of a 2-year-old from an early intervention program. What advice to the parents will MOST likely result in effective carryover of a therapeutic home program?
A. Set aside a certain time daily to focus on therapeutic activities.
B. Incorporate therapeutic activities into family routines.
C. Provide therapeutic activities on an as-needed basis.
D. Do therapeutic activities daily, but vary the time of day.

49. What extracurricular activity should a COTA recommend for a 12-year-old who will be discharged after having received treatment for anxiety disorder?
A. Competitive gymnastics team.
B. Debating club.
C. School newspaper.
D. Basketball team.

50. A COTA is discharge planning with the family of a 3-year-old with developmental delay. What toys would the COTA recommend to promote beginning symbolic play?
A. Busy box, nesting toys, blocks.
B. Board games.
C. Craft kits.
D. Doll house, dress-up clothes.

PHYSICAL DISABILITY QUESTIONS

Data Collection

51. An individual who had a myocardial infarction (MI) has been transferred from acute care to a rehabilitation unit. During the initial interview, he displays good memory of information processed before the MI but poor recall of the period spent in the acute facility. He is able to recall information since the transfer. The COTA should document this as:
A. impaired orientation.
B. impaired long-term memory.
C. anterograde amnesia.
D. retrograde amnesia.

Questions 52-54 pertain to this case study:

Mrs. B is a 79-year-old woman with RA. The COTA is contributing to the initial evaluation by performing a functional assessment of her upper extremities.

52. The COTA observes that Mrs. B has limited internal rotation when she is unable to touch:
A. the back of her neck.
B. the top of her head.

C. her lower back.
D. her opposite shoulder.

53. Mrs. B also demonstrates functional limitations in shoulder abduction and external rotation. She is MOST likely to have difficulty with:
A. buttoning her shirt.
B. combing her hair.
C. tucking in her shirt in the back.
D. tying shoelaces.

54. The COTA notes AROM is limited to slightly less than 90 degrees of shoulder flexion. While in this position, Mrs. B is able to tolerate moderate resistance. The COTA observes PROM to be the same as AROM. The patient's manual muscle test score would be:
A. normal (5).
B. good (4).
C. fair (3).
D. fair minus (3-).

55. An individual with arthritis has a total range of shoulder flexion from 0 to 90 degrees. During manual muscle testing of the pain-free range, the individual is able to take moderate resistance. The individual's manual muscle grade is:
A. poor.
B. fair.
C. good.
D. normal.

56. The COTA asks an individual to repeat a list of random numbers 1 minute after hearing the list. This would be accurately documented as which performance component?
A. Short-term memory.
B. Attention.
C. Hearing.
D. Orientation.

57. An alert, motivated individual who had a cerebral vascular accident affecting the parietal lobe is unable to learn compensation techniques for neglect after many ADL training sessions. The COTA would document this condition as:
A. a visual field cut.
B. apraxia.
C. aphasia.
D. anosognosia.

58. The COTA has been assigned to administer part of a sensory evaluation to a newly admitted patient who has experienced a CVA. The purpose of the sensory evaluation is to determine the degree of impairment in all of the following areas EXCEPT:
A. light touch.
B. temperature.
C. shoulder subluxation.
D. proprioception.

59. A COTA is assessing hand function in a man with arthritis by observing him as he makes a peanut butter sandwich. The individual is unable to remove the lid from a 28-ounce peanut butter jar but is able to stand at the counter, spread peanut butter on bread with a knife, and replace the lid when he has finished making the sandwich. The COTA would recognize this as a deficit in:
A. range of motion.
B. coordination.
C. endurance.
D. strength.

60. A young mother with rheumatoid arthritis has difficulty managing home and child-care responsibilities. The BEST interview for the COTA to use to obtain information about how this young mother spends and manages her time is the:
A. Role Checklist.
B. Activity Configuration.
C. Interest Checklist.
D. Occupational History Interview.

Treatment Planning

61. While completing the assessment and treatment planning process, the OTR and COTA confer with the individual to establish program goals. These goals should be:
A. specific measurable statements with time frames.
B. time frames for what will be accomplished.
C. specific measurements of the individual's skill/performance.
D. activities to be completed that correspond with the goals and objectives.

62. Proper use of body mechanics when lifting objects from the floor would be a primary goal for individuals who have:
A. chronic obstructive pulmonary disease.
B. fibromyalgia.
C. carpal tunnel syndrome.
D. low back pain.

Questions 63-65 pertain to this case study:

Maggie is a deconditioned 60-year-old woman with diabetes and a history of cardiac disease. She lives alone and is planning on returning home. The COTA is working with her to increase standing tolerance and UE strength and endurance. Maggie is looking forward to a visit from her granddaughter, whose birthday is tomorrow.

63. The COTA would like to plan an endurance activity in which Maggie can work, seated, on grasp and release for 5 minutes. She is interested in

baking something for her granddaughter's birthday. The MOST appropriate activity is:

A. blueberry muffins mixed from scratch with a hand-powered mixer and scooped into muffin tins with a cup.
B. an angel-food cake from a box mix using an electric mixer and pouring the mix into a pan.
C. cold chocolate-chip cookie dough mixed using a spatula with a built-up handle and dropping dollops onto a tray using an ice cream scoop.
D. sugar cookies sliced from a roll of dough at room temperature and placed on a tray using a spatula.

64. Maggie's long-term goal is to prepare three meals a week. The MOST relevant short-term goal would focus on:

A. energy conservation.
B. work hardening.
C. standing tolerance.
D. safety in the kitchen.

65. Maggie has opted to make a macramé planter as a way of increasing her standing tolerance. The MOST important factor for the COTA to take into consideration is the:

A. length of the cords Maggie will start with.
B. thickness of the cords Maggie will be using.
C. texture of the cords Maggie will be using.
D. type of surface Maggie will be standing on.

66. A COTA working in a hand center is implementing a desensitization program with an individual following an injury. The MOST appropriate way for the COTA to grade the stimuli used in the program is from:

A. soft to hard to rough.
B. tapping to rubbing to touching.
C. light to medium to heavy.
D. rough to hard to soft.

67. A COTA works with a 16-year old boy with C5 quadriplegia at lunchtime each day to develop independence in feeding. Which type of equipment would be MOST appropriate for this individual?

A. A wrist-driven flexor hinge splint.
B. A mobile arm support.
C. An electric self-feeder.
D. Utensils with built-up handles.

68. A long-term goal for Mrs. J. following a hip arthroplasty is independence in lower-extremity dressing. A related short-term goal would be:

A. "Mrs. J. will increase standing tolerance to 10 minutes."
B. "Mrs. J. will increase hip flexion to 90 degrees."
C. "Mrs. J. will demonstrate appropriate hip precautions."
D. "Mrs. J. will apply energy-conservation techniques during dressing activities."

69. A COTA provides a leather-working activity to a man with a C7 spinal cord injury. The aspect of the activity that requires the GREATEST degree of fine motor coordination is:

A. lacing with a whipstitch.
B. punching holes for lacing with a rotary hole-punch.
C. lacing with a double cordovan stitch.
D. measuring and cutting the exact length of leather lacing.

70. A COTA is working with a group of individuals with Parkinson's disease in an aquatic exercise program. The three performance components MOST important for successfully walking across the pool are:

A. strength, fine motor coordination, and kinesthesia.
B. visual motor integration, postural control, and gross motor coordination.
C. vestibular processing, postural control, and muscle tone.
D. range of motion, praxis, and crossing the midline.

71. The COTA is working on sequencing skills with a young woman who is s/p TBI. The activity that would BEST address this goal is:

A. leather stamping using tools in a random design.
B. stringing beads for a necklace, following a pattern.
C. putting together a 20-piece puzzle.
D. playing "Concentration," a card-matching game.

72. An individual with a C6 spinal cord injury is unable to button his shirt. The MOST appropriate piece of adaptive equipment for the COTA to provide him with is a buttonhook:

A. with an extra-long, flexible handle.
B. with a knob handle.
C. on a ½-inch diameter, 5-inch long wooden handle.
D. attached to a cuff that fits around his palm.

Treatment Implementation

73. The COTA has completed patient education with an individual who has just received a splint for carpal tunnel syndrome. When documenting this session, the COTA will indicate that the patient was instructed in precautions, wearing schedule, and care of a:

A. wrist cock-up splint.
B. thermoplastic splint.
C. resting hand splint.
D. dynamic MP flexion splint.

74. The COTA is performing AROM exercises with an individual with left hemiparesis following a CVA. She observes that AROM is limited throughout

the LUE. Reasons for limited AROM in this individual are MOST likely to include:
A. muscle tone, edema, sensation, and diadokinesis.
B. edema, proprioception, and muscle tone.
C. edema, contracture, muscle tone, and pain.
D. contracture, stereognosis, and sensation.

75. The COTA is working on sitting balance with an individual with C6 quadriplegia. The BEST position for the individual's hands to be in when using them for support is with the fingers:
A. extended and adducted.
B. flexed at all joints.
C. extended and abducted.
D. adducted and flexed only at the metacarpal-phalangeal joints.

76. When instructing a man with swan-neck deformities in a self-ROM program, the COTA will include exercises designed to prevent further:
A. hyperextension of the PIP and DIP joints.
B. hyperextension of the PIP joint and flexion of the DIP joint.
C. flexion of the PIP joint and hyperextension of the DIP joint.
D. hyperextension of the MP joint and flexion of the PIP joint.

77. The BEST way to instruct an individual with hemiparesis to button a shirt is to:
A. button all the buttons before putting the shirt on.
B. get the shirt all the way on, then line up the buttons and holes and begin buttoning from the top.
C. get the shirt all the way on, then line up the buttons and holes and begin buttoning from the bottom.
D. use a buttonhook with a built-up handle.

78. When instructing a man with hemiplegia in how to remove a front-opening shirt, the COTA should train him to use the following sequence:
A. (1) pull the shirt off over the head; (2) remove the affected arm; (3) remove the unaffected arm; (4) unbutton the shirt.
B. (1) pull the shirt off over the head; (2) remove the unaffected arm; (3) remove the affected arm; (4) unbutton the shirt.
C. (1) unbutton the shirt; (2) pull the shirt off over the head; (3) remove the unaffected arm; (4) remove the affected arm.
D. (1) unbutton the shirt; (2) pull the shirt off over the head; (3) remove the affected arm; (4) remove the unaffected arm.

79. A COTA is instructing a man with hemiplegia and good standing balance in how to don his trousers. The appropriate sequence for him to use is:
A. (1) seated, slip trousers over affected foot; (2) cross the unaffected leg over the affected leg; (3) place affected leg into trousers; (4) uncross legs, stand, and pull up trousers.
B. (1) seated, cross the affected leg over the unaffected leg; (2) slip affected foot through leg of trousers and uncross; (3) place unaffected leg into trousers; (4) stand and pull up trousers.
C. (1) seated, slip trousers over unaffected foot; (2) cross the affected leg over the unaffected leg; (3) slip affected foot through leg of trousers and uncross; (4) uncross legs, stand and pull up trousers.
D. (1) seated, cross the unaffected leg over the affected leg; (2) slip unaffected foot through leg of trousers and uncross; (3) place affected leg into trousers; (4) stand and pull up trousers.

80. A woman is beginning to demonstrate return in the right upper extremity following a CVA, but has mildly impaired proprioception in her right hand, which results in uneven letter formation during writing activities. Which of the following would BEST improve her letter formation?
A. The COTA verbally describes to her how to make a letter as she writes.
B. She watches her grip on a felt-tip pen while writing.
C. She works with thera-putty to strengthen her hand.
D. She traces letters through a pan of rice with her fingers.

81. A good way for an individual with arthritis to maintain range of motion while performing housework is:
A. use short strokes with the vacuum cleaner.
B. keep elbow flexed when ironing.
C. keep lightweight objects on low shelves.
D. use dust mitt to keep fingers fully extended.

82. An OTA student needs to design an adaptation in order to complete his level II fieldwork experience. He decides to focus on gardening for a client with a low-back injury. The MOST appropriate adaptation for him to design would be:
A. ergonomically correct hand tools.
B. a wheelbarrow with elongated handles.
C. a 12-inch-high seat with tool holders.
D. a raised-bed garden.

83. Carolyn is s/p TBI and exhibits good strength with ataxia in both upper extremities. The writing adaptation that would be MOST appropriate for her is:
A. a keyboard.
B. a universal cuff with pencil-holder attachment.
C. a balanced forearm orthosis with built-up felt-tip pen.
D. a weighted pen and weighted wrists.

84. After wearing a new splint for 20 minutes, an individual develops a reddened area along the ulnar styloid. The correct modification for the COTA to make to the splint is to:

A. line the splint with moleskin.
B. line the splint with adhesive-backed foam.
C. flange the area around the ulnar styloid.
D. reheat and refabricate the entire splint.

85. The COTA is carrying out a dressing program with a woman who is s/p LCVA. The MOST appropriate way for this individual to don a blouse that buttons down the front is to:
A. button it up and put it on over her head.
B. get assistance.
C. place her left arm in the left sleeve first.
D. place her right arm in the right sleeve first.

Evaluating the Treatment Plan

86. After the OTR has fabricated a splint for an individual with a hand injury, he asks the COTA to monitor the patient's splint use. It is MOST important for the COTA to make certain that:
A. the individual's fingers are flexed in a functional position.
B. the individual's thumb is opposed and abducted.
C. the splint is being worn at all times.
D. pressure marks or redness disappear after 20 minutes.

87. When documenting patient progress in a weekly note, the COTA should include:
A. concise objective information.
B. speculative and judgmental information.
C. objective and speculative information.
D. subjective information and personal opinions.

88. The subjective section of the SOAP format includes:
A. measurement results.
B. analysis of measurements recorded.
C. speculative information.
D. quotes from the individual.

89. During a home visit, a woman with rheumatoid arthritis informs the COTA that her joints have recently become very painful and inflamed. She reports she has been performing her exercise program despite the pain and demonstrates a series of briskly executed AROM exercises to the COTA. The COTA should instruct her to:
A. continue performing her program as she has been.
B. instruct her to perform gentle AROM with weight as tolerated.
C. eliminate all ROM exercises for a week.
D. instruct her to perform only gentle AROM.

90. A woman with quadriplegia was unable to grasp a toothbrush with a built-up handle, using tenodesis, at the time of her initial evaluation. After working on upper-extremity strengthening and grooming skills for 2 weeks, the COTA needs to determine the degree of progress that has been achieved in this area. Using a functional method of evaluation, the COTA evaluates progress by:
A. measuring the patient's grip strength with a goniometer.
B. measuring the patient's pinch strength with a pinch meter.
C. assessing the patient's ability to hold the toothbrush with a built-up handle.
D. assessing the patient's ability to hold the toothbrush using a universal cuff.

91. Carol is a 25-year-old single female 4 months s/p TBI. She requires minimal assistance in most self-care activities and moderate assistance for transfers. Her progress has plateaued and a family meeting is scheduled for next week. What type of response should the COTA anticipate from the family members?
A. They are likely to react with anger, anxiety, and depression.
B. They will probably be anxious to take Carol home as soon as possible.
C. They will schedule family members to provide the necessary round-the-clock care.
D. They will probably request family/caregiver training.

92. Rachel is a 45-year-old woman with COPD. A long-term goal is to be able to shop independently for groceries. She has achieved the short-term goal of going to a convenience store and purchasing three items. Which statement is the BEST example of a revised short-term goal?
A. "Pt. will purchase 10 items at the supermarket with supervision."
B. "Pt. will cook a one-dish meal."
C. "Pt. will shop independently for a birthday present for her daughter."
D. "Instruct patient in energy conservation techniques that apply to grocery shopping."

93. The outcome that would be MOST appropriately anticipated after a carpenter has learned how to use proper body mechanics is:
A. the ability to work a full day without becoming fatigued.
B. the ability to install a door without reinjury.
C. minimization of joint damage.
D. the ability to hammer for sustained periods of time.

Discharge Planning

94. An individual with left hemiparesis and impaired balance wishes to vacuum the floors upon return home. The BEST type of vacuum cleaner for the COTA to recommend is a(n):

A. canister vacuum cleaner.
B. upright vacuum cleaner.
C. self-propelled vacuum cleaner.
D. handheld cordless vacuum cleaner.

95. Which of the following precautions should be included in a home program for an individual who had a total knee replacement?
A. Avoid hip flexion past 80 degrees and internal rotation.
B. Avoid full knee extension.
C. Limit weight bearing on involved lower extremity.
D. Limit full weight bearing on the uninvolved lower extremity.

96. Which features are necessary when ordering a wheelchair for an individual who will be performing a sliding board transfer with assistance of the family upon discharge?
A. Lightweight frame, swing-away leg rests.
B. Reclining back rest, elevating leg rests.
C. Swing-away leg rests, removable arm rests.
D. Elevating leg rests, removable arm rests.

97. How much space is needed around the front door to allow easy access by a standard wheelchair?
A. 3 feet by 5 feet.
B. 4 feet by 4 feet.
C. 4-1/2 feet by 3 feet.
D. 5 feet by 5 feet.

98. Following surgery to remove a malignant tumor, Mr. S. is being discharged to home from an acute care hospital. He is very weak and will continue to receive intravenous chemotherapy with the help of a home health nurse. He was seen once by OT as an inpatient. The COTA/OTR team believe he would benefit from additional OT treatment to increase independence in ADLs. The MOST appropriate way for him to receive OT services would be:
A. from a home health OTR or COTA.
B. staying in the hospital a little longer.
C. going to a rehabilitation center.
D. coming back for outpatient OT.

99. Nick uses a wheelchair and is independent in transfers and basic ADLs. With continued occupational therapy intervention, he is expected to be able to function independently in the community. The MOST appropriate community living option for him, at this time, would be a(n):
A. cradle-to-grave home.
B. transitional living center.
C. adult day program.
D. clustered independent living arrangement.

100. Which of the following is the BEST example of an excerpt from the "Objective" section of a discharge summary?
A. "Pt. reports he can work at the computer much longer and more comfortably than he could initially."
B. "Pt. was initially able to work at the computer for only 10 minutes. Upon discharge, he can work at the computer for 3 hours with stretch breaks every 30 minutes."
C. "Pt. has improved significantly in his ability to work at the computer."
D. "Pt. reports he is now able to work at the computer for 3 hours, where initially he was only able to tolerate 10 minutes."

PSYCHOSOCIAL QUESTIONS

Data Collection

101. A COTA is working with a 35 year-old woman with a personality disorder. Deficits in the following area should be expected:
A. sensorimotor skills.
B. activities of daily living.
C. relationships with others.
D. instrumental activities of daily living.

102. The COTA is working in a long-term psychiatric inpatient setting for adults. He is asked by the treatment team to assess a patient's ability to maintain his clothing, get dressed, eat a meal, and bathe, because these are required skills for discharge to a group home. The MOST appropriate assessment to use to obtain this information is the:
A. Milwaukee Evaluation of Daily Living Skills (MEDLS).
B. Allen Cognitive Level (ACL).
C. Kohlman Evaluation of Living Skills (KELS).
D. Barthel Self-Care Index.

103. When a new patient is referred for psychiatric services, the COTA and OTR both review the chart. Then the OTR completes performance measures, and the COTA performs an interview. The COTA/OTR team will rely on the interview part of this assessment to address the individual's:
A. diagnosis.
B. current medications.
C. ability to concentrate and solve problems.
D. view of the problem and an overall goal.

104. A COTA working in an eating disorders treatment program for individuals with bulimia is MOST likely to treat:
A. women over the age of 30.
B. men under the age of 30.
C. individuals who weigh less than their normal body weight.
D. individuals who are at or above their normal body weight.

105. The assessment that provides the COTA with a computer-generated summary of an individual's overall occupational performance functioning is:
A. OT FACT.
B. Occupational History Interview.
C. RIC Functional Assessment Scale.
D. Assessment of Motor and Process Skills (AMPS).

106. The OTR has asked the COTA to conduct a structured interview to determine the patient's ability to function within the community. Which of the following is the COTA MOST likely to use?
A. Comprehensive Occupational Therapy Evaluation (COTE).
B. Milwaukee Evaluation of Daily Living Skills (MEDLS).
C. Moorhead's Occupational History.
D. Allen's Routine Task Inventory.

107. The OTR has asked the COTA to identify how the patient spends his leisure time, which leisure activities he especially enjoys, and which others he has participated in that he would be interested in renewing. The MOST appropriate tool for the COTA to use is the:
A. Kohlman Evaluation of Living Skills (KELS).
B. NPI Interest Checklist.
C. Activity Configuration.
D. Scorable Self-Care Evaluation.

108. Which of the following documented statements provides an objective basis for judgment?
A. "Patient enjoys reading photography magazines."
B. "Patient likes news magazines."
C. "Patient obviously likes to read *People* magazine."
D. "Patient stated that he likes to read sports magazines."

109. "The patient refused to participate in the group activity." This statement is an example of which of the following portions of a SOAP note?
A. Subjective.
B. Objective.
C. Assessment.
D. Plan.

110. The COTA is working with an individual who demonstrates vacillation between grandiosity and hostility several times within one group session. This individual is demonstrating behaviors associated with:
A. mania.
B. emotional lability.
C. paranoia.
D. denial.

Treatment Planning

111. Comprehensive psychiatric rehabilitation services often include recreational therapy. The primary role of recreational therapy is to:
A. provide a variety of therapeutic sports, arts, crafts, music, and recreation activities to develop and reinforce healthy interest patterns.
B. use heat, light, and sound to increase function of a body part.
C. provide acting-doing experiences that enable the individual to acquire leisure, work, and self-care skills at a maximal level of independence and a sense of self-satisfaction and personal worth.
D. provide aptitude testing and job placement.

112. The COTA is planning to use remedial strategies to prepare individuals treated in a psychosocial setting for job hunting. The activity MOST consistent with this approach is:
A. reviewing the NPI Interest Checklist.
B. a class about job-seeking strategies.
C. modification of the work environment to reduce stress.
D. an expressive group magazine collage using pictures of different types of workers.

113. The COTA is working with a group of individuals with substance-abuse disorders. He wants to use an activity that will allow the individuals both to experience success after making a mess and to delay gratification. The activity process that BEST provides this experience is:
A. working in a group with three other individuals.
B. selecting the design pattern for a tile trivet.
C. applying grout to a tile trivet and waiting for it to dry.
D. cleaning off the table at the end of the group.

114. A COTA is working with an individual who is building a wooden birdhouse. An adapted sequencing approach is being used for this particular project. Which of the following is the BEST example of adapted sequencing?
A. The individual kneels in front of the supply cabinet to obtain the craft kit, proceeds to sitting in a chair with the materials placed to the right and left of midline, and stands up to sand and glue the pieces together.
B. The small wood pieces are precut by the OT aide, and the patient uses a template for cutting the large straight-edged pieces then uses step-by-step directions and photographs to put it together.
C. The individual measures and saws all the needed pieces, sands the pieces, assembles the pieces with glue, sands the pieces again, assembles the birdhouse, and applies a coat of stain.
D. Gross-motor movements are used initially with sawing and sanding, then fine-motor coordination is used for assembling and painting the birdhouse.

115. Directive group treatment is the MOST appropriate approach in acute care mental health for individuals with:
A. substance abuse.
B. eating disorders.
C. adjustment disorders.
D. disorganized psychosis.

116. The COTA is planning to demonstrate and then practice "broken record" behaviors with group members as part of:
A. music therapy activities.
B. self-awareness activities.
C. assertiveness training.
D. psychodrama activities.

117. The COTA has administered the Activity Configuration as part of an initial evaluation of a 28-year-old man with a substance abuse problem. The COTA's report indicates that the patient's leisure-time activities consist of drinking and playing billiards. The MOST appropriate goal for this patient would be:
A. The client will be able to identify two activities that are of interest to him within 2weeks.
B. The client will concentrate and attend to a task long enough to complete it.
C. The client will be able to identify his likes and dislikes within 2 weeks.
D. The client will participate in at least one AA meeting per week.

118. The goal of an arts and crafts group for chronically mentally ill individuals is to improve their decision-making abilities. The MOST appropriate level at which to begin a mosaic activity would be:
A. providing patients with individual projects and having them choose a tile color for their projects.
B. having the patients choose from a variety of projects.
C. having the patients decide on the design, size, shape, and colors for a group mosaics project.
D. having each patient decide on a pattern and two tile colors to use in his or her mosaic project.

119. In the arts and crafts group cited in question 118, the COTA can upgrade the degree of decision-making ability to the next level by having the patients:
A. decide on the design, size, shape, and colors for a group mosaics project.
B. select their individual projects, designs, and materials from a wide sampling of projects.
C. select a new project from three options.
D. design their individual projects.

120. The COTA is leading an activity-based group for clients who are at risk for acting out sexually. The environmental modification that would BEST reduce this risk is:
A. provide a relatively active and stimulating environment with opportunities for the at-risk individuals to engage in real-life activities.
B. stand to the side of at-risk individuals instead of face to face during interactions with them.
C. avoid having at-risk individuals in close proximity to others to reduce opportunities for physical contact.
D. advise at-risk individuals in a calm, nonjudgmental manner about the behavior you expect.

121. The COTA is running a cooking group for four women with schizophrenia who are all functioning at a parallel level. The MOST appropriate goal for members of this group is:
A. each member will take a leadership role within the session.
B. members will share materials with at least one other group member.
C. each member will express two positive feelings about herself within the group session.
D. each member will remain in the group without disrupting the work of others for 30 minutes.

122. The COTA is working in a psychosocial setting with clients who are classified as having some suicide risk. In selecting craft media, the activity that would be MOST safe is a:
A. leather checkbook cover with single cordovan lacing.
B. macramé plant hanger.
C. ceramic ash tray.
D. decoupage wood key fob.

Treatment Implementation

123. A young woman diagnosed with depression confides to the COTA that she feels very alone and afraid. Chart review reveals that the woman leads a very isolated lifestyle. The BEST way for the COTA to respond is:
A. reassuring the woman that she is her friend.
B. telling the woman, "I know how you feel."
C. encouraging the woman to socialize more often.
D. using active listening techniques.

124. A COTA running a stress management group explains to the members that stress is the:
A. process by which individuals adjust to daily stressful events within their environments.
B. body's reactions to threat, often described as "fight or flight."
C. precipitating conditions and events that elicit stress reactions.
D. process of "fit" between the individual and his or her environment.

125. The COTA has planned a community outing that involves walking outdoors from the bus stop to the bank, the utility company, and the grocery

store on a hot summer day. Several individuals in the group take neuroleptic medications. The COTA will need to take precautions for which of the following possible side effects?
A. Hypotension.
B. Photosensitivity.
C. Excessive perspiration.
D. Weight gain..

126. When leading groups, the COTA should demonstrate consistency from day to day. Inconsistent behavior could result in:
A. overdependence of group members.
B. group members knowing what to expect from the group leader.
C. anxiety and confusion among group members.
D. group members receiving too much praise.

127. A 14-year-old boy is attending a COTA's woodworking group for the first time. The COTA is observing him closely for signs of aggressive and violent behavior, as he has been diagnosed with:
A. hyperactivity.
B. attention deficit disorder.
C. conduct disorder.
D. oppositional defiant disorder.

128. An example of a group norm is when:
A. one member contributes superficial comments.
B. members role play.
C. there is improved self-esteem among members.
D. smoking during the group session is prohibited.

129. The COTA is planning a meal preparation activity for a 42-year-old woman with attentional and organizational deficits secondary to alcohol abuse. The treatment goals address her difficulties in properly sequencing tasks. The MOST appropriate activity to use initially is:
A. setting the table.
B. planning an entire meal.
C. baking cookies using a recipe.
D. preparing a shopping list.

130. The COTA is selecting treatment activities to use with a 28-year-old man diagnosed with schizophrenia, undifferentiated type, that would help to increase his ability to receive, process, and respond to sensory information. The MOST suitable activities for this patient include:
A. social skills training.
B. vestibular stimulation and gross-motor exercise.
C. role playing.
D. discussion group.

131. A COTA is running a discharge planning group where individuals discuss their personal feelings and concerns about returning to the community. Which is the BEST method to use?
A. Patients write fears and concerns on index cards. The COTA collects and reads the cards to the group for discussion.
B. Patients write fears and concerns on index cards and then take turns reading their cards to the group.
C. Patients each take a turn verbalizing their fears and concerns to the group.
D. The psychologist speaks to the group about discharge fears in general.

132. While in the hospital, Mr. Rodriguez, a 48-year-old roofing contractor, experienced extrapyramidal syndrome after he began taking neuroleptic medication. He is to continue taking the medication after discharge from the hospital. It is MOST important to advise Mr. Rodriguez:
A. to keep time in the sun as brief as possible.
B. to avoid use of power tools and sharp instruments.
C. to get up slowly from a standing, sitting, or lying position.
D. about the dehydrating effects of caffeinated drinks and alcohol.

133. The COTA is leading a grooming group for female clients in a psychosocial treatment setting. In order to comply with universal precautions, the COTA should:
A. use disposable cotton swabs and have clients bring their own cosmetics.
B. use disposable gloves when combing client's hair.
C. wash and dry makeup brushes between uses.
D. avoid bringing cosmetics with glass containers to the group.

134. The COTA is working with a man with impaired memory. When the client is unable to follow verbal instructions, the COTA changes her approach to demonstration. This is an example of:
A. activity analysis.
B. activity adaptation.
C. grading the activity.
D. clinical reasoning.

135. The COTA has been assigned to develop an expressive activity group for women who have experienced emotional and physical abuse. The BEST choice would be:
A. meditation and yoga exercises.
B. writing a soap opera.
C. personal hygiene and grooming classes.
D. aerobics and fitness program.

Evaluating the Treatment Plan

136. While running a nutrition awareness group, the COTA observes that one member tends to monopolize the discussion. Which intervention would be BEST to implement after other, more conservative, approaches have been unsuccessful?

A. Sit beside the person who is monopolizing and touch his or her hand or arm as a reminder not to interrupt others who are talking.
B. Confront the individual's behavior: "Are you aware that your frequent interruptions prevent others from having a chance to contribute?"
C. Redirect the individual: "Now, let's hear what others have to say about this."
D. Restructure the task: select a group activity that requires sequential turn taking.

137. The COTA is conducting a predischarge interview with a female patient who has been treated on the psychiatric unit for schizophrenia. The COTA asks, "Are you ready to go home today?" This question is an example of a(n):
A. open question.
B. closed question.
C. directed or leading question.
D. double question.

138. At the end of each day, the COTA documents treatment sessions in each client's chart. The purpose of this documentation includes all of the following EXCEPT:
A. facilitating communication with the client's family.
B. satisfying accrediting agencies.
C. providing data for research.
D. facilitating effective treatment.

139. Wendy is participating in an assertiveness training group. The expected outcome of this intervention is that Wendy will improve her ability to:
A. engage in relevant conversations with her coworkers.
B. use appropriate facial expressions when disagreeing with her coworkers.
C. express disagreement with her coworkers in a productive manner.
D. use courteous behavior when disagreeing with her coworkers.

Questions 140-142 are based on this case study:

Isadore is a 65-year-old man with impulsive behavior, poor table manners, and very few teeth. He mumbles when he speaks and rarely makes eye contact. He eats with his fingers, and at meals the entry-level COTA has observed him stuffing an entire sandwich into his mouth at one time. The COTA observes that when she cuts Isadore's sandwich into bite-sized pieces and gives him no more than two pieces at a time, he slows his eating pace to a safe level.

140. Which of the following is the MOST appropriate new short-term goal for Isadore?
A. Isadore will demonstrate good table manners at four out of five meals.
B. Isadore will demonstrate decreased impulsivity at three out of five meals.
C. Isadore will make eye contact with three individuals during current events group.
D. Isadore will chew and swallow each piece of sandwich before placing the next piece in his mouth four out of five times.

141. The FIRST thing the COTA should do after formulating a new short-term goal for Isadore is:
A. document the goal in Isadore's chart.
B. introduce the new feeding program to other staff involved in Isadore's care.
C. present the new goal and treatment plan to the OTR.
D. implement the new feeding program.

142. When working on table manners with Isadore, the FIRST item to address would be:
A. using the appropriate utensil for specific foods.
B. taking portions of food of the appropriate size while using utensils.
C. eating the meal in a reasonable amount of time.
D. using eating utensils when appropriate.

143. Mary has moved to a community residential center after 30 years in a state hospital. She has mild mental retardation and engages in self-abusive behavior when she becomes anxious. After participating in craft group for 2 months, she has achieved her goal of engaging in a simple craft activity for up to 10 minutes before demonstrating self-abusive behavior. Which statement is the MOST appropriate revised short-term goal for Mary?
A. Mary will engage in a simple craft activity for 15 minutes without demonstrating self-abusive behavior.
B. Mary will engage in a craft activity of moderate complexity for 10 minutes without demonstrating self-abusive behavior.
C. Mary will engage in a craft activity of moderate complexity for 15 minutes without demonstrating self-abusive behavior.
D. Mary will engage in a complex craft activity for 10 minutes without demonstrating self-abusive behavior.

Discharge Planning

144. The community vocational services that adults with mental retardation are MOST likely to be referred to in order to learn and master basic work skills are:
A. adult activity centers.
B. supported employment.
C. fast-food restaurants with supervision from job coaches.
D. sheltered workshops.

145. The legal principle that affects the occupational therapy discharge planning process within all mental health practice areas is:
A. least restrictive environment.
B. state licensure/regulation of occupational therapy practitioners.
C. Public law 94-142.
D. the Tarasoff decision.

146. Mr. Gonzalez, 72 years old, was hospitalized for an episode of acute depression following the death of his wife. He is preparing for discharge and would like to return to his own home but is fearful of spending his days alone. The BEST way for Mr. Gonzalez to continue socialization and participation in meaningful occupation would be:
A. partial hospitalization.
B. adult day care.
C. home health care.
D. psychosocial rehabilitation center.

147. The husband of a woman being treated for bipolar disorder describes his frustration with the ups and downs of his wife's condition. The BEST support group to refer this man to is:
A. Al-Anon.
B. family therapy.
C. National Alliance for the Mentally Ill.
D. Recovery, Inc.

Questions 148-150 refer to this sample document:

Section I: James D. Smith
#54321
11/1/97

Section II: Mr. Smith attended a total of 24 occupational therapy groups throughout his hospitalization for depression 10-15-96 to 11-1-96.

Section III: Patient achieved the following goals:

1. Pt. has demonstrated four alternative effective coping strategies for restating negative automatic thoughts.

2. Pt. identified three former interests and specified plan for gradually resuming involvement in these after discharge.

3. Pt. has demonstrated improved assertiveness skills in refusing unreasonable requests from boss in simulated experiences.

Section IV: Pt is capable of resuming role of parent and spouse and part-time worker at discharge. Mr. Smith will gradually resume his work activities to full time (40-45 hours/week) over the course of 2 weeks. On final evaluation, Mr. Smith's leisure interest checklist showed a 15% increase in quantity of interests and included three interests that he upgraded from casual to strong. Mr. Smith has agreed to take his journal of automatic thoughts, restatements, and activities for his first week after discharge to the outpatient group at the community mental health center. Mr. Smith has been scheduled to attend the outpatient support group next Tuesday at 7:00 PM. Mr. Smith has completed the authorization to transfer occupational therapy treatment records to the CMHC.

148. The sample documentation above is an example of a(n):
A. progress note.
B. initial note.
C. discharge summary.
D. treatment plan.

149. In the sample documentation, the section that contains Mr. Smith's follow-up plan is:
A. Section I
B. Section II
C. Section III
D. Section IV

150. In the preceding documentation sample, the section that contains Mr. Smith's home program is:
A. Section I
B. Section II
C. Section III
D. Section IV

PROFESSIONAL PRACTICE QUESTIONS

Promote Professional Practice

151. The program that ensures that disabled children receive educational services in the LEAST restrictive environment is:
A. the Americans with Disabilities Act.
B. the Education for All Handicapped Children Act.
C. Children's Protective Services.
D. Medicare.

152. Current trends in the provision of health care will result in a(n):
A. reduction in home health services.
B. increase in the amount of hospitalizations.
C. reduction in the need for nursing homes.
D. increase in outpatient services.

153. COTAs employed in community settings are MOST likely to be employed in:
A. private practice.
B. school systems.
C. home health agencies.
D. independent living centers.

154. The MOST severe sanction that the National Board for Certification in Occupational Therapy (NBCOT) may apply against a COTA who has demonstrated misconduct is:
A. a reprimand.
B. a censure.
C. probation.
D. revocation.

155. In order to provide direct supervision for a Level II OTA fieldwork student, the supervisor should:
A. be an OTR with 6 months of experience.
B. have at least 1 year of experience as a COTA.
C. have at least 2 years of experience as a COTA.
D. have supervised a Level I student before supervising a Level II student.

156. A COTA violates the Occupational Therapy Code of Ethics and is censured by the NBCOT. A censure is:
A. a formal written expression of disapproval against a practitioner's conduct that is issued and retained in the NBCOT's files.
B. a formal, public disapproval of a practitioner's conduct .
C. when a practitioner is given a period of time to retain the counseling or education required to remain certified.
D. permanent loss of NBCOT certification.

157. An OTR asks a COTA to provide a paraffin bath to an individual with arthritis. The COTA has never had training in the use of physical agent modalities and recognizes that her lack of competence could result in harm to this client. The COTA's obligation to avoid doing harm to the client is referred to as:
A. informed consent.
B. fidelity.
C. beneficence.
D. nonmaleficence.

158. A COTA on a rehabilitation unit is working on LE dressing with a 23-year-old man with a spinal cord injury. As the client tries to put on his underwear, he notices an erection and asks the COTA how it is possible for him to have an erection and if he will be able to have sex. The COTA is slightly embarrassed and uncomfortable with the question. The BEST action for the COTA to take is to:
A. tell him she will find out the answers to his questions and get back to him with an answer by the next morning.
B. answer his questions to the best of her ability and quickly return to the LE dressing program.
C. refer him to his physiatrist.
D. refer him to her OTR supervisor, who has attended a workshop on sexuality and spinal cord injury.

159. A paraffin bath is ordered for a nursing home resident with arthritis in her hands. The COTA's supervising OTR is not on site that day, and he asks advice from the PT. The PT shows the COTA how to administer a paraffin bath, and a few hours later the COTA administers a paraffin bath to the resident. That evening, a nurse notices second-degree burns on the residents hand's in the area where the paraffin was applied. Who would MOST likely be held accountable for the resident's burns?
A. The physical therapist.
B. The supervising OTR.
C. The COTA.
D. Both the COTA and supervising OTR.

160. A COTA arrives for a home health visit on a Thursday morning, 11/14/96, but the client is not feeling well. They reschedule for the following day. The COTA's charges for the week are due on alternating Thursday afternoons. Knowing she will see the client the next day (11/15/96), and reluctant to wait another 2 weeks to submit for payment, she bills for treatment using the 11/14/96 date. This COTA's action is:
A. acceptable, because treatment has been scheduled for the next day.
B. acceptable if the agency she works for allows it.
C. unacceptable, because it violates the Code of Ethics.
D. unacceptable, because if the patient is still ill and unable to participate in therapy on 11/15/96, a delay of more than 1 day is unacceptable for billing purposes.

161. A certified occupational therapy assistant has recently attained the skill level at which it is appropriate for her to develop and supervise a volunteer program in an inpatient occupational therapy department. This practitioner MOST likely is operating at which skill level?
A. Entry level practice.
B. Intermediate level practice.
C. Advanced level practice.
D. Educator level practice.

162. Most COTAs are employed in:
A. rehabilitation hospitals.
B. school systems.
C. skilled nursing facilities.
D. psychiatric hospitals.

163. An entry-level COTA is completing designated areas of the discharge report. The section that the COTA would MOST likely leave to be completed by the OTR is the:
A. discharge recommendations.
B. patient's current level of independence in activities of daily living.
C. patient's most recent strength and coordination measurements.
D. patient's discharge disposition.

164. A COTA/OTR team wants to establish service competency providing facilitation and inhibition techniques for normalizing tone. They decide to do this by cotreating. Service competency will be established when the OTR and COTA obtain:
A. the same results in three successive treatment trials.
B. similar results in a treatment session.

C. the same results in two consecutive treatment trials
D. similar results in three treatment sessions.

165. An OTR/COTA team needs to report discharge information and document the information in the patient's chart. At what level does the COTA participate in making discharge recommendations?
A. An entry-level COTA may perform the task independently.
B. An intermediate-level COTA may perform the task independently.
C. A COTA contributes to the process but does not complete the task independently.
D. A COTA cannot perform the task.

166. While documenting the week's OT sessions in an individual's chart, the COTA notices that a progress note from 2 weeks ago was not completed. The COTA recalls providing treatment that week and how the patient responded. The ONLY appropriate action for the COTA to take is to:
A. complete the note using the original date.
B. document services provided and date the note as a late entry.
C. leave the chart as is without documenting services provided.
D. write a brief note stating that documentation was not completed for the specified dates.

167. An OTR asks a COTA to provide a paraffin bath to an individual with arthritis. The COTA has never had training in the use of any heat modalities. Which of the following is NOT one of the reasons that it would be a violation of the OT Code of Ethics for the COTA to use the paraffin bath with the patient?
A. Physical agent modalities are not within the scope of practice of COTAs.
B. She would risk harming the patient.
C. She does not have service competency in this area.
D. She did not refer the patient to a qualified provider.

168. A COTA who has demonstrated service competency in the use of physical agent modalities (PAMs) may:
A. use only such PAMs as paraffin and whirlpool but no electrical modalities.
B. use PAMs only under direct supervision.
C. use PAMs only in preparation for or as an adjunct to purposeful activity.
D. use PAMs only if an OTR is on-site.

169. A COTA who has demonstrated service competency in the use of paraffin baths moves from one state to another to take a position in a hand rehabilitation center. The licensure act in her new state prohibits OT practitioners from using physical agent modalities (PAMs). The MOST appropriate action for her to take is to:
A. use PAMs only under the supervision of a licensed physical therapist.
B. use PAMs only under the supervision of a doctor.
C. use only paraffin.
D. not use physical agent modalities in the new state.

170. A COTA finds herself staying late every day because she is constantly behind with paperwork and preparation for the following day. The MOST professional action for the COTA to take is to:
A. continue to stay late so that she will not fall behind.
B. develop and implement time management strategies.
C. develop assertiveness skills to "just say no" to her supervisor.
D. leave at the end of the scheduled day in order to avoid burnout.

171. A COTA observes an OT practitioner locked in a passionate embrace with one of his female patients after work. The MOST responsible action for the COTA to take would be to:
A. remain quiet about it because the incident occurred after working hours.
B. find out if the patient and therapist have a "serious" relationship.
C. ignore the incident because there was no misconduct involved.
D. report the incident to the state licensure board.

172. COTAs are MOST frequently found working with which age group?
A. up to 3 years of age.
B. 6–12 years of age.
C. 19–64 years of age.
D. 75–84 years of age.

173. Continued professional education after certification is required by:
A. the AOTA.
B. the NBCOT.
C. some state occupational therapy associations.
D. some state regulatory acts.

174. An instructor from a local nursing school has asked a COTA to speak about occupational therapy to a class of first-year nursing students. The COTA feels uncertain about speaking in front of a group and decides to discuss the situation with her supervisor. The supervisor shares with the COTA public relations information provided by AOTA that may be shared with the nursing students. The MOST appropriate action for the COTA to take is:
A. recommend to the nursing course instructor that she call AOTA and obtain public relations information to share with her students.
B. send the information provided by the supervisor to the instructor.

C. decline to do the inservice.
D. use the brochures, posters, videotapes, and films available from the association to enhance her presentation to the nursing students.

175. A COTA is stopped in the hallway of an acute-care hospital by the family of a patient she is treating. The family asks if she will answer some of their questions while their mother is in the radiology department. The COTA spends a total of 15 minutes with the family, answering questions and describing their mother's OT program and progress. When submitting billing charges at the end of the day, the MOST ethical action for the COTA to take is to:
A. charge the patient an additional 15 minutes of treatment for the time spent with the family.
B. reduce the woman's time in therapy in the afternoon by 15 minutes, but charge for a full session to cover the time spent with the family.
C. call the finance department and ask their advice.
D. charge only for the amount of time spent with the patient directly that day.

176. The COTA on an inpatient psychiatric unit calls in sick to work. Her schedule includes a task group and coping-skills group. The only other person available to lead groups on that day is the certified therapeutic recreation specialist (CTRS). The COTA should request that the:
A. art therapist lead two task groups and bill for occupational therapy.
B. CTRS lead leisure-awareness and skills groups and bill for occupational therapy because the groups were held during the regularly scheduled occupational therapy group time.
C. CTRS substitute recreational activities during the occupational therapy time, without billing for occupational therapy services.
D. nurse have patients work on tasks they were given by the COTA during this time; the COTA will bill for occupational therapy services when she returns to work.

177. The document that provides occupational therapy guidelines for screening, referral, evaluation, treatment planning, implementation, discontinuation of services, quality assurance, indirect services, and legal and ethical issues is called:
A. Uniform Terminology for Reporting Occupational Therapy Services.
B. Standards of Practice.
C. licensure regulations.
D. AOTA Policies and Procedures.

Support Service Management

178. The COTA is treating an adult whose medical coverage is provided by a state payment system. The system MOST likely to be involved is:
A. Medicare.
B. Worker's compensation.
C. Blue Cross.
D. Education for All Handicapped Children.

179. An OTR and an entry-level COTA both work on an inpatient psychiatric unit. They each work 4 days a week, overlapping schedules only on Mondays. Which of the following tasks would be inappropriate for the OTR to ask the COTA to perform?
A. Lead the daily craft group.
B. Begin the assessment process when individuals are admitted on the weekends. The OTR will finish the assessment on Monday.
C. Work with individuals requiring ADL training on Saturday and Sunday mornings.
D. Carry out a leisure-planning group on Saturday afternoon.

180. A COTA is working with a 14-year-old boy with AIDS. She should use universal precautions to protect herself from contact with the patient's:
A. blood.
B. nasal secretions.
C. tears.
D. urine.

181. A COTA is responsible for supervising volunteers in an occupational therapy department. The MOST appropriate task for a volunteer is:
A. transporting patients to and from therapy.
B. working with a patient once the OT practitioner has set up the activity.
C. assisting with stock and inventory control.
D. completing chart reviews.

182. Studies that evaluate patient care, identify problems with patient care, and seek to resolve those problems are MOST accurately described as:
A. program evaluation.
B. quality assurance.
C. research.
D. cost-effectiveness studies.

183. The term given to the arrangement for delivery of health care in which an organization acts as an intermediary between an insurance agency and a hospital is:
A. managed care.
B. utilization review.
C. peer review.
D. prospective payment.

184. An advanced-level COTA who has worked at an independent living center for the past 7 years has been offered the position of Director of the program. There are no funds to pay for OTR supervision. According to the AOTA, can the COTA accept the position?
A. Only if the COTA can find some way to fund OTR supervision.

B. Yes, as long as state regulations allow autonomous practice and the COTA recognizes situations that require consultation with or referral to an OTR.
C. No. The COTA cannot work in this practice setting without OTR supervision.
D. Only if the COTA relinquishes use of the credentials "COTA."

185. "10-27-96: ADL evaluation and treatment for diagnosis of RCVA. Three times a week for 1 month. Signed, Malcolm Johnson, MD." This is an example of:
A. a referral.
B. screening.
C. goal setting.
D. treatment planning.

186. The first step a COTA should take upon receiving a written referral for OT services for an acute care patient being discharged in 2 days is to:
A. initiate the ADL component of the evaluation.
B. begin a chart review.
C. notify the OTR.
D. screen the patient.

187. Forms for making referrals to occupational therapy are often developed within the occupational therapy department. Which of the following documents would be helpful in developing a referral form?
A. Standards of Practice.
B. Uniform Terminology.
C. Role Delineation.
D. Code of Ethics.

188. During a group community reentry outing, one of the individuals complains of chest pain. The COTA monitors his heart rate and blood pressure. His resting heart rate is 120 beats per minute, and his blood pressure is 220/180. The MOST appropriate action for the COTA to take is to:
A. continue the community reentry outing.
B. return all the patients immediately to the hospital.
C. help the patient lay down and wait until his vital signs return to normal.
D. call 911.

189. A COTA is working in a psychiatric occupational therapy department that uses lots of craft paints, stains, and sharp tools. In order to ensure patient safety, the COTA will routinely complete which one of the following activities?
A. Label and store chemicals used within the department.
B. Complete a tool count of departmental sharps.
C. Obtain a locked storage cabinet for sharps.
D. Dispose of hazardous chemicals and substances per facility procedure.

190. A senior COTA has been given the responsibility of supervising staff COTAs in an OT department. This means that the:
A. staff COTAs will require only minimal supervision from an OTR.
B. senior COTA's caseload will be reduced.
C. senior COTA can redefine the role of COTAs in the department.
D. senior COTA will evaluate, guide, and teach the staff COTAs.

191. A new employee is becoming acquainted with the OT department's policy and procedure manual during her first week on the job. Which of the following is the BEST example of a statement that would be found in the "Procedures" section of the manual?
A. "The OT department will provide inservices on relevant information on a regular basis."
B. "All OT personnel are required to participate in continuing education at least annually."
C. "Individuals presenting inservices must sign up for the conference room at least 2 weeks in advance."
D. "Employees are entitled to 1 continuing education day per year."

192. Chloe, who has been attending a stress management group led by an OTR/COTA team in private practice, brings along her friend, Jordan, one day. Jordan would like to attend the group to learn how to better handle her own stress. Jordan does not have a physician referral. The fee is reasonable, and Jordan, like the others, will pay for it herself. Will the OT practitioners be able to accept Jordan into the stress management group?
A. No, OT cannot be provided without a physician referral.
B. Only if Jordan brings a prescription with her on her next visit.
C. Yes, since it is a group and not individual treatment.
D. Yes, if state law does not require a physician referral.

193. During toilet transfer training an individual's external catheter is dislodged and urine spills onto the floor. The therapist observes there is no blood in the urine. The COTA recognizes that an exposure has:
A. occurred and she should use universal precautions.
B. NOT occurred so she does not need to use universal precautions.
C. occurred but is not severe enough to require universal precautions.
D. NOT occurred, but she should use universal precautions anyway.

194. The mechanism to review the results of service interventions for a population is referred to as:
A. a process.
B. an outcome.

C. program evaluation.
D. utilization review.

195. When transferring an individual from one seat to another, the COTA can BEST protect herself from injury by:
A. stepping back from the patient.
B. keeping her back in a flexed position.
C. keeping her knees bent.
D. maintaining a narrow base of support.

196. The COTA should use protective eyewear when:
A. applying oil-based stains to wood projects.
B. using a band saw.
C. applying liver of sulfate to a copper-tooling project.
D. soldering metal.

197. A COTA is coordinating a cooking group. As a part of the competency training program for leading the group, the COTA must be aware of policies and procedures that relate to the storage and maintenance of staple products as well as the handling of food. This policy will MOST likely be a part of the facility's:
A. Infection Control plan.
B. Risk Management plan.
C. Emergency Procedures plan.
D. Environmental Survey plan.

198. A basic request for occupational therapy services that may come from a nurse, social worker, or teacher is referred to as a(n):
A. recommendation
B. plan of treatment
C. intervention strategy
D. referral

199. An occupational therapy department is understaffed and the hospital administrator recommends that OTRs only do evaluations and allow COTAs to provide all of the treatment and discharge planning independently. The BEST response to give to the administrator is:
A. this is an appropriate solution to the problem of being understaffed.
B. this does not provide for adequate supervision of COTAs. However, the OT department will follow the administrator's recommendation.
C. this does not provide for adequate supervision of COTAs. However, if the OTRs are allowed time to provide general or routine supervision to the COTAs, the COTAs would then be able to treat the patients and write the progress notes and discharge summaries.
D. this is not an appropriate solution. The OTRs must do the evaluation, progress, and discharge documentation on all patients.

200. A staff entry-level COTA is MOST likely to be assigned all of the following quality assurance activities except:
A. collecting data from patient charts.
B. administering patient interviews at discharge.
C. administering family interviews at discharge.
D. designing the patient discharge interview.

ANSWERS FOR SIMULATION EXAMINATION 1

1. (D) determine the need for further occupational therapy evaluation. The purpose of screening is to determine whether further assessments are needed, and if so, which tests would be appropriate for that child. Screening tests are not designed for planning programs or consultation, nor do they test any skills in a comprehensive way. See reference: Dunn (ed): Collier, T: The screening process.

2. (C) ulnar palmar. Ulnar palmar grasp precedes the other types of grasp. The infant first grasps on the ulnar side of the hand against the palm, then with all four fingers against the palm (palmar grasp) (answer D), and finally the grasp moves to the radial side of the hand (radial grasp) (answer A). The highest level of grasp is pincer grasp (answer B), when the pad of the index finger meets the opposed thumb. See reference: Case-Smith, Allen, and Pratt (eds): Exner, CE: Development of hand skills.

3. (D) home visit and interview with the parents. "To write functional goals, the therapist evaluates the child's performance areas and asks meaningful questions to the caregivers regarding the child's functional performance... Although the assessment of performance areas is of primary concern for the occupational therapist, most of the evaluation tools used currently by therapists measure children's performance components." Meaningful questions and observation of the child in his or her natural environment will provide information about individual variations of function within the child's environment, such as family expectations, parenting styles, and cultural context. Answers A, B, and C are incorrect because they provide information about performance components only, not overall function. See reference: Case-Smith, Allen, and Pratt (eds): Stewart, KB: Occupational therapy assessment in pediatrics.

4. (C) lower extremities, trunk, and mild upper extremities. The correct answer is C because diplegia refers to these specific areas of the body. Involvement of both lower extremities is called paraplegia (answer C), and involvement of all upper and lower extremities is called quadriplegia (answer D). Answer A is also incorrect as there is no specific classification or name for involvement of both upper limbs when describing cerebral palsy. See reference: Case-Smith, Allen, and Pratt (eds): Gordon, CY, Schanzenbacher, KE, Case-Smith, J, and Carrasco, R: Diagnostic problems in pediatrics.

5. (B) structured. "Structured interviews . . . consist of sets of questions, which are to be asked in a given order. Furthermore, the interviewer must adhere to the questions as they are written. In a semistructured interview (answer A), the questions may be rephrased and more questions added." Criterion-referenced tests (answer C) compare the performance of the child to a set standard or criterion. This information is usually obtained through direct observation of the child. Open-ended interviews (answer D) are designed to facilitate the expression of feelings or associations and usually have no set format aside from an opening statement. See reference: Early: Data gathering and evaluation.

6. (D) ability to relate to others. "Autism is a pervasive developmental disorder characterized by severe permanent behavioral and cognitive disabilities. . . particularly associated with autism are the inability to relate to others and the display of ritualistic, repetitive behaviors." The degree of the child's ability to relate is directly related to function. Answers A, B, and C may be normal in a child with autism, but because of his inability to relate, these skills may be nonfunctional splinter skills. See reference: Case-Smith, Allen, and Pratt (eds): Gordon, CY, Schanzenbacher, KE, Case-Smith, J, and Carrasco, R: Diagnostic problems in pediatrics.

7. (B) structured. This type of checklist is structured, and can give useful information for treatment planning. The questions have not been tested on a large normal population, so there are no normative data (answer A). Therefore, this checklist cannot be used to distinguish between normal/abnormal responses. The checklist is structured, not unstructured (answer C), because it requires the tester to adhere to the given questions. The intent of the questions is not projective (answer D), as they do not ask about symbolic content that could be interpreted as representing projections from the patient's unconscious. See reference: Early: Data gathering and evaluation.

8. (A) age appropriate. At 5 years, a typical child can dress unsupervised. She can tie and untie knots but generally does not know how to tie a bow independently. See reference: Case-Smith, Allen, and Pratt (eds): Shepherd, J, Procter, SA, and Coley, IL: Self care and adaptations for independent living.

9. (C) age appropriateness, functionality of skills, family priorities. "Critical questions to ask when making decisions about intervention are: 'How do the skills compare with those of same age peers? How functional is the child? What are the main preferences/concerns of the child and the family?'." Answers A and B are relevant for general treatment planning, not specifically for dressing. Answer D describes specific concerns that should be addressed only if they are consistent with the child's priorities. See reference: Case-Smith, Allen, and Pratt (eds): Shepherd, J, Procter, SA, and Coley, IL: Self care and adaptations for independent living.

10. (B) echolalia. "Classic echolalia consists of parrot-like repetitions of phrases immediately after the child has been exposed to them." Echolalia is a disturbance of communication commonly seen in children with autism. Rigidity (answer A) refers to a lack of flexibility or ability to adjust to changes, a commonly seen behavioral response in individuals with autism, mental retardation, and head injury. Learned helplessness (answer C) is a type of depression developed in children who are exposed to unsolvable problems and have learned that they fail, no matter how hard they try. Nystagmus (answer D) refers to rapid involuntary movement of the eyes. The quality and the duration of a nystagmus following spinning may be interpreted as an indication of CNS processing of vestibular information by a tester trained in sensory integration assessments. See reference: Case-Smith, Allen, and Pratt (eds): Gordon, CY, Schanzenbacher, KE, Case-Smith, J, and Carrasco, R: Diagnostic problems in pediatrics. Also: Cronin, AS: Psychosocial and emotional domains of behavior; also Parham, LD, and Mailloux, Z: Sensory integration.

11. (B) public school system. Answer B is correct because the Individual Education Plan (IEP) is the required plan for children receiving special education in public school systems. This document describes the child's goals and the services to be received. The occupational therapist contributes an evaluation of the child as well as educational objectives. Answers A, C, and D are incorrect because each of these settings has different methods of coordinating a plan for a child, none of which are called an IEP. See reference: Hopkins and Smith (eds): Kaufmann, NA: Occupational therapy in school systems.

12. (D) child, caregiver, and therapist priorities. The problems established in the OT evaluation are not the only base for writing OT goals and objectives. The child's priorities as well as the caregiver's needs and concerns must be addressed so that immediate needs are met and there is a commitment on everyone's part to the success of the program. See reference: Case-Smith, Allen, and Pratt (eds): Case-Smith, J: Planning and implementing services.

13. (C) wheeling efficiency. Answer C is correct because the light weight of this type of wheelchair allows the child with weakness to be independent for longer periods of time. This type of chair is also easier for parents to handle when lifting it in and out of a car. Answer A is not correct because the removable armrest wheelchair feature is helpful in sliding transfers. Answer B is not correct because the desk arm feature allows children to sit closer to tables for school work and other table-top activities. Answer D is not correct because it is the adjustable arm rest feature that allows adjustment for varying heights of lap trays or work surfaces. See reference: Case-Smith, Allen, and Pratt (eds): Wright-Ott, C, and Egilson, S: Mobility.

14. (B) individual family service plan. The IFSP is a comprehensive written plan that identifies desired outcomes and delineates services the child and the family will need. The plan is developed in collaboration with the family and any health care providers, social services providers, and educators. The IFSP is required in the provision of early intervention services under PL 99–457, the Education of the Handicapped Act Amendment of 1986. See reference: Case-Smith, Allen, and Pratt (eds): Stephens, LC, and Tauber, SK: Early intervention.

15. (D) Removing a nut from a bolt. Answer D describes rotation, one type of in-hand manipulation. Rotation is the movement of an object around one or more of its axes, where objects may be turned horizontally or end-over-end with the pads of the fingers. Answers A, B, and C are incorrect because they describe hand activities that do not require manipulation but keep the object in one position as it is grasped, released, or carried. See reference: Case-Smith, Allen, and Pratt (eds): Exner, CE: Development of hand skills.

16. (C) an adequate attention span. This skill is the most important one for a child to benefit from educational services offered in kindergarten. In order for OT to qualify as a "related service," intervention goals must be directly related to education. While skills listed in answers A, B, and D are usually developed during the time a child enters kindergarten, they are not essential for the child to benefit from education. See reference: Case-Smith, Allen, and Pratt (eds): Case-Smith, J, and Shortridge, SD: The developmental process. Also: Dubois: Preschool services.

17. (C) provide enjoyable activities in a safe and accepting environment. Answer C is correct because children who learn to enjoy activities alone will be more likely to cooperate with peers in a group activity. Answer A is not correct because the child will not initiate and develop social interaction in an environment that inhibits independence (such as an authoritarian environment). Answer B is not correct because children with peer interaction problems will need to be taught some basic social skills in order to increase peer interaction. Answer D is not correct because the children will more likely learn and accept rules and limits established by their group. See reference: Kramer and Hinojosa (eds): Olson, L: Psychosocial frame of reference.

18. (C) elbow and wrist stability, by wheelbarrow-walking ten steps while being held at the knees." Answer C is the only one that relates directly to the long-term goal. The delayed grasp pattern may due to poor wrist stability, which can be enhanced by weight bearing in prone position. Answers A and B address visual perceptual skills. Answer D deals with an unrelated UE motor pattern. See reference: Case-Smith, Allen, and Pratt (eds): Amundsen, SJ, and Weil, M: Pre-writing and handwriting skills. Also: Case-Smith, J: Planning and implementing services.

19. (A) pull-to-sit, leaning back against therapy ball. While all answers involve anti-gravity control, answer A addresses beginning control in neck and shoulders. Because control develops cephalocaudally, neck and shoulder control should be addressed first. By using an incline, the pull of gravity can be reduced, thus facilitating maximum control. See reference: Case-Smith, Allen, and Pratt (eds): Nichols, DS: The development of postural control.

20. (C) reduce competing sensory input—use head phones during work. Reducing competing sensory input is helpful in increasing visual attention. Increasing competing input (answers A and B) or reducing the amount of visual input (answer D) may serve to reduce the ability to attend. See reference: Case-Smith, Allen, and Pratt (eds): Schneck, CM: Visual perception.

21. (D) involve the children in the rule-making process. If children are involved in the rule-making process, they are more likely to value the rules and adhere to them. This also provides them with a sense of control over their environment, leading to a feeling of mastery. Aversive consequences (answer A) may be effective in behavior management but may also increase behavior targeted at avoidance of "being found out." Ignoring transgressions (answer B) may not be appropriate for dangerous or socially unacceptable behavior. Enlisting the help of families (answer C) is helpful but secondary to the establishment of rules. See reference: Case-Smith, Allen, and Pratt (eds): Cronin, AS: Psychosocial and emotional domains of behavior.

22. (A) performing regular weight shifts. Although all of the answers may be appropriate for many individuals using wheelchairs, skin inspection takes priority because of the seriousness of the consequences of skin breakdown. Skin breakdown is most likely to occur over bony prominences and can develop within 30 minutes. Therefore, frequent weight shifts and regular skin inspection are essential. Wheelchair gloves (answer B) are useful in improving grip on the wheels of the chair for wheelchair propulsion and can also protect the skin on the hands. Keeping wheelchair speed moderate (answer C) protects the wheelchair user and those around him. Avoiding sandy surfaces (answer D) keeps the wheelchair cleaner and in better working order. See reference: Pedretti (ed): Adler, C: Spinal cord injury.

23. (A) Exploratory. Exploratory play provides the child with experiences that develop body scheme, sensory integrative and motor skills, and concepts of sensory characteristics and actions on objects. Therefore the obstacle course is an example of exploratory play. Symbolic play (answer B) is associated with the development of language and concepts (use of "dress-up" materials would be an example of this type of play). Creative play (answer C) and interests are characterized by refinement of skills in activities that allow construction, social relationships, and dramatic play (finger painting is an example of creative play). Recreational play (answer D) involves play-leisure experiences that allow exploration of interests and roles such as arts and crafts or sports. See reference: Case-Smith, Allen, and Pratt (eds): Stewart, KB: Occupational therapy assessment in pediatrics: Purposes, process, and methods of evaluation.

24. (A) forward and backward chaining. Chaining with the child who demonstrates a cognitive disability shows the entire process of a task with all sequences. Initially, the child performs only the beginning or end of the task. Thus, the child concentrates on only a small part of the task but gradually increases participation in all sequences in their correct order. Answers B, C, and D are other methods that can be used, but forward and backward chaining are instructional methods that have been particularly successful with individuals who are mentally retarded. See reference: Hopkins and Smith (eds): Humphry, R, and Jewell, K: Mental retardation.

25. (A) transitional movements to sitting are restricted. Answer A is correct because children are unable to rotate onto their buttocks or sit back on lower legs when using such an adaptive device. Answers B, C, and D are incorrect because all of these movements are incorporated in the use of an adaptive device for support of creeping. See reference: Case-Smith, Allen, and Pratt (eds): Wright-Ott, C, and Egilson, S: Mobility.

26. (C) Handle the child slowly and gently. Answer C is correct because the child with hypertonicity will be most relaxed, and easier to handle, if tone is inhibited by the therapist's slow and gently handling of his body. Answer A is incorrect because adaptive equipment is frequently needed to provide a child with a sense of security during bathing. Answer B is not correct because a full explanation of the procedure will also increase a child's sense of security during bathing. Answer D is not correct because it provides the parent with a poor model of good body mechanics; rather, the therapist should kneel or sit on a stool. See reference: Case-Smith, Allen, and Pratt (eds): Hunter, JG: The neonatal intensive care unit.

27. (D) picking up raisins with a pair of tweezers. While all answers describe methods to promote some aspect of handwriting skills, this activity is the only one that targets isolated finger use. Drawing on sandpaper (answer A) can be used to increase kinesthetic awareness and finger strength. Copying shapes (answer B) is primarily a perceptual-motor task. Rolling out Play Doh (answer C) is an activity that can promote bilateral hand use and the development of palmar arches. See reference: Case-Smith, Allen, and Pratt (eds): Amundsen, SJ, and Weil, M: Pre-writing and handwriting skills.

28. (A) Physical guidance. The correct answer is A, because physical guidance requires the least cognitive ability and provides the child the opportunity to learn through a sensory-motor experience. Answer B is not correct because verbal cues require understanding of language. Answer C is not correct because visual cues, such as pictures, require understanding the meaning of pictures. Answer D is not correct as forward chaining requires the first step of a sequence be completed by the child. See reference: Hopkins and Smith (eds): Humphry, R, and Jewell, K: Mental retardation.

29. (A) A prone scooter. Spastic diplegia is defined as abnormal tone affecting primarily the lower extremities; therefore, Joey may use his upper extremities to propel himself through space while having his lower extremities positioned on the scooter. The airplane mobility device (answer B) is designed for children with good lower extremity function who need support in the upper body. A tricycle (answer C) requires good lower extremity control, including reciprocal movement. A power wheelchair (answer D) is designed for individuals with limited upper and lower extremity function. See reference: Case-Smith, Allen, and Pratt (eds): Wright-Ott, C, and Egilson, S: Mobility.

30. (A) What type of chair he should sit in. Correct postural alignment and postural stability are essential to a child's self-feeding skills. Children with abnormal muscle tone often lack the stable postural base required for distal control of the arm and hand in self-feeding; therefore, seating during feeding should be addressed first. Answers A, B, and D are also important considerations but should be addressed after the seating position has been successfully solved. See reference: Case-Smith, Allen, and Pratt (eds): Case-Smith, J, and Humphry, R: Feeding and oral motor skills.

31. (A) Applesauce. Foods with even consistency and uniform texture are the easiest to control and swallow. Foods with multiple textures like chicken noodle soup (answer A), sticky foods like peanut butter (answer B), and foods that are fibrous or break up in the mouth like carrot sticks (answer C) should be avoided. See reference: Case-Smith, Allen, and Pratt (eds): Case-Smith, J, and Humphry, R: Feeding and oral motor skills.

32. (C) Wheelbarrow race. The shunt serves to reduce fluid in the head by means of a catheter that runs from the ventricles to the abdominal cavity, where the fluid can be safely absorbed. Any upending of the child, i.e., any activity that involves positioning the head lower than the rest of the body, will interrupt this flow and is therefore contraindicated. Answers A, B, and D involve upright positioning and are therefore fine for Mikey to participate in. See reference: Case-Smith, Allen, and Pratt (eds): Gordon, CY, Schanzenbacher, KE, Case-Smith, J, and Carrasco, R: Diagnostic problems in pediatrics.

33. (D) blowing cotton balls into a target. Children with ADD have difficulty with sustained attention and effort. Answers A, B, and C require sustained visual vigilance and involve delayed gratification. By contrast, blowing cotton balls into a target is a short-term activity with immediate reward for successful completion. This activity is therefore the most appropriate one, responding to Jamie's dual needs. See reference: Logigian and Ward (eds): Ward, JD: Attention Deficit Disorder/Hyperactivity.

34. (C) oversized tee-shirts and elastic-top pants. For a child with difficulty in self-dressing due to incoordination (as seen in athetoid cerebral palsy), clothing should be loose fitting with simple or no fasteners. Oversized clothing is preferred to tight-fitting garments (answers A and B). Garments with elasticized waist bands are better than those using zippers (answer B) or snaps and buttons (answer D). See reference: Logigian and Ward (eds): Logigian, MK: Cerebral palsy.

35. (C) Pencil gripper. These are all adaptive devices that can be used with a child who has juvenile rheumatoid arthritis for various reasons. However, the correct answer is C, because the pencil gripper will probably make grasping the pencil easier and reduce hand grasp fatigue. Because of weak hands, and because printing and handwriting is a common task for children this age, it is important that fatigue be reduced. The reacher (answer A) is not correct because it frequently requires grip strength, although it is an important piece of equipment for children who have problems with extended reach. The jar opener (answer B) is not incorrect in terms of its adaptation for hand-strength problems, but jar opening is not a task frequently performed by a school-aged child (as is handwriting). The plate guard (answer C) will provide adaptation for incoordination, one-handedness, and limitations in hand/arm function but is not particularly necessary when hand strength is decreased (adapting the utensil would be more reasonable). See reference: Case-Smith, Allen, and Pratt (eds): Gordon, CY, Schanzenbacher, KE, Case-Smith, J, and Carrasco, R: Diagnostic problems in pediatrics.

36. (B) raising the handle bars. The correct answer is B because raising the handle bars demands that the arms are raised, thus bringing the child to the upright posture. Answers A and D are not correct because the hips and lower extremities are already positioned correctly and this positioning would be disrupted. Answer D is not correct because the arms would be lowered and trunk forward flexion would be increased. See reference: Kramer and Hinojosa: Colangelo, CA: Biomechanical frame of reference.

37. (B) Extension. Protective arm reactions allow one to return to a support base or to protect the body when there are environmental changes. Answer B is the correct answer because the arms extend during this protective movement. Facilitation of protective reactions may be a beginning point for the development of arm extension in treatment. Answers A, C, and D are incorrect because these movements are not the major movement component of protective arm reactions. See reference: Gilfoyle, Grady, and Moore: Strategies for developmental and purposeful sequences.

38. (C) snipping the edge of a paper ("making fringes"). Snipping is considered the first scissors skill, preceding other scissors skills such as cutting on a line. Snipping, or initial cutting, is the process of simply closing the scissors on the paper, but with no ongoing adjustment of the paper by the other hand. Snipping may also be done while the child's forearm is still pronated, i.e., in an earlier developmental position than the more mature forearm-in-midposition required for coordinated cutting. Answers A and B may be used for further skill development once cutting on a line has been established. Answer D is probably not effective, since Ida will most likely choose her dominant hand for a skilled activity such as cutting. If Ida has a clearly preferred hand, switching dominance is contraindicated. See reference: Case-Smith, Allen, and Pratt (eds): Exner, CE: Development of hand skills.

39. (C) a set of cymbals. Cymbals are played by holding one in each hand and bringing them together at midline for a clashing sound—a direct extension of the clapping at midline skill that Michelle has just mastered. Symmetrical midline manipulation represents the first step in functional bilateral hand use. Bells on wrist straps (answer A) do not require any bilateral activity to be activated, and therefore represent a level of skill Michelle has surpassed. Answers B and D represent skills that are too advanced for Michelle at this point. The drum (answer B) necessitates stabilization in one hand and manipulation in the other. The piano (answer D) requires simultaneous asymmetrical bilateral manipulation. See reference: Case-Smith, Allen, and Pratt (eds): Exner, CE: Development of hand skills.

40. (B) acknowledges his efforts and encourages his active experimentation. In order to develop task competence, Sebastian should be allowed to persist in the activity as long as he is interested. An important part of task mastery is the challenge and practice leading to success based on one's own behavior. If the COTA were to provide the solution by giving him the correct block (answer A), explaining his difficulties to him (answer C), or changing the whole task (answer D), she would deprive him of the opportunity to achieve task competence needed to develop further his play skills. See reference: Case-Smith, Allen, and Pratt (eds): Cronin, AS: Psychosocial and emotional domains of behavior.

41. (C) supervision. At this level, the child performs the task on his or her own but is unsafe to be left alone or may need verbal cuing or physical prompts for 1–24% of task. At the independent level (answer A) the child performs the complete task, including the setup. At the independent-with-setup level (answer B) the child performs the task after someone sets it up. Minimal assist (answer D) signifies that the child performs half to three quarters of the task independently, but needs physical assistance or other cuing for the remainder of the task. See reference: Case-Smith, Allen, and Pratt (eds): Shepherd, J, Procter, SA, and Coley, IL: Self care and adaptations for independent living.

42. (A) The time he spends at the computer. As computer work requires very little active movement, and lower extremities, trunk, and neck are generally held in a static position, it is essential to assess the time Ricardo spends in this position. The COTA must instruct Ricardo to take regular breaks and maintain proper positioning while at the computer to avoid further strain. Answers B, C, and D address other relevant factors in computer use but none that would directly produce the symptoms described. See reference: Ryan (ed): Ryan SE, Ryan BJ, and Walker, JE: Computers. *The Certified Occupational Therapy Assistant.*

43. (C) prevent deformity. The most correct answer is C because a child with juvenile rheumatoid arthritis (JRA) will need splinting to prevent deformity and maintain range of motion. Answer A is not correct because hypertonus is not a characteristic of JRA. Answer B is not correct because, owing to the active nature of JRA, increasing range of motion may be contraindicated. The correction of deformity may also be contraindicated with this child because of the active nature of her disease. Therefore, answer D is not correct. See reference: Case-Smith, Allen, and Pratt (eds): Gordon, CY, Schanzenbacher, KE, Case-Smith, J, and Carrasco, R: Diagnostic problems in pediatrics.

44. (B) manual rocking while in prone on a therapy ball. Answer B is correct because it employs slow, regular vestibular input in a comfortable and safe position, which is inhibitory. Answers A, C, and D are vestibular activities, but they involve fast or irregular movements that will increase the level of arousal. See reference: Hopkins and Smith: Kinnealey, M, and Miller, LJ: Sensory integration/learning disabilities.

45. (A) Matthew should participate in preparatory vestibular activities to enable him to concentrate on simple activities. The discharge summary is a summary of an individual's course of treatment and includes recommendations for further services. Answer B is a treatment goal that reflects the action the individual is to take, as well as a specific time frame, and is included in the treatment plan. Answers C and D reflect the subjective reports/observations of Matthew and his parents and are more appropriate for initial or discharge notes. See reference: Ryan (ed): Backhaus, H: Documentation. *Practice Issues in Occupational Therapy.*

46. (B) give praise for completed dressing; do not help him get dressed. Since Ross has achieved dressing independence, he does not need assistance (answer A), clothing adaptations (answer C), or verbal prompts (answer D) to complete the task. In fact, assisting him now may cause him to lose his independence and regress to relying on his parents again. See reference: Ryan (ed): McFadden, SA: The child with mental retardation. *Practice Issues in Occupational Therapy.*

47. (C) attainment of kindergarten readiness skills. The primary focus of intervention is to prepare the student for the transition to kindergarten. Readiness for kindergarten includes academic skills as well as ADL (answers A and D) and social skills (answer B). Once a student has achieved age-level skills in all these areas, she may benefit fully from the educational program and OT services can be discontinued. See reference: Case-Smith, Allen, and Pratt (eds): Dubois, SA: Preschool services.

48. (B) Incorporate therapeutic activities into family routines. Separate "therapy routines" (answers A and D) can take up an excessive amount of time and energy and may interfere with family life; therefore long-term follow-through may not be as effective as when activities can be made to fit the existing daily routines and developed into habits. Activities provided on an as-needed basis (answer C) will never become habits, and therefore follow-through is less effective. See reference: Case-Smith, Allen, and Pratt (eds): Stephens LC, and Tauber, SK: Early intervention.

49. (C) School newspaper. Anxiety disorder is characterized by extreme self-consciousness and anxiety about competence. Public exposure and pressure for on-the-spot performance heighten the felt anxiety. By becoming involved in the newspaper preparation, the student will have an opportunity to develop a sense of competence without the pressure of a face-to-face audience and judged competition, as represented by activities described in answers A, B, and D. See reference: Case-Smith, Allen, and Pratt (eds): Davidson, DA: Programs and services for children with psychosocial dysfunction.

50. (D) Doll house, dress-up clothes. To encourage symbolic play, the child should be exposed to toys offering imaginative, open-ended play opportunities, encouraging formulation of ideas and feelings. Answers A, B, and C are not only representative of the younger (answer A) or older child (answers B and C), but they also offer more defined, closed-ended play opportunities with predictable results. See reference: Case-Smith, Allen, and Pratt (eds): Morrison, CD, Metzger, P, and Pratt, PN: Play.

51. (C) anterograde amnesia. Anterograde amnesia is the inability to recall events after a trauma. Retrograde amnesia (answer D) is the inability to recall events prior to trauma. Long-term memory (answer B) is the storage of information for recall at a later time. Orientation (answer A) is the awareness of person, place, and time. See reference: Trombly (ed): Quintana, LA: Evaluation of perception and cognition.

52. (C) her lower back. Touching the lower back requires shoulder abduction and internal rotation. Answers A and B are incorrect because they require external shoulder rotation. Touching the opposite shoulder (answer D) demonstrates horizontal adduction. See reference: Trombly (ed): Evaluation of biomechanical and physiological aspects of motor performance.

53. (B) combing her hair. An individual normally abducts and externally rotates the shoulder to comb his or her hair. Shoulder abduction is not required for buttoning a shirt (answer A) or tying a shoe (answer D). Tucking in her shirt in the back (answer C) requires shoulder abduction and internal rotation. Tying shoelaces (answer D) is less dependent on shoulder motion than on hip and spine flexibility. See reference: Pedretti (ed): Foti, D, Pedretti, LW, and Lillie, S: Activities of daily living.

54. (B) good (4). The individual's "available" range is the range the joint may be moved through passively. Therefore, if an individual is able to move the joint actively through the entire movement that is completed passively and then take maximum resistance, the grade is normal (5). Good (4) is the grade given when a part moves through the available range but against gravity and is able to sustain moderate resistance. Fair (3) is the grade given when an individual is able to move a part through full range against gravity but lacks strength for any resistance. Fair minus (3–) is the grade given when an individual moves a part against gravity through less than full range of motion. Fair minus is the last graded range for movement against gravity. Grades poor and trace are for gravity-eliminated movements. See reference: Trombly (ed): Evaluation of biomechanical and physiological aspects of motor performance.

55. (C) good. The individual demonstrates good muscle strength because moderate resistance is taken in the pain-free range. Individuals with arthritis should always be tested in the pain-free range of active range of motion. Testing in a painful position may limit the effort the individual is able to produce against resistance. This may yield a false assessment of the individual's functional strength and could also damage arthritic tissues. Individuals with poor (answer A) or fair (answer B) strength would be unable to sustain any resistance in the pain-free range. A individual with normal strength (answer D) would be able to take full resistance against gravity in the pain-free range. See reference: Trombly (ed): Evaluation of biomechanical and physiological aspects of motor performance.

56. (A) Short-term memory. Short-term memory is the ability to recall information that has just been received and hold it in temporary use from 1 to 5 minutes or more. Attention (answer B) refers to the ability to focus on a stimulus for a period of time without being distracted. In assessing attention, the COTA would ask an individual to repeat numbers presented by the therapist immediately, without the 1–5-minute delay used for assessing memory. A person who is being evaluated for hearing (answer C) would be checked for the accuracy of sound at different pitches, not a specific sound. Orientation (answer D) refers to the accurate awareness of person, place, and time. See reference: Trombly (ed): Quintana, LA: Evaluation of perception and cognition.

57. (D) anosognosia. Anosognosia is a form of neglect in which the individual denies any deficits. Compensation techniques cannot be taught to someone who has no awareness of his or her deficits. A person with a visual field cut (answer A) has a loss of a specific area of vision related to an area of the visual system that has been damaged. When there is an awareness of the loss, compensatory techniques can be taught. A person who has apraxia (answer B) is unable to perform a purposeful movement on command but is able to understand a loss of ability and can perform activities spontaneously or follow some cues. Aphasia (answer D) is an impairment of receptive or expressive communication verbally, but a person with aphasiais able to comprehend gestures or pictures and use them as a compensatory technique. See reference: Trombly (ed): Quintana, LA: *Evaluation of perception and cognition.*

58. (C) shoulder subluxation. Shoulder subluxation is a condition in which the humerus is partially dislocated as a result of weakness of the muscles surrounding the shoulder joint. It is evaluated by manual palpation of the shoulder joint. Answers A, B, and D are all sensory processing components, according to AOTA Uniform Terminology, and are evaluated during a sensory evaluation. See reference: Ryan (ed): Larson, BA, and Watson, PM: The adult with a cerebral vascular accident. *Practice Issues in Occupational Therapy.*

59. (D) strength. Exerting enough pressure to twist off the lid requires strength. He demonstrates adequate range of motion (answer A) when he grasps the knife. He demonstrates adequate coordination (answer B) by spreading peanut butter on bread and accurately positioning the lid onto the jar opening. He demonstrates adequate endurance (answer C) by standing during the entire activity of making a peanut butter sandwich. See reference: AOTA: Uniform Terminology for Occupational Therapy, third edition.

60. (B) Activity Configuration. The Activity Configuration asks the individual to break down the week into days and hours and indicate the types of activities being performed as well as the meaning of each activity to that individual. This is the only tool that addresses time management. The Role Checklist (answer A) asks the individual to indicate past, present, and future roles and examines the values of the various roles to the individual. The Interest Checklist (answer C) lists dozens of activities and asks the individual to indicate his or her degree of interest in each. The Occupational History Interview (answer D) asks questions about an individual's life roles, interests, values, and goals. Answers A, B, and D are all useful tools for collecting information concerning the roles of homemaker and parent. See reference: Hopkins and Smith (eds): Culler, KH: Home and family management.

61. (A) specific measurable statements with time frames. Goals can be either short-term (meaning in the immediate future) or long-term (meaning over an extended period of time). The purpose of a goal is to provide a specific statement that is measurable and indicates what is to be accomplished. Patients and significant others play a vital role in working with the therapist to establish goals that are meaningful and realistic. Time frames, answer B, may only be a part of a measurable goal/objective. Specific measurements of the patient's skill and performance (answer C) is a part of the assessment information that assists the therapist in establishing appropriate goals and objectives for treatment. Activities to be completed that correspond with the goals (answer D) is part of the treatment plan. See reference: Jacobs and Logigian (eds): Pagonis, J: Documentation.

62. (D) low back pain. A low back injury requires body mechanics training to prevent further injury to the area and to allow healing. People with chronic obstructive pulmonary disease (answer A) and fibromyalgia (answer B) generally benefit from energy conservation techniques to prevent further depletion of their limited energy. Individuals with carpal tunnel syndrome (answer C) need to position the wrist and restrict lifting to light-weight items because of pain and weakness in the wrist and hand. See reference: Pedretti (ed): Smithline, J: Low back pain.

63. (D) sugar cookies sliced from a roll of dough at room temperature and placed on a tray using a spatula. The sugar-cookie dough would be soft enough to provide minimal resistance without causing immediate fatigue and provide isotonic contractions during the repetitive grasp and release of the knife and the spatula. Although muffin and cake batter (answers A and B) provide the least amount of resistance, the hand is using sustained isometric grasp on the electric or hand-powered mixer, which combined with the minimal resistance of the batter and mixer weight is fatiguing. The chocolate-chip-cookie dough (answer C) is resistive whether it is warm or cold, and to maintain an isometric grasp while mixing with a spatula or scooping with an ice-cream scooper would cause the individual to tire before the activity is finished. If the individual becomes fatigued while performing any of the activities, only the sugar cookies or the chocolate-chip cookies would allow the individual time to rest without affecting the final product. See reference: Trombly (ed): Stewart, C: Retraining housekeeping and child care skills.

64. (A) energy conservation. Energy conservation techniques reduce the amount of energy expenditure an individual requires to perform various activities. Energy conservation techniques should be taught early so they can be implemented and reinforced while performing other activities, such as standing tolerance activities (answer C). Safety in the kitchen (answer D) would be more relevant to individuals with sensory or balance loss than limited endurance. Work hardening (answer B) is not relevant to the goal of meal preparation. See reference: Hopkins and Smith (eds): Pizzi: HIV infection and AIDS.

65. (C) texture of the cords Maggie will be using. Coarse materials like jute may shred and give Maggie splinters or injure the skin on her hands and fingers. This is particularly important for individuals with diabetes who frequently have poor sensation and circulation in their extremities. Skin damage must be avoided since healing is compromised. The length of the cord (answer A) would be significant for an individual with limited range of motion. The thickness of the cord (answer B) would be significant for an individual with limited hand function. The type of surface the individual stands on (answer D) would be important to an individual with back pain. See reference: Reed: Diabetes mellitus - type II.

66. (A) soft to hard to rough. Desensitization stimuli are graded by texture and force. Texture begins with soft and progresses to hard and finally to rough. The force begins with touching and progresses to rubbing and then tapping (opposite of answer B). The texture and force of the stimuli are graded together. Answer C does not clearly specify the degree or type of texture and force. A person with hypersensitivity would be unable to tolerate training beginning with a rough texture (answer D). See reference: Trombly (ed): Bentzel, K: Remediating sensory impairment.

67. (B) A mobile arm support. An individual with C5 quadriplegia typically has fair strength in shoulder flexion and abduction and at least poor– strength in the biceps, upper trapezius, and external rotators. With this level of strength, he will be able to operate a mobile arm support for self-feeding and facial hygiene activities. A wrist-driven flexor hinge splint (answer A) would be used by an individual with a lower-level spinal cord injury (C6-C8) who has functional use of the shoulder and arm muscles and has fair+ or better wrist-extension strength. This splint is indicated for individuals who lack prehension power. An electric feeder (answer C) is indicated for individuals with a higher level of involvement (C4) who demonstrate poor+ or weaker shoulder strength. Built-up utensils (answer D) may be indicated for individuals with C8 or T1 injuries who may lack the strength to tightly grasp regular utensils. See reference: Trombly (ed): Hollar, LD: Spinal cord injury.

68. (C) "Mrs. J. will demonstrate appropriate hip precautions." The ability to stand for 10 minutes (answer A) or flex her hip to 90 degrees (answer B) is not necessary for independence in dressing. Use of appropriate hip precautions, however, is mandatory. Energy-conservation techniques (answer D) are appropriate for individuals who demonstrate very low endurance levels, which is not an issue for most individuals following hip replacement surgery. See reference: Ryan (ed): Gower, D, and Bowker, M: The elderly with a hip arthroplasty. *Practice Issues in Occupational Therapy.*

69. (C) lacing with a double cordovan stitch. The double cordovan stitch is a complex stitch requiring good fine motor coordination. The whipstitch (answer A) is simpler and does not require the same level of coordination. Punching holes with the rotary punch (answer B) requires grip strength. Measuring and cutting the leather lacing (answer D) requires range of motion and gross motor coordination. See reference: Breines: Folkcraft.

70. (C) vestibular processing, postural control, and muscle tone. Vestibular processing and postural control are required for maintaining balance. Muscle tone that is too high or too low will limit the individual's ability to move the lower extremities for ambulation; hence, these three components are important for successfully walking in the pool. Fine motor coordination (answer A) is not required to walk across the pool. In addition, while walking in the water requires some strength, it can still be successfully performed with significantly decreased strength because the body weighs significantly less when submerged. Answer B includes postural control and gross motor coordination, which are both important to walking in the pool, but it also includes visual motor integration, which is not. Answer D includes range of motion and praxis, both of which are required to some degree for walking in the pool, but it also includes crossing the midline, which is not required. See reference: AOTA: Uniform Terminology for Occupational Therapy, third edition.

71. (B) stringing beads for a necklace, following a pattern. This is the only activity of those listed that requires the woman to follow a sequence in order to achieve the desired outcome. Leather stamping in a random design (answer A) does not require sequencing skills but does require coordination, visual-motor integration, and strength. Putting together a puzzle (answer C) requires perception of spatial relations. Playing "Concentration" (answer D) requires memory and attention span. See reference: AOTA: Uniform Terminology for Occupational Therapy, third edition.

72. (D) attached to a cuff that fits around his palm. Individuals with C6 quadriplegia may have a tenodesis grasp or no grasp at all available to them. Therefore, a buttonhook that fits onto the palm or a buttonhook with a built-up handle are the only appropriate choices. A buttonhook with a knob handle (answer B) or on a 1/2-inch dowel (answer C) is appropriate for an individual with a functional grasp but limited dexterity. A buttonhook with an extra-long, flexible handle benefits an individual with limited range of motion. See reference: Trombly (ed): Retraining basic and instrumental activities of daily living.

73. (A) wrist cock-up splint. Carpal tunnel syndrome is a condition that results from compression of the median nerve at the wrist. A wrist cock-up splint positions the wrist in 10 to 20 degrees of extension to alleviate symptoms and prevent further damage. Answer B refers to splints made out of thermoplastic materials and does not indicate a splint type specific to carpal tunnel syndrome. Resting hand splints (answer C) are typically used to prevent development of deformity in individuals with arthritis or quadriplegia. Dynamic MP flexion splints (answer D) are used to assist flexion at the MP joints when this motion is weak or absent. See reference: Ryan (ed): Schober-Branigan, P: Thermoplastic splinting of the hand. *The Certified Occupational Therapy Assistant.*

74. (C) edema, contracture, muscle tone, and pain. Edema limits range of motion because of the increase of fluid in the extremity. A contracture can result when joint motion is limited by a by prolonged spasticity or change in the tissues, causing resistance to passive stretch. Muscle tone may also be a limiting factor in one's ability to complete range of motion. If an individual is unable to move a part through full range against gravity, the therapist may put the individual in a gravity-eliminated position to attempt the same movement. Finally, pain may be a limiting factor. This may be seen particularly in individuals with arthritis or shoulder subluxation. Pain generally occurs in the end ranges of motion. Other options listed in this answer (proprioception, diadokinesis) may affect the quality of active movement or coordination but do not limit active or passive range of motion. See reference: Trombly (ed): Evaluation of biomechanical and physiological aspects of motor performance.

75. (B) flexed at all joints. When weight bearing, the fingers should be flexed at all joints (the fisted position). This preserves the tenodesis function by protecting the finger flexors from over-stretching, which could result if fingers are positioned as described in answers A, C, and D. Another reason for this position is to prevent claw-hand deformity by protecting the intrinsic hand muscles from over-stretching. See reference: Hill (ed): Farmer, A: Setting goals.

76. (B) hyperextension of the PIP joint and flexion of the DIP joint. Answer B is the only answer provided that describes a swan-neck deformity. The pattern of hyperextension of the PIP and DIP joints (answer A) may be seen in lower-motor-neuron palsies. Flexion of the PIP joint and hyperextension of the DIP joint (answer C) is descriptive of a boutonniere deformity. An individual who has over-stretched the volar plates at the PIP and DIP joints would have hyperextension of the MP joint and flexion of the DIP joint (answer D). See reference: Pedretti (ed): Hittle, JM, Pedretti, LW, and Kasch, MC: Rheumatoid arthritis.

77. (C) get the shirt all the way on, then line up the buttons and holes and begin buttoning from the bottom. It is easier to see the buttons and buttonholes at the bottom of the shirt than at the top (answer B); therefore, beginning to button from the bottom is more likely to result in success for the individual with motor or visual-perceptual deficits. Buttoning first (answer A) may result in ripping off the buttons as the shirt is pulled over the head. Although a buttonhook may be helpful to the individual with hemiplegia, the built-up handle is not. A buttonhook with a built-up handle (answer D) would be helpful for an individual with finger weakness or incoordination (e.g., quadriplegia). See reference: Pedretti (ed): Foti, D, Pedretti, LW, and Lillie, S: Activities of daily living.

78. (C) (1) unbutton the shirt; (2) pull the shirt off overhead; (3) remove the unaffected arm; (4) remove the affected arm. Answers A, B, and D are examples of incorrect sequences that would result in failure to remove the shirt successfully. See reference: Pedretti (ed): Foti, D, Pedretti, LW, and Lillie, S: Activities of daily living.

79. (B) (1) seated, cross the affected leg over the unaffected leg; (2) slip affected foot through leg of trousers and uncross; (3) place unaffected leg into trousers; (4) stand and pull up trousers. Answers A, C, and D are examples of incorrect sequences that would result in failure to don the trousers successfully. See reference: Pedretti (ed): Foti, D, Pedretti, LW, and Lillie, S: Activities of daily living.

80. (D) She traces letters through a pan of rice with her fingers. This method involves greater input of sensory information to the brain by performing a gross movement in a more stimulating environment. A verbal description of how to make a letter (answer A), watching her grip (answer B), or performing strengthening exercises (answer C) would not give her proprioceptive feedback on her letter formation through tactile input. See reference: Trombly (ed): Bentzel, K: Remediating sensory impairment.

81. (D) use dust mitt to keep fingers fully extended. Using dust mitts "keeps fingers straight and prevents the static contraction and potentially deforming forces of holding a dust cloth." Pushing the vacuum (answer A) forward by straightening the elbow completely, then pulling it back close to the body uses *long* strokes and promotes good elbow and shoulder range of motion. When ironing (answer B), trying to get the elbow into full *extension* helps to maintain elbow range of motion. Keeping lightweight objects (answer C) on *high* shelves encourages reaching, which helps maintain shoulder range of motion. See reference: Pedretti (ed): Hittle, JM, Pedretti, LW, and Kasch, MC: Rheumatoid arthritis.

82. (D) a raised-bed garden. The individual with back pain must avoid activities that stress the lumbar spine such as "prolonged static postures with a flexed lumbar spine, repetitive bending with a flexed spine, and lifting and carrying when the normal lumbar curve is not maintained." A raised-bed garden would allow gardening without bending. A wheelbarrow with elongated handles (answer B) would be harder to control while pushing than would a wheelbarrow with normal handles and would place undue stress on the low back. A 12-inch-high seat with tool holders could benefit an individual with low endurance, but working the ground from that position would be very difficult for an individual with back pain. See reference: Pedretti (ed): Smithline, J: Low back pain.

83. (D) a weighted pen and weighted wrists. Weighting body parts and utensils (or writing tools) is effective with individuals with ataxia in improving control during performance of a task. Hitting the keys on a keyboard (answer A) would be difficult for Carolyn, although weighting her wrists could make performance of the activity possible. A keyboard is a good alternative for individuals with difficulty writing due to weakness, limited ROM, or incoordination. A universal cuff with a pencil-holder attachment (answer B) would be appropriate for an individual with hand weakness who uses a universal cuff for other tasks. A balanced forearm orthosis (answer C) is appropriate for individuals with severe muscle weakness. In addition, individuals with muscle weakness find felt-tip pens easier to write with than ballpoint pens. See reference: Pedretti (ed): Schlageter, K, and Zoltan, B: Traumatic brain injury.

84. (C) flange the area around the ulnar styloid. Reddened areas indicate the splint is too tight in a particular spot. "To reduce pressure, it is often helpful to flange splint edges." Lining the splint with any material, whether moleskin or foam (answers A and B), will only make a tight area tighter. Remaking the splint (answer D) is unnecessary and a waste of the COTA's time. See reference: Hopkins and Smith (eds): Fess, EE, and Kiel, JH: Upper extremity splinting.

85. (D) place her right arm in the right sleeve first. In upper-extremity dressing, the involved arm should always be dressed first. Buttons could be ripped of if the patient attempts to pull on a blouse on which the buttons have already been buttoned (answer A). Placing the left arm in the left sleeve first (answer C) would be appropriate for an individual with an RCVA resulting in left hemiplegia. Since the ability to don a front-opening blouse has been identified as an appropriate goal for this patient, getting assistance (answer B) is inappropriate. See reference: Pedretti (ed): Foti, D, Pedretti, LW, and Lillie, S: Activities of daily living.

86. (D) pressure marks or redness disappear after 20 minutes. All splints made or given to a patient are checked for correct fit by adjusting any areas that still have redness or pressure marks after the splint has been removed for 20 minutes. Many types of splints may be made with the fingers not flexed or the thumb opposed and abducted (answers A and B), for example, an antispasticity ball splint or a dynamic splint for extension. Most splints are not worn at all times (answer C) but removed for activities such as self-care or exercise. A wearing schedule is issued when a splint is fitted or given to a patient. See reference: Ryan (ed): Schober-Branigan, P: Thermoplastic splinting of the hand. *The Certified Occupational Therapy Assistant.*

87. (A) concise objective information. All medical documentation should be accurate, concise, and objective. Personal opinions and statements that are speculative, judgmental, or subjective (answers B, C, and D) are not appropriate for inclusion in the patient's chart. See reference: Jacobs and Logigian (eds): Pagonis, J: Documentation.

88. (D) quotes from the individual. SOAP is an acronym for Subjective, Objective, Assessment, and Plan. The SOAP format is a common format in the medical fields for documentation. The subjective portion of the SOAP note contains information found in the chart provided by the patient or family. Measurement results (answer A) are based on a patient's performance during the evaluation and are included in the objective section. Answer B, analysis of the measurements, is recorded in the assessment area of the SOAP note. Speculative information (answer C) should not be included in documentation. See reference: Hopkins and Smith (eds): Perinchief, JM: Service management.

89. (D) instruct her to perform only gentle AROM. Gentle active range of motion allows the individual to control the movement and avoid over-stretching of inflamed joint tissues. Brisk AROM (answer A) and the addition of resistance (answer B) are likely to cause further damage to the joints by increasing stress, which results in increased inflammation. The individual must be taught in therapy the importance of joint protection during exercise. Eliminating all ROM exercise (answer C) would result in further joint stiffness and loss of range of motion. See reference: Trombly (ed): Feinberg, JR, and Trombly, CA: Arthritis.

90. (C) assessing the patient's ability to hold the toothbrush with a built-up handle. Progress is demonstrated by the ability to successfully perform an activity that was previously unsuccessful. A patient who is initially unable to hold a built-up handle successfully may need to use a universal cuff (answer D); however, assessing her ability to use a universal cuff is not an appropriate method for determining if she has achieved progress in this area. Evaluation using tools such as a dynamometer and pinch meter (answers A and B) are formal, not functional methods of evaluation. In addition, an individual using tenodesis may not have the strength to actually register a reading on these tools. See reference: Trombly (ed): Hollar, LD: Spinal cord injury.

91. (A) They are likely to react with anger, anxiety, and depression. The news that a family member who has sustained a traumatic injury has plateaued is usually not welcome because it drives home the fact that she is not going to be the way she was. Family members often react to this news with "denial, . . . shock, disbelief, anger, anxiety, depression, mourning, and feelings of disassociation." They will most likely be fearful, not anxious (answer B), about taking the patient home. In today's society, where the husband and wife are often both employed, family members may not available to provide the care required by the individual (answer C). Caregiver/family training (answer D) will be necessary, but their initial reaction is most likely going to be emotional, not rational. See reference: Hopkins and Smith (eds): Versluys, HP: Family influences.

92. (A) "Pt. will purchase 10 items at the supermarket with supervision." Short-term goals must relate to the long-term goal being addressed. Since the long-term goal being addressed is independence in grocery shopping, the short-term goal must relate to grocery shopping. Answers B and C do not relate to grocery shopping. "Goals need to be written to show what the patient will accomplish, not what the therapist will do (p. 94)." Answer D is an appropriate treatment intervention but is written in a way that describes what the COTA, not the patient, will do. See reference: AOTA: Writing functional goals. *Effective Documentation for Occupational Therapy.*

93. (B) the ability to install a door without reinjury. Using proper body mechanics may enable the individual with a back injury to lift heavy objects and perform activities in a variety of potentially stressful positions without increasing pain or chance of reinjury. Using joint-protection techniques may reduce joint stress and pain and preserve joint structures (answer C). The ability to work a full day without becoming fatigued (answer A) may be an outcome of participating in a work-hardening program or using energy conservation techniques. The ability to use a hammer for a prolonged period of time (answer D) may result from a strengthening or conditioning program. See reference: Pedretti (ed): Smithline, J: Low back pain.

94. (A) a canister vacuum cleaner. A canister vacuum cleaner may be managed by someone with weakness and impaired balance while sitting down. The hose is light enough to be easily pushed, and the canister is on wheels and may be moved by a seated person by pushing it with the foot or having someone else move it. An upright vacuum cleaner (answer B) is too heavy for repetitive pushing and pulling and can cause exhaustion or pull the individual off balance. A self-propelled vacuum cleaner (answer C) could also pull the individual off balance by moving too fast for the individual to respond with appropriate postural adjustments. A hand-held vacuum cleaner (answer D) requires too much stooping to do anything but a very small area of the floor. Repetitive bending can cause fatigue quickly and challenges impaired balance. See reference: Trombly (ed): Stewart, C: Retraining housekeeping and child care skills.

95. (C) limit weight bearing on involved lower extremity. Precautions following a total knee replacement would include graded lower extremity weight bearing determined by the surgeon. This may range from non-weight bearing to toe touch, or partial or full weight bearing. The level usually changes between the day of surgery and discharge, according to the person's rate of healing as seen in x-rays. The individual usually has a course of physical therapy to practice the appropriate level of weight bearing during gait and may or may not be seen by an occupational therapist to receive self care or home management training. Following the knee surgery, a person is allowed full hip movement (answer A) and is allowed full weight bearing on the uninvolved lower extremity (answer D). Full knee extension is encouraged (answer B), and flexion exercises for the knee are part of the individual's physical therapy. See reference: Trombly (ed): Bear-Lehman, J: Orthopedic conditions.

96. (C) swing away leg rests, removable arm rests. After swinging away the leg rests and removing the armrests, the individual can move across the sliding board without being blocked by the wheelchair. Answers A and B are incorrect because they would not facilitate a sliding board transfer. Answer D is incorrect because a removable arm rest may make transfers easier, but elevating leg rest would not. A leg rest would need to be detachable or swing away in order for it to be moved out of the way. See reference: Pedretti (ed): Adler, C and Tipton-Burton, M: Wheelchair assessment and transfers.

97. (D) 5 feet by 5 feet. An outward opening door needs a space of 5 feet by 5 feet to allow the wheelchair to be maneuvered around the door. A standard wheelchair requires 5 feet of turning space for a 180 or 360 degree turn. An area that is 3 by 5 feet (answer A), 4 feet by 4 feet (answer B), or 4½ feet by 3 feet (answer C) would not provide enough space to allow the wheelchair to be turned. See reference: Rothstein, Serge, and Wolf: Wheelchairs and standards for access.

98. (A) from a home health OTR or COTA. Home health services, which may include nursing, OT, PT, and speech therapy, are provided in the patient's home. Individuals who require continued care following discharge from the hospital may be appropriate for home health services if they are unable to travel to the hospital for outpatient services. If the decision to discharge Mr. S. has already been made, recommendations for a continued stay in the acute care hospital or transfer to a rehabilitation center (answers B and C) are not appropriate. His weakness and continuing requirement for intravenous drug therapy would make it extremely difficult for Mr. S. to return to the hospital for outpatient therapy (answer D). See reference: Hopkins and Smith (eds): Levine, RE, Corcoran, MA and Gitlin, LN: Home care and private practice.

99. (B) transitional living center. Transitional living centers "provide temporary living arrangements for individuals who are in a transitional phase between hospital or institution and independent community living. Professional staff, including occupational therapy practitioners, assist the residents in gradually assuming responsibility in self-maintenance." Cradle-to-grave homes (answer A) are houses designed with accessibility in mind at the time of construction. Should an individual begin to use a wheelchair later in life, his home would already be wheelchair accessible. Adult day programs (answer C) are rehabilitation oriented day programs for clients who live in the community. They are not residential. Clustered independent living arrangements (answer D) are usually comprised of "apartment clusters or other types of housing in close proximity to each other, in which groups of residents with disabilities share services such as attendants and transportation." See reference: Trombly (ed): Law, M, Stewart, D and Strong, S: Achieving access to home, community, and workplace.

100. (B) "Pt. was initially able to work at the computer for only 10 minutes. Upon discharge, he can work at the computer for 3 hours with stretch breaks every 30 minutes." The "objective" section of the discharge summary should summarize the patient's condition upon discharge from the facility. Some facilities compare initial and final evaluation, while others only address progress from the time of the previous note. Answers A and D are subjective reports. Answer C is an example of a statement that belongs in the "assessment" section of a discharge summary. See reference: Kettenbach: Writing objective (O).

101. (C) relationships with others. The primary problem area for most individuals with personality disorder is their interactions with others. Specific personality disorder categories indicate that there is some variation among the types of relationships that are impacted. Individuals with mood and thought disorders often have problems with ADLs (answers B and D). Individuals with schizophrenia often demonstrate deficits in sensorimotor skills (answer A). See reference: Early: Understanding psychiatric diagnoses.

102. (A) Milwaukee Evaluation of Daily Living Skills (MEDLS). The MEDLS was designed specifically for long-term psychiatric settings, whereas the KELS (answer C) was designed for acute-care settings. The areas described in the question are contained in the MEDLS. The ACL (answer B) is an indirect measure of self-care abilities. The Barthel Self-Care Index (answer D) was designed for physically impaired individuals. See reference: Hemphill (ed): Leonordelli, C: The Milwaukee Evaluation of Daily Living Skills (MEDLS).

103. (D) view of the problem and an overall goal. The interview is generally the component of the assessment process where the OT practitioner asks about the individual's goals for treatment and gains an understanding of the problems from the person's perspective. Diagnoses and medications (answers A and B) are most often found in a review of the chart. Abilities (answer C) are determined through performance measures. See reference: Denton: Assessment.

104. (D) individuals who are at or above their normal body weight. Most people with eating disorders, bulimics and anorexics, are between adolescence and adulthood and are female. Only one third of all individuals with bulimia weigh less than their normal body weight. Occupational therapy treatment usually focuses on body image, nutrition and food management, social and sexual relationships, interpersonal communication skills, and work and leisure skills. See reference: Hopkins and Smith (eds): Beck, NL: Eating disorders: Anorexia nervosa and bulimia nervosa.

105. (A) OT FACT. OT FACT stands for Occupational Therapy Functional Assessment Compilation Tool. It is a computer software program designed to organize and summarize occupational performance information obtained through a variety of evaluation strategies. The other items are not computerized. The Occupational History Interview (answer B) addresses the patient's life roles, interests, values and goals, and the effect of environment on function. The RIC Scale (answer C) addresses ADL performance in patients with physical disabilities. The AMPS (answer D) addresses ADL performance and the underlying motor and organizational skills. It can be used with a wide range of patient populations. See reference: Hopkins and Smith (eds): Culler, KH: Home and family management.

106. (D) Allen's Routine Task Inventory. This tool assesses an individual's independent living skills. The structured interview format can be used with either the patient or his caregiver. The MEDLS (answer B) is a standardized evaluation; the COTE (answer A) evaluates the patient's general, task and interpersonal behaviors; and the Occupational History (answer C) addresses the patient's occupational role development. See reference: Early: Data gathering and evaluation.

107. (B) NPI Interest Checklist. This tool is frequently used to initiate discussion of how a patient usually spends his leisure time and to identify areas of specific interest. While the KELS and the Scorable Self-Care Evaluation (answers A and D) address the use of leisure time, they are used primarily to assess skills in personal care, safety and health, money management, transportation, use of the telephone, and work. The Activity Configuration (answer C) is used to assess the patient's use of time and his feelings about all of the activities he performs in a typical day or week. See reference: Early: Data gathering and evaluation.

108. (D) "Patient stated that he likes to read sports magazines." This statement provides a basis for an objective judgment on what the patient likes because it has been made by the patient. Answers A, B, and C are examples of assumptions by the practitioner. See reference: Early: Medical records and documentation.

109. (B) Objective. The objective portion of a SOAP note describes observable behavior noted by the COTA. "I don't want to attend..." would indicate what the patient said and would be placed in the subjective portion. The subjective portion of a SOAP note (answer A) refers to what the patient reported or comments about the treatment. The assessment part of a SOAP note refers to the effectiveness of treatment and any changes needed, the status of the goals, and justification for continuing occupational therapy treatment. The plan section of a SOAP note includes statements related to continuing treatment; the frequency and duration of the treatment; suggestions for additional activities or treatment techniques; the need for further evaluations; and, when needed, recommendations for new goals. See reference: Early: Medical records and documentation.

110. (B) emotional lability. Emotional lability is the rapid shifting of moods. Emotional lability may be one of the symptoms observed with individuals experiencing mania (answer A), but it may be seen in non-manic conditions, such as confusion and stroke, as well. Paranoia (answer C) describes enduring beliefs about being harmed. Denial (answer D) is not acknowledging the presence of information. See reference: Early: Responding to symptoms and behaviors.

111. (A) provide a variety of therapeutic sports, arts, crafts, music, and recreation activities to develop and reinforce healthy interest patterns. Differences among psychiatric service providers should be based on roles versus the media and modalities used. Answer B is the role of physical therapy, answer C is the role of occupational therapy, and answer D is the role of vocational rehabilitation. Effective program planning is based on a clear understanding of the contributions of all the service providers within a team. See reference: Ryan (ed): Blechert, TF, Christiansen, MF, and Kari, N: Teamwork and team building. *Practice Issues in Occupational Therapy.*

112. (B) a class about job seeking strategies. The purpose of applying remedial strategies is to enhance underlying abilities. Teaching and training methods are commonly used techniques. Answer A, the NPI Interest Checklist, is a tool used to identify the degree of an individual's interest in a variety of leisure areas. Answer C is an example of a compensatory strategy. Answer D provides opportunities for exploration and expression. See reference: Early: Cognitive and sensorimotor activities.

113. (C) applying grout to a tile trivet and waiting for it to dry. Activities provide a variety of opportunities for therapeutic gains. The process of grouting a tile trivet involves covering the individual's tile design with the grout mixture, which is a messy step. The individual then sees that the tile pattern is emphasized with the addition of the grout. Waiting for the grout to dry requires an individual to delay gratification. Working in a group (answer A) promotes cooperation. Selecting a tile design (answer B) involves decision making. Cleaning off the table (answer D) may promote the experience of success after a mess but does not involve delayed gratification. See reference: Hopkins and Smith (eds): Simon, CJ: Use of activity and activity analysis.

114. (B) The small wood pieces are precut by the OT aide, and the patient uses a template for cutting the large straight-edged pieces and then uses step-by-step directions and photographs to put it together. Adapted sequencing involves using steps that have been adapted to enhance success or completion. Precutting pieces, which decreases the number of steps required while using templates and picture directions, simplifies the task. Answers A and D are examples of developmental sequencing. Answer C is an example of normal sequencing. See reference: Denton: Treatment planning and implementation.

115. (D) disorganized psychosis. Directive group treatment is a highly structured approach that is used in acute care psychiatry for minimally functioning individuals. This approach is useful for individuals with psychoses and other neurological disorders who demonstrate disorganized and disturbed functioning. Task groups involve working on simple tasks for the purpose of developing basic performance skills and are more appropriate for individuals with substance abuse (answer A). Psychoeducation groups are appropriate for those with eating disorders and adjustment disorders (answers B and C). See reference: Hopkins and Smith (eds): Beck, NL: Substance Abuse: Drug addiction and alcoholism.

116. (C) assertiveness training. "Broken record" is a specific assertiveness skill concerned with repeating your position without losing control. Music therapy (answer A) is a creative arts discipline. Psychodrama (answer D) is a group technique for expressing catharsis. Self-awareness groups (answer B) tend to focus on feeling identification and expression versus skill building. See reference: Posthuma: Appendix A- Small group programs.

117. (A) The client will be able to identify two activities that are of interest to him within 2 weeks. Goals for treatment should be relevant to the patient's needs, contain some criterion against which success can be measured, and indicate the behavior the patient is to perform. See reference: Early: Treatment planning.

118. (A) providing patients with individual projects and having them choose a tile color for their projects. The activity should begin with the most basic level of decision making. Each of the other choices requires increasingly more challenging decision-making abilities. Choosing from an assortment of projects (answer B) requires higher-level decision-making ability than selecting a color. Answer C requires not only decisions on design, color, size, etc., but also involves decision making among group members. Answer D involves decision making on two separate aspects, pattern and colors, resulting in a higher level of complexity than answer A. See reference: Early: Analyzing, adapting, and grading activities.

119. (C) having the patients select a new project from three options. Choosing from a limited selection of projects encourages the patient to make a decision without being overwhelmed by a large number of choices. Answers A, B, and D all involve more challenging levels of decision making and should be considered as the patient improves in his decision-making ability. See reference: Early: Analyzing, adapting, and grading activities.

120. (C) avoid having at-risk individuals in close proximity to others to reduce opportunities for physical

contact. Avoiding close proximity situations is the recommended environmental modification for sexually acting out behaviors. Advising the client of your expectations (answer D) is an appropriate use of self in such situations. Standing to the side (answer B) is a recommended environmental modification for highly aggressive and hostile behavior risks. Providing real-life activities in a stimulating environment (answer A) has been found to be helpful with reducing some delusions. See reference: Early: Safety techniques.

121. (D) each member will remain in the group without disrupting the work of others for 30 minutes. People functioning at a parallel level do not have the ability to interact with the other group members beyond some casual greetings. Therefore, appropriate expectations for parallel groups focus on remaining in the group and working alongside others. Taking leadership roles (answer A) is a goal consistent with egocentric-cooperative groups. Sharing materials (answer B) is a project group goal. Expressing feelings within a group (answer C) is consistent with a cooperative group. See reference: Early: Group concepts and techniques.

122. (D) decoupage wood key fob. A wood key fob with a decoupage finish is the safest craft choice since it is free of sharp, toxic, and cord-like materials. A ceramic object (answer C) could be broken into sharp pieces that an individual could use to harm herself. Craft projects that contain rope or cord-like materials that can be used in hanging (answers A and C) should also be avoided. See reference: Early: Safety techniques.

123. (D) using active listening techniques. Active listening is an effective listening response that enables the patient to know that her message has been communicated. Behaviors listed in answers A, B, and C can be counterproductive to developing a therapeutic relationship. Answers A and B may be perceived as enhancing a friendship, rather than a therapeutic, relationship. Answer C is inappropriate for someone who doesn't have adequate social skills to begin with. See reference: Ryan (ed): Blechert, TF and Kari, N: Interpersonal communication skills and applied group dynamics. *The Certified Occupational Therapy Assistant.*

124. (C) precipitating conditions and events that elicit stress reactions. The conditions and events that elicit stress reactions are known as stressors. Stressors can be both short term or long term. Answer A describes coping. Answer B describes stress. Answer D describes adaptation. See reference: Christiansen and Baum (eds): Christiansen, C: Performance deficits as sources of stress.

125. (B) Photosensitivity. Photosensitivity is a side effect of neuroleptic medications that increases sensitivity to the sun, resulting in sunburn. Hypotension (answers A) and weight gain (answer D) are also known to be side effects of neuroleptics but would generally not be problematic for a community outing. Excessive perspiration (answer C) is not a side effect of these medications. See reference: Early: Psychotropic medications and somatic treatments.

126. (C) anxiety and confusion among group members. It is important for the group leader to demonstrate consistency by showing the same degree of respect, interest, and authority toward every group member. Overdependence (answer A) would be a result of the group leader not giving group members enough autonomy. Group members know what to expect from the group leader (answer B) when the group leader demonstrates consistent behavior. Too much, too little, or inappropriate praise are aspects of nurturing behavior, which supports growth and development of group members. See reference: Early: Group concepts and techniques.

127. (C) conduct disorder. Conduct disorders often involve aggression toward people and/or animals and property destruction. Individuals with hyperactivity, (answer A) demonstrate extremely high energy and activity levels. Answer B, attention deficit disorders, involve impulsive but not typically violent behaviors. Answer D, oppositional defiant disorders, involve similar but less severe behaviors as conduct disorders. See reference: Early: Understanding psychiatric diagnosis.

128. (D) smoking during the group is prohibited. Norms are guidelines for behavior in groups, whether stated explicitly or implicitly, shared by the members. Answer A is an individual's behavior versus the groups guidelines. Role playing (answer B) is a group activity. Improved self-esteem (answer C) is a general group goal or outcome. See reference: Early: Group concepts and techniques.

129. (C) baking cookies using a recipe. This is a well-delineated meal preparation activity that provides structure with a specific sequence of tasks. Setting a table or preparing a shopping list (answers A and D) do not necessarily require sequencing of tasks. Planning a meal (answer B) involves a great deal of organizational ability and would not be an appropriate choice for an initial activity to address goals relating to sequencing tasks. See reference: Early: Responding to symptoms and behaviors.

130. (B) vestibular stimulation and gross motor exercise. The sensory integration treatment approach, which aims to improve the reception and processing of sensory information within the central nervous system, utilizes both vestibular stimulation and gross motor exercises. Social skills training (answer A), role-playing activities (answer C) and discussion groups (answer D) might be used when an individual needs help in relating appropriately and effectively with others. While these interventions may be a part of the overall treatment program, this type of individual must be able to receive and process sensory information before embarking on a higher level of social interaction. See reference: Early: Models for Occupational Therapy in Mental Health.

131. (A) Patients write fears and concerns on index cards. The COTA collects and reads the cards to the group for discussion. This method allows for anonymity by having each patient write down concerns without including his or her name, thereby eliminating any fear of embarrassment. Answers B and C require patients to make public their concerns, which might prevent complete openness when attempting to express concerns and fears. While there are certain concerns that might be common to a large number of patients, and having a team member address these concerns in general would be helpful (answer D), this approach would not address the specific concerns of the patients in this group. See reference: Early: Expressive and coping skills.

132. (B) to avoid use of power tools and sharp instruments. Individuals experiencing extrapyramidal syndrome, which may cause muscular rigidity, tremors, and/or sudden muscle spasms, should avoid using power tools or sharp instruments. Photosensitivity, an increased sensitivity to the sun, is another side effect often associated with neuroleptic medications that can be addressed by limiting sun exposure (answer A). Answer C is a strategy that can be used to avoid postural hypotension, a sudden drop in blood pressure resulting in feeling faint or loss of consciousness when moving from lying or sitting to standing. Dry mouth is a common side effect of many drugs and can be intensified by the dehydrating effects of caffeinated drinks and alcohol (answer D). All of the above are possible side effects of neuroleptic medications, but answer C is most important because it is the only one Mr. Rodriguez has experienced. See reference: Early: Psychotropic medications and somatic treatments.

133. (A) use disposable cotton swabs and have clients bring their own cosmetics. Universal precautions are related to the prevention of the spread of infection. Using disposable cotton swabs and having clients use their own cosmetics would be effective in reducing the risk of infection. Combing someone's hair (answer B) does not usually involve risks related to blood or bodily fluids. Washing equipment (answer C) that is used near eyes and mouths by several individuals is inadequate. Avoiding glass containers (answer D) is a safety precaution that is related to self-harm and not universal precautions. See reference: Early: Safety techniques.

134. (B) activity adaptation. Modifying how directions are provided is one way to adapt activities. Activity analysis (answer A) is the process of identifying the aspects, steps, and materials used in performing the activity. Grading activities (answer C) is a gradual progression of steps toward a goal. Clinical reasoning (answer D) is the problem-solving process that practitioners use in thinking about a client's treatment. See reference: Early: Analyzing, adapting, and grading activities.

135. (B) writing a soap opera. While answers A, C, and D would benefit the self-confidence and stress management needs of women struggling with the issues associated with emotional and physical abuse, they are not expressive group activities. Writing a soap opera is a creative approach used to help individuals express their inner thoughts, feelings, anxieties, and beliefs. See reference: Early: Expressive and coping skills.

136. (B) confront the individual's behavior: "Are you aware that your frequent interruptions prevent others from having a chance to contribute?" In general, the group leader should try A, C, or D before confronting the individual who is monopolizing. Confrontation within a group setting is difficult for many individuals to accept. See reference: Posthuma: What to do if....

137. (B) closed question. Closed questions can be answered with one word responses such as "yes" or "no." Open questions (answer A) are very broad and can be answered many different ways. Leading questions (answer C) suggest the desired response. A double question (answer D) asks two questions at once and forces a choice. See reference: Denton: Effective communication.

138. (A) facilitating communication with the client's family. A medical record is confidential and would not be shared with a patient's family. The primary purposes of documentation include: facilitate the treatment process; provide a record of evaluations and treatments performed; serve as legal documentation; facilitate communication between staff; provide information that can be used in accreditation, research and quality assurance; and report services provided for reimbursement. See reference: Hopkins and Smith (eds): Perinchief, JM: Service management.

139. (C) express disagreement with her coworkers in a productive manner. Assertiveness is the ability to express feelings in an appropriate and productive manner. Answers A, B, and D are examples of other types of social interaction skills. Answers A and B are examples of good conversation. Answer D is an example of proper social conduct. See reference: Hemphill, BJ, Peterson, CQ, and Werner, PC: Social interaction skills.

140. (D) Isadore will chew and swallow each piece of sandwich before placing the next piece in his mouth four out of five times. Goals must be objective and measurable. Five components should be included when writing goals: the behavior that is desired (chewing and swallowing); the condition of performance (in this case it is independently, since no level of assistance is indicated); frequency or duration (four out of five times); criteria for moving to next level (successful performance of the stated goal); and time frame (not indicated in this goal). Answer A does not define "good table manners." Answer B does not indicate what criteria will be used to measure impulsivity. Answer C is not appropriate since we have no information about Isadore's current level of eye contact. See reference: Hemphill, BJ, Peterson, CQ, and Werner, PC: How to write behavioral goals and objectives.

141. (C) present the new goal and treatment plan to the OTR. COTAs may write goals and implement treatment under the supervision of an OTR. Before documenting a new goal in the permanent medical record, introducing a new program to the staff, or implementing treatment (answers A, B, and D), the entry-level COTA should present the new goal and treatment plan to the OTR for approval. See reference: AOTA: Occupational therapy roles.

142. (D) using eating utensils when appropriate. Using utensils rather than fingers is the most basic of the skills listed. Progressing from simple to complex, the next skill would be using the appropriate utensil (answer A), followed by taking portions of the appropriate size (answer B), and finally eating the meal in a reasonable amount of time (answer C). See reference: Hemphill, BJ, Peterson, CQ, and Werner, PC: Social interaction skills.

143. (A) Mary will engage in a simple craft activity for 15 minutes without demonstrating self-abusive behavior. One may correctly deduce that it is more important for Mary to reduce the amount of self-abusive behavior than to learn increasingly complex craft activities. Once a significant reduction in self-abusive behavior has been achieved, attempting to maintain that level while gradually increasing the level of stress through increasingly complex tasks may be attempted. This would progress Mary toward tolerating greater levels of stress without becoming self-abusive. Answers B, C, and D all emphasize increasing the complexity of the task rather than extending the length of time without self-abusive behavior. See reference: Early: Analyzing, adapting, and grading activities.

144. (D) sheltered workshops. Sheltered workshops are designed to help individuals master basic work skills. Working with supported employment or in a fast-food setting with a job coach (answers B and C) are similar in that they incorporate actual job sites for developing work skills. Adult activity centers (answer A) focus on work-related and leisure activities. See reference: Hopkins and Smith (eds): Humphry, R and Jacobs, K: Mental retardation.

145. (A) least restrictive environment. Mental health services are organized along a continuum of care ranging from highly restrictive (i.e. hospitalization) to less restrictive (i.e. community mental health centers). Since 1970 (Wyatt v. Stickney), all psychiatric patients in the United States have had rights that protect them from receiving care that is more restrictive than their condition warrants. Occupational therapy practitioners should be aware of the restrictiveness of other treatment environments when planning for discharge. Professional licensure laws (answer B) protect consumers but do not define treatment settings. PL94–142 (answer C) enables handicapped children to receive educational services. The Tarasoff decision (answer D) describes rules for sharing confidential material involving threats of harm and is not specifically related to the discharge planning process. See reference: Hopkins and Smith (eds): Gibson, D: The evolution of occupational therapy.

146. (B) adult day care. This environment provides programming for the elderly that is psychosocial in nature and focuses on avocational skills and social activities. Partial hospitalization (answer A) is a type of outpatient program that serves as a transition to community living. It offers most of the structure and services available on an inpatient unit while allowing individuals to live in the community and to receive services by visiting the program. Home health care (answer C) provides treatment services to individuals in their own homes who have chronic or debilitating illnesses, in order to increase their functional independence. While most individuals who receive home health services have disabilities that are primarily physical, secondary psychiatric disorders are quite common. Psychosocial rehabilitation centers (answer D) focus on the social rather than the medical aspects of mental illness. The psychosocial club or rehabilitation center provides socialization programs, daily living skills counseling, pre-vocational rehabilitation, and transitional employment. See reference: Early: Treatment settings.

147. (C) National Alliance for the Mentally Ill. This is a support group that is open to clients and families and focuses on education and support related to all mental illnesses. Al-Anon (answer A) is a support group for family members of alcoholics. Family therapy (answer B) is not a support group. Recovery, Inc. (answer D) is a self-help support group for individuals with mental disorders. See reference: Hopkins and Smith (eds): Richert, GZ: Program planning, development, and implementation.

148. (C) discharge summary. The discharge summary includes a summary of the client's entire treatment and the goals achieved, and compares the initial and discharge status. Initial notes (answer B) record the OT practitioner's receipt of and response to the referral for service. Progress notes (answer A) contain information about the patient's performance since the previous note. Treatment plans (answer D) contain measurable goals, treatment procedures, and expected attainment dates. See reference: Early: Medical records and documentation.

149. (C) Section IV. Follow-up plans state the scheduled and specific plans upon discontinuation of services. Section I includes the patients name, the date of the note and the patient's case number. Section II indicates the amount of time the patient was involved in occupational therapy. Section III contains the summary of treatment sessions and the goals achieved. See reference: Early: Medical records and documentation.

150. (C) Section IV. Home programs are the written programs that the client will follow after discharge. Mental health approaches frequently incorporate journals as an effective way of following through with "exercises" or methods that were introduced in the hospital. See reference: Early: Medical records and documentation.

151. (B) the Education for all Handicapped Children Act. This bill was enacted in Congress in 1975. It requires that school systems receiving federal funds provide handicapped children with free appropriate education in the least restrictive manner. The Americans with Disabilities Act, answer A, was passed in 1990 and enacted in 1992 to provide accessibility to individuals with disabilities. Answer C, Children's Protective Services is an agency which investigates the home environment and removes children from families who neglect or abuse children. Medicare, answer D, was established in 1965 by an act of Congress as Title XVIII of the Social Security Act. The program consists of two parts. Medicare part "A" pays for inpatient hospitalization, skilled care, and hospice services. Medicare part "B" covers outpatient services, physician and other professional medical services. See reference: Bair and Gray (eds): Scott, S, and Somers, FP: Payment for occupational therapy services.

152. (D) increase in outpatient services. Current trends in health care are reducing inpatient hospital stays and increasing the types and amounts of services that are available on an outpatient basis. Answers A and C are incorrect because it is projected that with the population getting older and patients moving out of hospitals faster, utilization of nursing homes and home health services will increase. Answer B is incorrect because hospitalizations are anticipated to decrease as only individuals with more serious illnesses and higher acuities of illness will be admitted. See reference: Punwar: Current trends and future outlook.

153. (B) school systems. The primary place of employment for 14% of COTAs is in school systems. This is the largest percentage employed in a community-based practice setting. Other community-based settings include private practice (answer A), where 2.4% of COTAs practice; home health agencies (answer C), where 3.5% of COTAs practice; and residential care facilities, which include group homes, independent living centers (answer D), etc., where 3.8% of COTAs practice. See reference: AOTA: 1996 Member data survey.

154. (D) revocation. Revocation is the permanent loss of certification from the NBCOT. A reprimand (answer A) is a formal written expression of disapproval against an OT practitioner's conduct that is retained in the NBCOT's file. This information is also communicated privately with the individual. A censure (answer B) is a formal written expression of disapproval that is made public. Probation (answer C) is the period of time a therapist is given to retain the counseling or education required to remain certified. See reference: Hopkins and Smith (eds): Hansen, RA: Ethics in occupational therapy.

155. (B) have at least one year of experience as a COTA. Based on the Essentials, an OTR or COTA supervising a Level II student is required to have a minimum of 1 year of experience in a practice setting. Six months of experience is recommended for supervising Level I students. See reference: AOTA: Essentials and guidelines for an accredited educational program for the occupational therapy assistant.

156. (B) a formal, public disapproval of a practitioner's conduct. A censure differs from a reprimand in that it is more serious and is public. A reprimand is a formal written expression of disapproval against a practitioner's conduct that is retained in the NBCOT's files (answer A). This information is also communicated privately with the individual. Probation is when a practitioner is given a period of time to retain the counseling or education required to remain certified (answer C). Revocation is permanent loss of NBCOT certification (answer D). See reference: Hopkins and Smith (eds): Hansen, RA: Ethics in occupational therapy.

157. (D) nonmaleficence. Answer D, nonmaleficence, is defined as the obligation of the provider to avoid causing harm or injury to a patient. Informed consent (answer A) refers to the rights of individuals to be provided with information regarding their health care, as well as the right to make choices about their own health care. Fidelity (answer B) involves remaining faithful to the patient's best interests and observing confidentiality. Beneficence (answer C) is the duty to do what is best for the patient or client. See reference: Hopkins and Smith (eds): Hansen, RA: Ethics in occupational therapy.

158. (D) refer him to her OTR supervisor, who has attended a workshop on sexuality and spinal cord injury. Anyone providing sexuality counseling must not only be comfortable with his or her own sexuality but must have certain competencies as well. These competencies include awareness of personal and societal attitudes concerning sexuality, knowledge of male and female reproductive systems and how different disabilities affect sexuality, and the interpersonal skills to communicate with patients about sensitive and personal issues concerned with sexuality. When an occupational therapy practitioner who has developed these skills through continuing education is available to the patient, it is not necessary to refer the patient to his physiatrist (answer C). The COTA in this situation, who is unknowledgable and embarrassed by the patient's question (answers A and B), should not be the one to counsel him on these issues. See reference: Hopkins and Smith (eds): Neistadt, ME: Human sexuality and counseling.

159. (D) Both the COTA and OTR. According to the AOTA document "Supervision Guidelines for Certified Occupational Therapy Assistants," the "supervising OTR is legally responsible for the outcomes of all occupational therapy services provided by the COTA." The COTA should never have administered a procedure in which he had not demonstrated service competency. The responsibility of the physical therapist is somewhat less clear. Whereas it is not uncommon for physical therapists to instruct OT practitioners in the use of modalities, it would have been irresponsible for the PT to suggest it would be acceptable for the COTA to administer paraffin without much more knowledge and experience about heat modalities. See reference: AOTA: Supervision guidelines for certified occupational therapy assistants.

160. (C) unacceptable, because it violates the Code of Ethics. Whether or not an alternate date has been arranged (answer A) or the agency the COTA works for allows it (answer B), stating services were provided on a day when they, in actuality, were not, is falsification of documentation and violates the OT Code of Ethics. The client's inability to participate in therapy the next day due to illness (answer D) would only serve to further complicate an already compromised situation; however, this is not the reason why the action is unacceptable. See reference: Hopkins and Smith (eds): Hansen, RA: Ethics in occupational therapy.

161. (C) Advanced level practice. COTAs operating at this skill level have 3 or more years of experience and have demonstrated advanced clinical, administrative, or educational skills. Answers A and B, entry level and intermediate level, focus more on establishing service competency and the development of clinical skills. Certainly, someone at the educator level (answer D) would be able to coordinate a volunteer program. However, the question indicated that the therapist had recently attained the skill level to complete this activity. See reference: Ryan (ed): Ryan, SE: COTA supervision. *Practice Issues in Occupational Therapy.*

162. (C) skilled nursing facilities. The largest number of certified occupational therapy assistants (42.2%) work in skilled nursing facilities. School systems are next with 14%. Rehabilitation hospitals employ 9.3% and psychiatric hospitals 1.8%. See reference: AOTA: 1996 Member data survey.

163. (A) discharge recommendations. The COTA would contribute to the process of making discharge recommendations, but this section of the discharge evaluation is to be completed by the OTR. Answers B, C, and D may be completed independently by the COTA because these areas reflect factual data at the time of discharge. This information may include discharge disposition, and data on the patient's current status. See reference: AOTA: Occupational therapy roles.

164. (A) the same results in three successive treatment trials. Service competency is established when two occupational therapy practitioners obtain the same results on three successive trials. It is in this manner that the two professionals may identify if they are completing the procedure in the same manner. Answers B, C, and D either do not allow for enough successive trials or require that the occupational therapy practitioners have identical results. See reference: AOTA: Occupational therapy roles.

165. (C) A COTA contributes to the process but does not complete the task independently. The COTA participates in this process by providing factual information to the OTR and collaboratively identifying discharge needs. However, because of the analytical nature of discharge recommendations, the COTA does not complete this activity independently. Answers A and B are incorrect because they do not take into account the analytical nature of the task. Answer D is incorrect because it does not allow for the input of data from the COTA. See reference: AOTA: Occupational therapy roles.

166. (B) document services provided and date the note as a late entry. It is the responsibility of the occupational therapy practitioner to document services provided. Once the error was found, the therapist should document the services as she recalled. Therefore, answers C and D are incorrect because they do not provide for documentation of services. Answer A is unethical in that it is not appropriate for the practitioner to backdate the note. See reference: AOTA: Occupational Therapy Code of Ethics.

167. (A) Physical agent modalities are not within the scope of practice of COTAs. "Physical agent modalities may be used by occupational therapy practitioners when used as an adjunct to or in preparation for purposeful activity by a practitioner who has demonstrated service competency." Service competency in this area involves possessing the theoretical background and technical skills for the safe and effective use of the modality. Therefore, a COTA who has demonstrated service competency in this area may use physical agent modalities as part of OT intervention. Avoiding harm (answer B), possessing competence (answer C), and referral to appropriate providers when necessary (answer D) are all required by the OT Code of Ethics. See reference: AOTA: Occupational Therapy Code of Ethics. Also AOTA: Policy: Registered occupational therapists and certified occupational therapy assistants and modalities.

168. (C) Use PAMs only in preparation for or as an adjunct to purposeful activity. "Physical agent modalities may be used by occupational therapy practitioners when used as an adjunct to or in preparation for purposeful activity by a practitioner who has demonstrated service competency." Service competency in this area includes but is not limited to possessing the theoretical background and technical skills for the safe and effective use of the modality. While an appropriate level of supervision is required, no level is specified (answers B and D). The term "physical agent modalities" includes a wide variety of agents, and COTAs may use any PAM once service competency has been demonstrated. See reference: AOTA: Policy: Registered occupational therapists and certified occupational therapy assistants and modalities.

169. (D) not to use physical agent modalities in the new state. Although AOTA policy supports the use of PAMs by qualified practitioners as an adjunct to or in preparation for purposeful activity, state laws supersede AOTA policies. Answers A, B, and C all violate state law as well as the OT Code of ethics and could result in loss of licensure, loss of NBCOT certification, a fine, or imprisonment. See reference: AOTA: Occupational Therapy Code of Ethics.

170. (B) develop and implement time management strategies. It is usually possible to use time more efficiently. By analyzing how you spend your time, you may be able to eliminate or modify tasks that are unnecessary or overly time consuming. Continuing to stay late (answer A) will probably result in burnout. Before determining that the problem lies with the job or the supervisor, the COTA should determine what she can do to resolve the situation. Better time management skills could be the answer, and "saying no" to the supervisor (answer C) may not be appropriate or necessary. Answer D would result in falling behind with documentation and treatment planning and is not an acceptable option. See reference: Early: Organizing yourself.

171. (D) report the incident to the state licensure board. Reports of sexual misconduct are among the most common complaints received. The OT Code of Ethics specifically prohibits the sexual exploitation of patients/clients, and it is considered unacceptable for an OT practitioner to become sexually involved with an individual to whom he is providing treatment. The OT Code of Ethics also requires OT practitioners to report ethical violations. Answers A, B, and C do not recognize that sexual misconduct has occurred; only answer D addresses the duty of the COTA who observed the incident to report it. See reference: AOTA: Occupational Therapy Code of Ethics.

172. (D) 75–84 years of age. Recent studies show that 35% of employed COTAs work primarily with patients 75–84 years of age. Only 1.5% work with infants and children up to the age of three. Eleven percent work with children aged 6–12 and 15.9% work with adults aged 19–64. See reference: AOTA: 1996 Member data survey.

173. (D) some state regulatory acts. Many states are now requiring that a specified number of credits in continuing education be achieved for renewal of licensure. Even though it is recommended, it is not currently required by AOTA, NBCOT, or state associations. See reference: Hopkins and Smith (eds): Perinchief, JM: Service management.

174. (D) use the brochures, posters, videotapes, and films available from the association to enhance her presentation to the nursing students. This answer was hopefully clear and evident to all of those reading the question. The emphasis of this question is that it is every occupational therapy practitioner's responsibility to promote the profession. Simple, daily public relations activities occur each time an OT practitioner describes the services to be provided to patients and families. More complex public relations may include developing a plan to promote community awareness regarding the profession. A public relations program is designed to increase the public's awareness about the role and importance of occupational therapy services. See reference: Ryan (ed): Jones, RA: Service operations. *Practice Issues in Occupational Therapy.*

175. (D) charge only for the amount of time spent with the patient directly that day. This answer is correct because this meeting was not part of the planned intervention and occurred spontaneously and without measurable goals. Based on the Standards of Practice, if collaboration with the individual and/or significant others were included as a part of the intervention plan, the patient could be billed for the time. See reference: Hopkins and Smith (eds): Hansen, RA: Ethics in occupational therapy.

176. (C) CTRS substitute recreational activities during the occupational therapy time, but not bill for occupational therapy services. Answers A, B, and D are incorrect because they all involve billing for occupational therapy services when actual services performed by an OT practitioner were not completed. Therefore, the only correct answer is to not bill for occupational therapy. See reference: Hopkins and Smith (eds): Gibson, D and Richert, G: Mental health: The therapeutic process.

177. (B) Standards of Practice. These standards are a guide to the provision and management of occupational therapy services. The Uniform Terminology for Reporting Occupational Therapy Services (answer A) defines areas of practice and descriptors of services. This document assists in providing consistent documentation in occupational therapy throughout all areas of practice. Licensure regulations (answer C) vary from state to state and are not always consistent with the guidelines for practice. AOTA Policies and Procedures (answer D) guide the activities of the association but do not refer to the provision of services. See reference: AOTA: Uniform Terminology.

178. (B) Worker's compensation. Workers compensation is a state supported program into which employers pay. Medicare (answer A) is a federal program for health care coverage for individuals 65 years or older, disabled individuals, or people in end stage renal failure. The Education for All Handicapped Children is funded through the provision of state and federal grants. See reference: Bair and Gray (eds): Scott, S, and Somers, FP: Payment for occupational therapy services.

179. (B) Begin the assessment process when individuals are admitted on the weekends. The OTR will finish the assessment on Monday. The primary role of the COTA is to implement treatment such as that described in answers A, C, and D. A COTA may not independently evaluate patients. Working on weekends, the COTA would be independently initiating evaluations. See reference: AOTA: Occupational therapy roles.

180. (A) blood. OSHA has identified materials that require universal precautions to be blood, semen, vaginal secretions, cerebrospinal fluid, synovial fluid, pleural fluid, pericardial fluid, peritoneal fluid, amniotic fluid, any body fluid with visible blood, any unidentifiable body fluid, and saliva from dental procedures. Answers B, C, and D all contain fluids that are not on this list. Items that OSHA identified as not needing universal precautions are feces, nasal secretions, sputum, sweat, tears, urine, and vomitus. See reference: Occupational Safety and Health Administration.

181. (C) assisting with stock and inventory control. Volunteer performance within an occupational therapy department should be limited so that it is in the direct line of vision of the supervisor. Transporting patients (answer A) takes them out of view of the supervisor. In addition, it is not appropriate for volunteers to treat a patient (answer B) in that they lack the skill and expertise of an occupational therapy practitioner. Answer D is incorrect because it violates the confidentiality of the patient. See reference: Ryan (ed): Jones, RA: Service operations. *Practice Issues in Occupational Therapy.*

182. (B) quality assurance. Quality assurance is a "systematic approach to the evaluation of patient care that enables the identification, assessment and resolution of problems in order to improve health care benefits for patients." Program evaluation (answer A) is an ongoing method of examining a program's effectiveness. Research (answer C) refers to the formal investigation of an intervention and is not specific enough a term to be the correct answer. Cost effectiveness studies (answer D) examine the results of departmental activities in relationship to their cost. See reference: Early: Treatment planning. Also, Ryan (ed): Jones, RA: Service operations. *Practice Issues in Occupational Therapy.*

183. (A) managed care. These companies serve as the link between hospitals and insurance companies. Managed care providers identify the need for medical care of an individual by referring to the patient's medical information as it relates to preestablished criteria for services. Utilization review (answer B) compares the length of stay or duration of services provided with the cost to ensure efficiency. Peer review (answer C) is a form of quality improvement in which charts are reviewed for indicators that represent the level of quality of a service. Prospective payment (answer D) is system for payment of services based on DRGs (Diagnostic Related Groups). See reference: Hopkins and Smith (eds): Levy, LL: The health care delivery system today.

184. (B) yes, as long as state regulations allow autonomous practice and the COTA recognizes situations that require consultation with or referral to an OTR. Occupational therapy plays a significant role working with consumers in the independent living movement by working both with individuals and their environments. According to the AOTA position statement "The Role of Occupational Therapy in the Independent Living Movement," AOTA "supports the autonomous practice of the advanced COTA practitioner in the independent living setting." In this situation, it would be the responsibility of the COTA to recognize and seek out OTR consultation when appropriate. However, this does not supersede state regulations when they prohibit autonomous practice by the COTA. Other options for this COTA would be to find some way to fund the necessary OTR supervision (answer A), or to work as a program director, and not use the COTA credentials (answer D). See reference: AOTA: Statement: The role of occupational therapy in the independent living movement.

185. (A) a referral. A referral is a request for OT services. Occupational therapy services may be requested verbally or in writing, depending on the policies of the facility. Referrals from a physician typically include some or all of the following information: date of request, patient/client name, diagnosis and precautions, desired goals, duration and frequency of treatment, and physician signature. Screening (answer B), which may be performed by the OTR or COTA, is the process of observing and collecting information about the individual to determine the need for OT services. The OTR and COTA may collaborate to set goals (answer C) for an individual. Goals should be included in occupational therapy documentation and should be objective and measurable. The COTA and OTR may also collaborate in treatment planning (answer D), which is the process of analyzing and determining what the individual's problems are and deciding how to solve them. See reference: Early: Overview of the treatment process.

186. (C) notify the OTR. Regardless of the source of the referral or the anticipated length of stay, the COTA must first notify the OTR of the referral, because the OTR is ultimately responsible for any action taken. Under the supervision of the OTR, the COTA may then initiate screening, chart review, or ADL evaluation (answers A, B, and D). See reference: Ryan (ed): Ryan, SE: Therapeutic intervention process. *Practice Issues in Occupational Therapy.*

187. (B) Uniform Terminology. The Uniform Terminology specifically outlines the performance components and areas addressed by occupational therapy practitioners. Requests for occupational therapy services come in the form of referrals, consultations, or orders. These requests are generated by physicians, social workers, nurses, and psychologists. Answers A, C, and D relate more to professional behavior and activities. See reference: AOTA: Uniform terminology.

188. (D) call 911. The COTA should be knowledgeable of situations that may be potentially dangerous for patients. This question requires that the COTA be knowledgeable about the appropriate ranges for heart rate and blood pressure. Both of the measures exceed safe ranges and indicate that the patient is medically unstable. Therefore, immediate medical services would be necessary. Answers A, B and C do not recognize the seriousness of the situation and could delay the necessary medical attention. See reference: Ryan (ed): Jones, RA: Service operations. *Practice Issues in Occupational Therapy.*

189. (B) Complete a tool count of departmental sharps. While answers A, C, and D are all required and necessary, the only activity that would be done routinely is a tool count. It is recommended that tool counts be completed prior to and following patient activities. This ensures that sharps are not removed by patients as this may provide them the opportunity to harm themselves or others. See reference: Ryan (ed): Jones, RA: Service operations. *Practice Issues in Occupational Therapy.*

190. (D) the senior COTA will evaluate, guide, and teach the staff COTAs. A supervisor has administrative, evaluative, and teaching roles. COTAs always require at least a general level of supervision, never minimal (answer A). Under general supervision, contact is made monthly. Minimal supervision is provided on an "as needed" basis. It is possible that this may be less than once a month. Taking a supervisory position does not always result in a decreased caseload (answer B). If the role of COTAs in a department is to be redefined, all OT staff should participate in the process (answer C). See reference: Early: Supervision.

191. (C) Individuals presenting inservices must sign up for the conference room at least 2 weeks in advance. Procedures state how a policy is carried out, in what sequence, and by whom. A policy provides information about actions that need to be taken. Answers A, B, and D are all examples of policies. See reference: Hopkins and Smith (eds): Perinchief, JM: Service management.

192. (D) Yes, if state law does not require a physician referral. AOTA does not require individuals to have a physician referral or prescription (answers A and B) in order to receive OT services, whether group or individual (answer C). However, OT practitioners must be aware of and adhere to the requirements of local, state and federal laws; government agencies; third-party payers; and facilities. Since Jordan is going to pay for the services herself, third-party payer policy is not an issue. In private practice, the OTR/COTA team may establish their own facility policies and can accept self-referrals if they so choose. Therefore, as long as state law does not require a physician referral or prescription, Jordan can be accepted into the stress management group. See reference: AOTA: Statement of occupational therapy referral.

193. (B) NOT occurred so she does not need to use universal precautions. OSHA has identified materials that require universal precautions to be blood, semen, vaginal secretions, cerebrospinal fluid, synovial fluid, pleural fluid, pericardial fluid, peritoneal fluid, amniotic fluid, any body fluid with visible blood, any unidentifiable body fluid, and saliva from dental procedures. Since the urine did not have visible blood in it, it would not be considered an exposure. Answers A and C are incorrect because they indicate that an exposure has occurred. Answer D is incorrect because it is not necessary to use universal precautions unless exposure has occurred. In addition, it should be noted that items OSHA has identified as not needing universal precautions are feces, nasal secretions, sputum, sweat, tears, urine, and vomitus. See reference: Occupational Safety and Health Administration.

194. (C) program evaluation. Program evaluation is the compilation of the intervention results for a population of individuals. One of the most frequently used program evaluation systems is the Functional Independence Measure (FIM). FIM scores may be compiled and compared to regional and national norms. The process (answer A) is the manner in which services are rendered. Each process has a sequence in which activities occur. An example of the process of interaction between the consumer and therapist may the progression from initial interview to evaluation to treatment to family training to discharge. An outcome (answer B) is the result of the service intervention that an individual receives. These measures are taken at the completion of service intervention. Utilization review (answer D) examines the care that is provided to assure that services were appropriate and not overutilized or underutilized. Utilization review also analyzes the services to assure that the interventions were provided in an economical manner. See reference: Hopkins and Smith (eds): Perinchief, JM: Service management.

195. (C) keeping her knees bent. This is the only correct advice given. The opposite of all other answers will contribute to injury prevention for the COTA: standing close to the patient, keeping the back in a neutral position, and maintaining a wide base of support. See reference: Pedretti (ed): Adler, C and Tipton-Burton, M: Wheelchair assessment and transfers.

196. (B) using a band saw. Protective eyewear should be worn when using power tools such as a band saw, electric sander, or drill press. Fumes from liver of sulfate and oil-based stains (answers A and C) may be noxious and require good ventilation, but protective eyewear is not necessary. While caution should be observed when soldering (answer D), eye protection is not necessary. See reference: Ryan (ed): Jones, RA: Service operations. *Practice Issues in Occupational Therapy.*

197. (A) Infection Control plan. An infection control plan will most likely include appropriate techniques and procedures for storing and handling foods within the occupational therapy department. Such plans specify the shelf-life of certain foods, standards for food storage, use of hair nets, and cooking temperatures and times. A risk management plan (answer B) addresses the issue of liability in reference to negligence and malpractice issues. Emergency procedures (answer C) specify the procedures and techniques to be used in a critical situation (i.e., fire, code blue, severe weather alert, etc.). An environmental survey (answer D) is a plan that inspects a service area for potential hazards and dangers and corrects the situation. See reference: Ryan (ed): Jones, RA: Service operations. *Practice Issues in Occupational Therapy.*

198. (D) referral. A referral is a basic request for an individual to be assessed by an occupational therapist. A referral generally includes information such as the individual's name, age, date of birth, address, physician, and diagnosis. An individual may be referred to occupational therapy for deficits in occupational performance in the areas of work, play, or leisure. A recommendation (answer A) is an advisement that an individual may benefit from a service. Plans of treatment and intervention strategies (answers B and C) are completed by the OT practitioner following the assessment. See reference: Hopkins and Smith (eds): Spencer, E: Preliminary concepts and planning. Also AOTA: Statement of occupational therapy referral.

199. (C) this does not provide for adequate supervision of COTAs. However, if the OTRs are allowed time to provide general or routine supervision to the COTAs, the COTAs would then be able to treat the patients, and write the progress notes and discharge summaries. Occupational therapy departments frequently are understaffed and need to operate as efficiently as possible. The collaborative teamwork between an OTR and a COTA is vital in treatment planning and implementation. When a collaborative relationship is operational, the COTA may carry out the tasks of providing treatment and completing the progress notes and discharge summaries (contradicts answer D). When the COTA's documentation skills are adequate, the OTR frequently "signs off" on the COTAs notes, after reading and approving them. It is not within the COTAs scope of practice to provide all of the treatment and discharge planning independently (answer A). Answer B is incorrect in that it violates the standards of practice and Code of Ethics for an OT practitioner to agree to provision of inappropriate services. See reference: Hopkins and Smith (eds): Perinchief, JM: Service management.

200. (D) designing the patient discharge interview. The most common way for COTAs to participate in quality assurance programs is in data collection. This is typically accomplished through chart review, patient interview, and interviewing family members or significant others (answers A, B and C). COTAs may also contribute to "selecting measures for quality assurance and developing plans for actions to respond to areas that need improvement." The responsibility for designing an interview tool would not be appropriate to assign to an entry-level COTA. See reference: Early: Treatment planning.

SIMULATION EXAMINATION 2

Directions: Circle the correct answer to the following questions. When you have completed this examination, check your answers against the answer key that follows. As you will see, an explanation is given for each answer along with a reference for further study. The book author is listed as well as the chapter author. See the bibliography for complete references. Study the areas in which your comprehension was low, then test yourself again by taking Simulation Examination 3.

PEDIATRIC QUESTIONS

Data Collection

1. During assessment of a 10-month-old child with Down syndrome, the COTA notes hyperextensibility of all joints. This means that the child probably has:
A. increased muscle tone.
B. decreased muscle tone.
C. contractures.
D. clonus.

2. The COTA observes that a 5-year-old child with Down syndrome and low muscle tone sits on the floor exclusively using a "W" sitting position (buttocks between heels). This observation indicates to the COTA that the child is:
A. developing normally.
B. using a compensatory position to achieve stability.
C. using a compensatory position to achieve mobility.
D. using a position normal for a younger child, not for a 5-year-old child.

3. A standardized test is one that:
A. is subjective.
B. depends on the skill of the practitioner.
C. has stated instructions for administration and scoring.
D. depends on the judgment of the practitioner administering it.

4. The best way for the COTA informally to assess cognitive performance components in an 8-year-old child with a learning disability is to:
A. record attention span during classroom observation.
B. interview the parents regarding the child's social activities.
C. consult with the teacher about the child's handwriting skills.
D. observe the child's coordination during a physical education session.

5. Which method of data collection should the COTA choose as the most effective for learning about a family's values and priorities?
A. Interview.
B. Skilled observation.
C. Inventory.
D. Standardized test.

6. The COTA may do an informal assessment of visual form perception in an 8-year-old child by having him or her:
A. play a game of marbles.
B. match picture dominoes.
C. play a matching-by-memory game such as "Memory."
D. assemble a 16-piece puzzle.

7. During the interview with the parents of a 3-year-old child with mild cerebral palsy, the COTA learns that the child is regularly fed by his grandmother and does not have any independent feeding skills. The COTA should first address the following issue:
A. the degree of abnormal muscle tone in the UEs.
B. the possibility of developmental delay.
C. the cultural context and family interaction patterns.
D. the need for adapted equipment.

8. The COTA administers the Beery Developmental Test of Visual-Motor Integration to a 6-year-old client. The client is most likely to be referred for testing if he or she demonstrates difficulty in:
A. copying letters.
B. remembering letters.
C. recognizing letters.
D. sequencing letters.

9. The COTA observes a 4-year-old with autism waving his hand in front of his eyes repeatedly in an apparent purposeless manner. The most relevant observation to be reported to the supervising therapist is:
A. the ability of eyes to focus at close range.
B. the degree of wrist mobility.
C. the hand preference.
D. the presence of self-stimulatory behavior.

10. The COTA witnesses a seizure in an 8-year-old client with severe spastic cerebral palsy. The child's body becomes rigid, he loses consciousness, and then his extremities contract and relax in rhythmic clonic contractures. The seizure lasts about 5 minutes. This is an example of:
A. a grand mal seizure.
B. a petit mal seizure.
C. a psychomotor seizure.
D. status epilepticus.

Treatment Planning

11. When planning treatment for a child with cerebral palsy, quadriplegic athetoid type, the COTA should include activities addressing:
A. one upper limb.
B. one body side.
C. both lower extremities.
D. all extremities.

12. A COTA is about to begin working with a 2-year-old child with hypotonia and extremely poor head control who is unable to maintain a sitting position. The first pre-sitting activity the COTA should plan is:
A. forward and backward movement on a ball with the child in prone position
B. forward and side-to-side movement with the child sitting on a ball.
C. forward and side-to side movement on a tilting board with the child in quadruped position.
D. place the child supine on a mat and pull him or her into sitting position.

13. A 2-year-old child who is cognitively intact but has severe lower-extremity weakness and contractures has not developed any form of mobility. A powered wheelchair could first be considered for this child by the age of:
A. 2 years.
B. 4 years.
C. 6 years.
D. 8 years.

14. In planning a therapeutic dressing program for a 5-year-old child who is mentally retarded, the COTA's FIRST consideration should be the need for:
A. adaptive equipment.
B. adaptive clothing.
C. proper positioning.
D. adapted teaching techniques.

15. The COTA is assisting the OTR with the development of long-term goals for a 14-year-old client with moderate mental retardation. Goal setting should focus on:
A. attainment of motor milestones.
B. maximizing cognitive skills.
C. normalizing sensory integration.
D. developing vocational skills.

16. Poor impulse control has been identified as the primary deficit in a 12-year-old boy with conduct disorder. Which of the following is the most effectively written functional OT goal?
A. Within 6 months, Billy will participate in classroom activities for 1 hour without disruptive outbursts, twice a day.
B. Within 6 months, Billy will attend to an activity for 30 minutes, demonstrating improved impulse control.
C. Billy will show a 50% reduction in the frequency of disruptive outbursts within 6 months.
D. When presented with a new activity, Billy will follow directions without protest, four out of five times, within 6 months.

17. A child diagnosed with arthrogryposis has been referred for an occupational therapy evaluation. The COTA will focus on ADL training knowing that the child will have ongoing problems with:
A. obstetric paralysis.
B. hip dislocation.
C. joint inflammation.
D. joint contractures.

18. Jeremy's long-term goal is to increase bilateral use of his hands. A relevant short-term goal would be: "Within 2 months, Jeremy will:
A. play 'pat-a-cake' when prompted."
B. make Play Doh 'meatballs' using his index finger and thumb."
C. use an extended index finger to operate a busy-box dial."
D. tolerate fingerpainting using shaving cream."

19. Ashanti has poor independent-sitting skills owing to inadequate postural reactions. A good FIRST activity to promote the development of independent sitting is:
A. swinging on a playground swing with a bucket seat.
B. wide-base sitting on the floor while reaching for a suspended balloon.
C. straddling a bolster swing while batting a ball.
D. riding a hippity-hop, while using only one hand for support.

20. Jerry has a deficit in visual memory affecting his reading skills. The COTA recommends which game to promote visual memory?
A. Dominoes.
B. Concentration.
C. Pick-up sticks.
D. Checkers.

21. The COTA has received a referral for an 8-year-old girl with tactile defensiveness. Which of the following activities should be implemented FIRST?
A. Brushing of her neck and face by the COTA.
B. Balancing on a therapy ball.
C. Rolling in a carpeted barrel.
D. Swinging in a hammock swing.

Treatment Implementation

22. When treating a child with "tactile defensiveness," the COTA handles the child as if the child were:
A. underreactive to being touched.
B. overreactive to being touched.
C. craving touch.
D. unaffected by light touch.

23. The BEST way to adapt a chair in order to inhibit extensor tone and make sitting possible is to use a:
A. lateral trunk support.
B. seatbelt at the hips and ankle straps.
C. wedge-shaped seat insert that is higher in front.
D. lap board fastened to the arm rests of the chair.

24. The COTA is teaching a parent to change a diaper for a 2-year-old child who has spastic cerebral palsy. The child exhibits poor trunk balance and severe extensor and adductor patterns in the legs. The BEST method of inhibitory positioning to teach this parent is to place the child:
A. supine with neck extended, then flex and abduct both legs.
B. prone over the parent's thighs, then flex and abduct both legs.
C. in sitting position with back supported and resting against the parent's trunk, then flex and adduct both legs.
D. prone over his parent's thighs, then extend and adduct both legs.

25. The COTA teaches the parents of a child with cerebral palsy how to use therapeutic handling techniques designed to provide the child with opportunities to move with "more normal" movement patterns. This is an application of which theoretical frame of reference?
A. Neurodevelopmental.
B. Sensory integration.
C. Cognitive disabilities.
D. Biomechanical.

26. An infant has difficulty swallowing and chokes easily on foods. The COTA instructs the parent to avoid the following position during feeding:
A. supported sitting in an infant chair.
B. seated sideways in feeder's lap.
C. propped in beanbag chair, facing feeder.
D. held supine in feeder's arms.

27. A sixth-grader with a diagnosis of athetoid cerebral palsy needs an adapted computer for communication. Her upper-extremity control is poor owing to fluctuating muscle tone. The best way for her to operate her computer is a:
A. single-pressure switch firmly mounted within easy reach.
B. lightweight keyboard placed at midline.
C. low-resistance mouse and pad.
D. mercury-switch headband set to respond to minimal movement.

28. A child with deficits in sensory integration demonstrates hypersensitivity to movement activities by becoming nauseated and dizzy. The most appropriate movement to use with the large therapy ball for this child is:
A. movement in any position or direction.
B. no movement.
C. slow and predictable movement.
D. quick and unpredictable movement.

29. Judy is a fifth-grader with hypertonicity. When seated for schoolwork, she tends to adduct her legs and extend her hips and spine. In order to give her better postural control in sitting, the COTA positions her :
A. tilted forward 45 degrees.
B. upright.
C. reclining 45 degrees.
D. in a lateral tilt of 45 degrees.

30. Jerry has poor trunk stability and resultant poor hand-to-mouth patterns. In order to assist him with self-feeding, the COTA recommends the following adaptation to his wheelchair tray:
A. Lower it.
B. Tilt it toward him.
C. Raise it.
D. Tilt it away from him.

31. Jason is 1 year old and demonstrates respiratory difficulties and a tendency to choke on foods. His mother would like to know how to position him during feeding to minimize his chances of aspiration. Which position is CONTRAINDICATED for Jason?
A. Held supine in his mother's arms.
B. Upright in an infant seat.
C. Seated in a high chair.
D. Supported in sitting position in his mother's lap, facing her.

32. Which of the following toys would be LEAST appropriate to promote exploratory learning in a visually impaired toddler?
A. Teddy bear.
B. Play Doh.
C. Musical instruments.
D. Wind-up toys.

33. For treating a child with autism, the therapeutic environment should:
A. be lively and colorful, to facilitate active involvement.
B. provide many options, to encourage decision-making.
C. involve many available toys and activities, to promote exploratory learning.
D. be highly structured, to facilitate step-by-step learning.

34. What type of wheelchair seat is best for providing postural support for a child with abnormal muscle tone?
A. Hard and firm.
B. Soft cushion.
C. Sling seat.
D. Gel cushion.

35. A 4-year-old boy avoids play equipment whose use would cause his feet to be off the ground. This is best described as:
A. tactile defensiveness.
B. developmental dyspraxia.
C. gravitational insecurity.
D. intolerance for motion.

Evaluation of the Treatment Plan

36. An 8-year-old girl has achieved her goal of using a "dynamic tripod grasp" for writing with a pencil. When reassessing the child's performance, the COTA will indicate that:
A. the child's pencil skills continue to be delayed.
B. treatment for this problem may be discontinued.
C. treatment for this problem should continue.
D. other children her age have also just developed this pencil grasp.

37. While working with a 9-year-old boy in his classroom, the COTA notices that the boy is demonstrating a hypertonic extension pattern. The wheelchair adjustment that will correct this problem is:
A. lengthening back support.
B. use of a hip trap.
C. use of a shoulder harness.
D. increased angle of flexion at the hip.

38. Luis' short-term goal is to "demonstrate increased manipulation skills by opening a 3-inch screw-top jar independently." What tools will the COTA need to assess Luis' progress?
A. a goniometer.
B. a 3-inch screw-top jar.
C. a dynamometer.
D. the Peabody Fine Motor Scale.

39. Laurie is 3 years old and has been given a night splint to prevent abnormal hand and wrist posturing. The COTA instructs her parent to watch for signs indicating a need for reassessment. The first sign(s) they should look for is sustained redness:
A. of the skin in the morning.
B. and skin breakdown.
C. and reports of itching.
D. and complaints of discomfort.

40. Julia is 7 years old and has mastered brushing her teeth with the COTA giving verbal and physical cues. What is the NEXT stage in the process of reducing the intrusiveness of cues?
A. Verbal cues.
B. Verbal and gestural cues.
C. Physical cues.
D. Verbal and physical cues.

41. Trinidad is 5 years old and attending preschool, where she is working on perceptual motor skills in preparation for prewriting tasks. Her parents want to know when she will be ready to begin writing letters. The COTA replies:
A. "When she can scribble independently."
B. "When she can copy a circle."
C. "When she can imitate a cross."
D. "When she can copy a triangle."

42. Cari is 1 year old and has been diagnosed with mental retardation. She has been participating in a craft group structured as a parallel group. She is now developing skills such as sharing materials and interacting with other group members. The COTA recommends to the OTR that Cari be moved to the NEXT level of structured interaction, represented by a(n):
A. egocentric cooperative group.
B. project group.
C. cooperative group.
D. mature group.

43. An 8-year-old girl experiences a sensory overload and demonstrates an autonomic nervous system response when the COTA swings her on the hammock. Which of the following is an example of this type of response?
A. Suddenly scratching oneself.
B. Spinning oneself very fast.
C. Hitting one's head on the floor.
D. Flushing, blanching, or perspiring.

Discharge Planning

44. Parents will be more motivated to carry out treatment programs if the:

A. occupational therapy program works for the child.
B. parents are constantly challenged by the difficulty of the occupational therapy program.
C. OT practitioners have set the goals.
D. home program is separate from family daily routines.

45. A 4-year-old child with athetoid cerebral palsy is about to be discharged from a rehabilitation setting to home. The COTA is instructing the family how to use correct jaw control when feeding the child from the side. The best instructions are, "Control jaw opening and closing with your:

A. index and middle fingers; place your thumb on the child's cheek."
B. index and middle fingers; place your thumb on the child's larynx for stability."
C. whole hand on the child's jaw."
D. index and middle fingers; place your thumb on the child's ear for stability."

46. June is 5 years old and has been diagnosed with developmental delay. She has just achieved independence in self-feeding with a spoon. What should the COTA suggest to the parents in order for June to maintain her skill level at home after discharge?

A. Use hand-over-hand technique to reinforce correct technique.
B. Consistently point out incorrect hand placement and/or movement patterns.
C. Let June's older sister feed her occasionally as a reinforcement.
D. Praise her for what she does well; reinforce her independence.

47. To help determine a third grader's readiness for discharge from direct OT as a related service, what criteria should the COTA focus on?

A. Whether the disability interferes with the child's education.
B. The degree of functional skills.
C. Independence in ADLs.
D. Accessibility of the learning environment.

48. The COTA is preparing for the discharge of a 9-year-old with limited upper-extremity range of motion. The most important home adaptation to recommend concerning use of the toilet is:

A. installation of safety bars next to the toilet seat.
B. mounting of a wide-base toilet seat.
C. placement of a skidproof stepping stool next to the toilet.
D. installation of a bidet with a spray wash and air-drying mechanism.

49. What recreational activities should the COTA recommend for an 8-year-old boy who is being discharged after treatment for social withdrawal and depression?

A. Swimming lessons.
B. Boy Scouts.
C. Computer games.
D. Piano lessons.

50. Luke is 5 years old and is diagnosed as having athetoid cerebral palsy. Upon discharge from OT, his parents would like advice as to the BEST type of construction toy to buy Luke for Christmas. The COTA recommends a set with:

A. large, easily interlocking pieces.
B. blocks that are small and have a firm surface.
C. lightweight and soft-textured building blocks.
D. colorful blocks in a variety of shapes.

PHYSICAL DISABILITY QUESTIONS

Data Collection

51. The COTA is evaluating two-point discrimination in an individual with a median nerve injury. The COTA should:

A. apply the stimuli beginning at an area distal to the lesion progressing proximally.
B. test the involved area first, then the uninvolved area.
C. present test stimuli in an organized pattern to improve reliability during retesting.
D. allow the individual unlimited time to respond.

52. The instrument used to measure the strength of a three-jaw-chuck grasp pattern is a(n):

A. aesthesiometer.
B. pinch meter.
C. dynamometer.
D. volumeter.

53. An individual is able to complete full range of shoulder flexion while supine. However, when flexing the shoulder against gravity, she is only able to achieve 50% of normal ROM for shoulder flexion. The tester should record the grade for shoulder flexion as:

A. good (4).
B. fair (3).
C. fair minus (3–).
D. poor plus (2+).

54. When documenting, the COTA would record a client's inability to begin a task or activity as:

A. problems with attention.
B. problems with concentration.
C. problems with initiation.
D. apraxia.

55. Which of the following is a nonstandardized test used by occupational therapy practitioners in a physical disabilities setting?
A. The Motor Free Visual Perceptual Test.
B. The Minnesota Rate of Manipulation Test.
C. The Manual Muscle Test
D. The Purdue Pegboard Evaluation.

56. A COTA in a work-hardening program needs background information about an individual's work history. The best method for obtaining detailed information about the individual's job requirements is:
A. interviewing the individual.
B. examining an analysis of the individual's job.
C. looking up the individual's job in the Dictionary of Occupational Titles.
D. requesting information from the referring physician.

57. When administering the Purdue Pegboard Evaluation, the COTA must use all of the following skills except:
A. the ability to assess hand strength.
B. observation.
C. the knowledge of standardized evaluation techniques.
D. the ability to assess fine motor coordination.

58. A COTA is working with a young man with quadriplegia. During the initial interview, the COTA administers the Role Checklist. The primary purpose of this tool is to:
A. assess how successful the individual perceives he is at performing roles that are meaningful to him.
B. determine the roles the individual has performed in the past, is currently performing, and plans to perform in the future.
C. assess the individual's ability to follow directions.
D. establish rapport with the individual.

59. The COTA is observing dressing skills in an individual with COPD. While donning his shirt, the individual becomes short of breath and stops to rest before finishing with the shirt and going on to his trousers. The COTA would recognize this as a deficit in:
A. postural control.
B. muscle tone.
C. strength.
D. endurance.

60. The instrument used to measure edema in the hand is a(n):
A. goniometer
B. aesthesiometer
C. volumeter
D. dynamometer

Treatment planning

Questions 61-64 pertain to this case study:

Mrs. R. is a 65-year-old woman s/p CVA. She has recently been admitted to a long-term care facility, where the COTA is developing her treatment plan. Mrs. R. demonstrates left hemiplegia and moderate perceptual deficits, including unilateral neglect and difficulty with sequencing, figure-ground discrimination, position in space, and crossing the midline. Her initial evaluation revealed that she enjoys craft activities and socializing with others.

61. Mrs. R.'s writing sample illustrated her difficulty with crossing the midline. In planning activities to address this deficit to improve writing, the BEST activity for the COTA to use with Mrs. R. is to have her:
A. practice wheeling a wheelchair following a taped line on the floor.
B. place commonly used self-care items on her right side.
C. trace newspaper headlines across the page with her right index finger from left to right.
D. place playing cards in a horizontal row from left to right in sequence.

62. The COTA is planning to work on meal-preparation skills with Mrs. R. What item would be BEST for Mrs. R. to use to stabilize a potato when cutting it?
A. piece of nonskid backing under the cutting board.
B. plate guard around the edge of the board.
C. rocker knife.
D. cutting board with two nails in it.

63. Mrs. R. uses her unaffected right upper extremity to push her wheelchair. She sometimes slides to the left in her wheelchair, which causes her left upper extremity to dangle over the side of the wheelchair. The BEST positioning device for the COTA to use to support Mrs. R.'s affected arm is:
A. a half laptray.
B. the wheelchair armrest.
C. an arm sling.
D. an arm trough.

64. The COTA is planning a group activity during which the residents will make holiday decorations. Would making a chain out of green and red paper strips glued into loops be a successful activity for Mrs. R.?
A. Yes, if the COTA provides methods to enable one-handed participation.
B. Yes, because the activity is consistent with Mrs. R's interests.
C. No, primarily because of her difficulty with figure-ground discrimination.

D. No, primarily because of her difficulty with position in space.

65. A COTA working in a rehabilitation hospital goes to the wheelchair room to select a chair for a new patient. The patient is a 65-year-old man with left hemiplegia. His wheelchair must be equipped with all of the following except:
A. a left arm trough.
B. left footrest.
C. power mobility.
D. one-arm drive.

66. What is the purpose of a treatment plan, or "plan of care?"
A. To list specific directions for the COTA or OTR.
B. To measure the individual's progress towards a goal.
C. To organize the individual's priorities.
D. To summarize the approach to managing the individual's condition.

67. A COTA is working with an individual who demonstrates poor handwriting skills as a result of muscle weakness. The activity that represents a compensatory strategy is:
A. learning to type.
B. practicing fine motor coordination exercises.
C. practicing letter or shape formations.
D. strengthening the finger flexors and extensors.

68. An individual is unable to bring her hand to her mouth for feeding because of weakness in supination. The MOST helpful adapted utensil for her would be a:
A. spoon with an elongated handle.
B. spork.
C. spoon with a built-up handle.
D. swivel spoon.

69. A 60-year-old automobile mechanic with diabetes has been referred to occupational therapy following an above-knee amputation. He has impaired sensation in the remaining lower extremity and will be using a wheelchair for the foreseeable future. The FIRST patient education subject the COTA should cover is:
A. skin inspection.
B. grooming techniques (shaving, trimming toenails, etc.).
C. retirement planning.
D. returning to work.

70. A person with a spinal-cord injury at the C8 level will be able to perform self-feeding independently using:
A. a mobile arm support.
B. a universal cuff.
C. built-up utensils.
D. no adaptive equipment.

71. A long-term goal for an individual with T8 paraplegia is independence in transfers. All of the following are related short-term goals except:
A. "The patient will increase triceps strength to 5/5."
B. "The patient will manipulate wheelchair armrests and legrests independently."
C. "The patient will balance independently while sitting on the side of the bed."
D. "The patient will increase quadriceps strength to 5/5."

Treatment Implementation

72. The COTA is instructing a 41-year-old woman who has had a myocardial infarction in energy conservation techniques. The BEST example of limiting the amount of work needed for a task is:
A. using a side-loading washer.
B. wearing permanent press clothing.
C. using an extended-handle dustpan.
D. using good body mechanics.

73. When providing adaptive equipment to an individual with arthritis, the COTA explains that the purpose of the equipment is to:
A. prevent deforming stresses.
B. correct deformity.
C. simplify work.
D. decrease independence

74. What is the term for keeping a diary or log in response to memory deficits?
A. Problem solving.
B. Retraining.
C. Substitution.
D. Sompensation.

Questions 75–77 pertain to this case study:

Mr. J. has been admitted to a long-term care facility following a cardiovascular accident that resulted in left hemiplegia. He demonstrates unilateral neglect and mild difficulty with swallowing. His goals include independence with self-feeding and dressing activities.

75. When working on self-feeding with Mr. J., the COTA should teach him to hold his head in the following position:
A. 10 degrees of neck flexion
B. 10 degrees of neck extension
C. 30 degrees of neck flexion.
D. 30 degrees of neck extension.

76. A COTA is instructing Mr. J. how to don a teeshirt. The correct sequence is:
A. (1) place left hand into sleeve and pull up sleeve past elbow; (2) place right hand into sleeve and pull up sleeve; (3) pull shirt up over head; (4) pull shirt down over trunk.

B. (1) position shirt on lap; (2) place left hand into sleeve and pull up sleeve past elbow; (3) place right hand into sleeve and pull up sleeve; (4) pull shirt up over head.
C. (1) position shirt on lap; (2) place right hand into sleeve and pull up sleeve past elbow; (3) place left hand into sleeve and pull up sleeve; (4) pull shirt up over head.
D. (1) pull shirt up over head; (2) place left arm into sleeve; (3) place right arm into sleeve; (4) pull down shirt over trunk.

77. The MOST appropriate activity to use with Mr. J. to decrease his unilateral neglect would be:
A. rubbing lotion on the uninvolved limbs.
B. exercises using the uninvolved arm to move the involved arm across the midline.
C. participation in tasks that do not cross the midline.
D. participation in tasks involving materials placed on the uninvolved side.

78. The COTA is performing patient education with an outpatient who has received a resting hand splint. The COTA must be certain that the patient is able to:
A. identify landmarks on the hand/arm to align the splint.
B. discontinue use of the splint if redness occurs.
C. describe the wearing schedule in general terms.
D. remove and replace the splint with verbal cues from the COTA.

79. During lower-extremity dressing training, a woman with right hemiplegia and good balance is ready to pull her slacks up over her hips. The COTA should instruct her to:
A. use a dressing stick to pull the pants up over her hips.
B. remain seated and pull the slacks over her hips by leaning back against the wheelchair and elevating her hips.
C. remain seated and lean to the left, using her right hand to pull up the slacks past the right hip. Then, lean to the right, using the left hand to pull the slacks up past the left hip. Continue with this method until the slacks are all the way up.
D. place her left index finger through a belt loop, then stand and pull the slacks up past her hips.

80. A COTA needs an easily-graded activity designed to promote shoulder strengthening. The BEST activity would be:
A. passive range of motion.
B. Codman's exercises.
C. popping a balloon.
D. batting a balloon.

81. A COTA applies weights to the wrists of a woman who is making a macramé planter to improve strength in her shoulders. This treatment approach would be considered:
A. neurophysiological.
B. neurodevelopmental.
C. biomechanical.
D. rehabilitative.

82. A COTA in a work-hardening program is working with a man with an excessive anterior pelvic tilt. Instruction in proper body mechanics should emphasize correction of:
A. stenosis.
B. scoliosis.
C. kyphosis.
D. lordosis.

83. A COTA making a bedside visit finds her patient slouched over between the mattress and the bed rail. To address his edematous left upper extremity appropriately, she should:
A. elevate the arm on pillows so it rests higher than the heart.
B. massage the arm gently, stroking toward the fingers.
C. instruct him to avoid active range of motion.
D. instruct him to avoid passive range of motion.

84. In the middle of a wheelchair-to-bed transfer, an obese patient begins to slip from the grasp of an average-size COTA. The BEST action for the COTA to take is to:
A. ease the patient onto the floor, cushioning his fall.
B. reverse the transfer, getting the patient back in the wheelchair.
C. continue the transfer, attempting to get the patient to the bed.
D. call next door for assistance.

85. An individual with a weak grasp has difficulty holding a fork. The COTA wants to assess whether providing a fork with a built-up handle would be beneficial to this individual. The BEST way for the COTA to fabricate the equipment needed is to:
A. slip a piece of cylindrical foam onto the fork handle.
B. fabricate a built-up handle out of a thermoplastic material.
C. wrap the fork handle with adhesive-backed foam.
D. use a plastic fork and wrap a washcloth around the handle.

Evaluating the Treatment Plan

86. A COTA observes that a nonspeaking man using a wheelchair is suddenly making many errors on his augmentative communication device, although he had experienced no difficulty the previous day. The FIRST step the COTA should take to correct this problem is:

A. refer him to a physician for a physical exam.
B. reposition him in the wheelchair to allow optimal range of motion.
C. reassess his communication abilities.
D. replace his communication device.

87. As part of an initial evaluation of an individual with carpal tunnel syndrome, the OTR evaluates light touch sensation using a cotton ball. After wearing a wrist splint for 2 weeks, the patient returns for a reevaluation, which the COTA performs. The MOST appropriate method for the COTA to use is:
A. a tissue or cotton ball.
B. an aesthesiometer.
C. Semmes-Weinstein monofilaments.
D. the same method used initially.

88. A COTA providing home-based care to an individual with AIDS learns from his care giver that he has become too weak to turn himself in bed. What is the MOST important modification to the treatment plan for the COTA to recommend?
A. To begin a strengthening program.
B. To begin a bed-mobility program.
C. To teach the care giver how to lift and turn the client safely.
D. To provide an environmental control unit to the client.

89. Aaron is 2 weeks s/p CVA and has developed a two-finger subluxation in the left shoulder. The COTA thinks that wearing a sling will help to protect Aaron's arm when he propels his wheelchair and during transfers. Which aspect of the treatment process must the COTA attend to FIRST, in view of this new development?
A. Evaluation.
B. Treatment planning.
C. Treatment implementation.
D. Referral.

90. The most important information for the COTA to communicate to family members at an initial family meeting is:
A. information about the patient's prognosis.
B. information about the effect the individual's illness will have on role performance.
C. options concerning discharge.
D. anticipated equipment needs.

91. A patient with C4 quadriplegia informs his COTA that he will commit suicide if he is never able to walk again. The BEST response for the COTA to give is:
A. "Don't worry, you never know how things might turn out."
B. "You'll feel better if you start to talk with some of the other patients on your unit."
C. "You sound like things are looking pretty bad to you right now."
D. "Most individuals with quadriplegia can lead very fulfilling lives."

92. Margie is a 60-year-old woman with back pain. A long-term goal is to be able to return to her job as an illustrator. She has achieved the short-term goal of sitting at a work table for 20 minutes. Which statement is the BEST example of a revised short-term goal?
A. "Pt. will draw sitting at work table."
B. "Pt. will draw for 1 hour, taking stretch breaks every 20 minutes."
C. "Instruct patient in stretching techniques to be performed every 20 minutes."
D. "Instruct patient in the use of proper body mechanics that apply to prolonged sitting."

93. The expected outcome after a homemaker with severe back pain has completed a work-hardening program is:
A. acquisition of a part-time job out of the home.
B. acquisition of a full-time job out of the home.
C. decreased pain levels.
D. resumption of the homemaker role.

Discharge Planning

94. An individual begins taking a blood-thinning medication after surgery for an endarterectomy. What grooming tool should the COTA recommend for use in the hospital and after discharge?
A. An electric razor
B. A single-blade safety razor
C. A straight razor
D. A double-blade safety razor

95. An individual is about to be discharged to home following a hip arthroplasty. He is able to ambulate with a quad cane, but his balance remains slightly impaired. When preparing a home evaluation, which is the most important safety recommendation for the COTA make?
A. Remove all throw or scatter rugs.
B. Place lever handles on faucets.
C. Install a ramp where there are steps.
D. Install a handheld shower.

96. The COTA is teaching a client with chronic obstructive pulmonary disease how to modify his bathing techniques when he goes home from the hospital. What is the best method?
A. A tub bath using hot water.
B. A hot shower using a bath chair.
C. A lukewarm shower using a bath chair.
D. A tub bath using lukewarm water.

97. Sam is being discharged after hospitalization for a cardiovascular accident and a 2-week inpatient rehabilitation program. He requires minimal assistance in advanced ADLs but is independent in

most basic ADLs, and his RUE function is improving. He plans on eventually returning to work as a cashier. What should the OTR/COTA team recommend concerning occupational therapy services?
A. Home health OT.
B. Outpatient OT.
C. A work-hardening program.
D. Discontinuation of OT services.

98. Mrs. Z. is about to be discharge following rehabilitation for an acute arthritic flare-up. The COTA's contributions to the discharge plan include all of the following except:
A. instructing Mrs. Z. in joint-protection techniques.
B. summarizing Mrs. Z.'s progress in the discharge summary.
C. giving Mrs. Z. a handout that describes the exercises prescribed for her.
D. recommending that Mrs. Z. participate in local Arthritis Association activities.

99. Rita is about to be discharged after completing a rehabilitation program following a total hip replacement. In assessing her home environment, the COTA takes into consideration Rita's poor visual acuity. The MOST appropriate adaptation to ensure Rita can go up and down the stairs safely is:
A. installation of a stair glide.
B. installation of hand rails on both sides of the steps.
C. marking the end of each step with high-contrast tape.
D. instructing her to take only one step at a time when going up or down.

100. Jasmine and her sister are planning an outing into the community for the week after Jasmine is discharged from the rehabilitation center. The location at which she is most likely to run into barriers to wheelchair accessibility is the:
A. post office.
B. public library.
C. doughnut shop.
D. new multiplex cinema.

PSYCHOSOCIAL QUESTIONS

Data Collection

101. As part of a structured assessment, the COTA objectively assess a client's general behaviors (e.g., appearance), interpersonal behaviors (e.g., self-assertion), and task behaviors (e.g., following directions). The psychosocial assessment instrument that provides this information is the:
A. Milwaukee Evaluation of Daily Living Skills (MEDLS).
B. Kohlman Evaluation of Living Skills (KELS).
C. Comprehensive Occupational Therapy Evaluation (COTE) Scale.
D. Allen Cognitive Level (ACL).

102. The COTA is working with an elderly client who has been taking antipsychotic medications for many years. The side effects experienced by this individual include impaired swallowing and involuntary, jerky arm and leg movements. These behaviors are best described as:
A. Parkinsonian syndrome.
B. antipsychotic medication overdose.
C. tardive dyskinesia.
D. lithium toxicity.

103. The COTA has been assigned a patient who is mentally retarded and emotionally disturbed. This patient:
A. has a dual diagnosis.
B. is multiply handicapped.
C. has axis I and II duplicity.
D. has primary and secondary diagnoses.

104. "Self-concept," according to Uniform Terminology, is categorized as which type of performance component?
A. Sensory-perceptual.
B. Cognitive.
C. Social .
D. Psychological.

105. The advantage of asking a closed question is that the question:
A. allows the COTA to obtain facts.
B. avoids emphasizing feelings being expressed by the patient.
C. can help the COTA who is in a hurry.
D. forces the person to give the answer that the COTA needs.

106. The COTA, under the supervision of an OTR, is going to administer a projective assessment to an inpatient on a psychiatric unit. The MOST appropriate tool is:
A. the Magazine Picture Collage.
B. the Rorschach Ink Blot test.
C. proverb interpretation.
D. the House-Tree-Person Test (H-T-P).

107. Dana, a COTA, is interviewing a new patient to obtain general information about the patient. What is the BEST way for her to promote trust and encourage a relationship with the patient?
A. Introduce herself and explain why and how she became a COTA.
B. Introduce herself, explain why she wants to get to know the patient, briefly describe what the patient might gain from occupational therapy, and set a time for the next meeting.

C. Ask the patient to tell her what the patient hopes to achieve and how occupational therapy can help him or her.
D. Introduce the patient to the activities available in the OT clinic and inform the patient that he or she will have an opportunity to choose and to participate in any of the activities observed.

108. At the completion of the first interview, the patient asks the COTA, "What happens next?" What is the MOST appropriate response?
A. "The OTR and I will discuss your problems and decide on a treatment plan and the best activity groups to meet your needs."
B. "I will analyze our conversation and assign you to an appropriate group."
C. "The OTR and I will review the information you have given me and meet with you tomorrow afternoon to plan an activity program that best meets your needs."
D. "I'll be back."

109. When reporting data collected to the OTR, it is important for the COTA to:
A. observe everything the patient said and did during the interview and provide extensive notes for the OTR to read.
B. provide the OTR with a comprehensive treatment plan based on the results of the evaluation.
C. provide a summary of observations of the patient's behavior, including what the patient said and did during the interview.
D. provide an interpretation of how the patient behaved during the interview.

110. Which of the following is the most appropriate documentation of an initial observation?
A. "I think the patient is confused and would benefit from occupational therapy."
B. "Patient demonstrates possible cognitive disability, indicated by numerous errors in task execution."
C. "Patient displays poor planning, disorientation, psychomotor retardation, and generalized confusion."
D. "Patient attempted to assemble a woodworking kit. He didn't have a clue as to what was expected or how to do it."

Treatment Planning

111. The COTA wants to use a drawing activity with adolescent girls diagnosed with eating disorders. Which of the following would be the MOST appropriate activity?
A. The COTA asks a group member to lean against a wall where a large piece of paper had been posted. She then outlines the girl's body shape with a marker. She then asks the other group members to draw clothes and accessories on the silhouette.
B. The COTA asks members of a small group to draw pictures of themselves on a piece of paper. The COTA then leads a discussion about body-image concerns and links the discussion to the groups members' drawings.
C. The COTA asks all group participants to draw pictures of their current families. The COTA leads a discussion that focuses on the underlying family dynamics symbolized in the drawings.
D. The COTA meets separately with each girl and asks her to draw a picture of a person doing an activity. After the girl draws the picture, the COTA asks the girl to describe what the person in the drawing is doing; the COTA also asks the girl what skills she used while drawing this picture.

112. Which of the following groups is MOST likely to result in too much focus on the group leader and not enough interaction among group members?
A. A group consisting of fewer than five members.
B. A group made up of members of differing ages.
C. A group size consisting of between 7 and 10 members.
D. A group made up of members with similar goals and abilities.

113. The COTA is selecting an activity to use with a woman with paranoid schizophrenia. Which of the following activities is contraindicated for this client?
A. Playing "Whisper Down the Lane."
B. Making jewelry out of paper clips and contact paper.
C. Putting together puzzles of geometric designs.
D. Organizing files for the OT department.

114. The COTA is working with a young adult with a behavior disorder. When selecting computer software to use with the client, the most important consideration is:
A. whether the program offers simulations of social skills.
B. whether the program allows the "teacher," i.e., the COTA, to adjust the number, type, and frequency of attempts the individual can make to use the program.
C. whether, if it is game software, the game requires the cooperative efforts of two or more persons to achieve a successful outcome.
D. whether, in the case of game software, the games are noncompetitive in nature.

115. The COTA is arranging seating to facilitate communication among members of a group. The best arrangement is to:
A. provide enough chairs around a rectangle table.
B. provide enough chairs around a round table.
C. provide enough pillows to sit on the floor.

D. use the couches and chairs that are already in the room.

116. The COTA is working with a 32-year-old woman who has difficulty with self-expression. What is the MOST appropriate goal for this client?

A. The client will identify and pursue activities that give her pleasure.
B. The client will use facial expressions and gestures that are consistent with stated emotions during assertive, passive, and aggressive role-playing situations.
C. The client will recognize the nature of her behavior and understand the possible negative and positive consequences.
D. The client will identify her assets and limitations after participating in a movement group.

117. Goals for treatment should be:

A. written by the COTA independently.
B. relevant to the patient's needs and values.
C. limited by the patient's cognitive impairments.
D. left flexible, so as not to pressure the patient to perform.

118. The COTA is working with a patient who has difficulty attending to a task and sustaining attention for a reasonable length of time. Which of the following activities would be most appropriate for the patient?

A. a mosaic tile project.
B. ceramics using a potter's wheel.
C. leather carving.
D. creating jewelry with pliable wire.

119. The COTA has been asked to select activities for a patient with manic behavior. Which type of activities would be contraindicated with this patient?

A. Small leather projects.
B. Small group exercise class.
C. Oil painting on a large canvas.
D. Copper tooling with a template.

120. The COTA is planning a game activity for a group in a psychosocial treatment setting. It is important to select a game that provides equal opportunities to win and can be played by people at a variety of functional levels. The best game type to select is:

A. games of strategy.
B. hobbies.
C. games of chance.
D. puzzles.

121. The COTA is working with a client to develop her work potential in a prevocational program. The psychosocial performance components that are most important to emphasize are:

A. punctuality, accepting responsibility for oneself, accepting directions from a supervisor, and appropriately interacting with peer co-workers.
B. memory, sequencing of the work tasks, and making decisions.
C. standing tolerance, eye-hand coordination, and endurance.
D. meeting workplace grooming requirements and adherence to safety procedures.

Treatment Implementation

122. The COTA selects a pie-of-life activity to use with a stress management group. The COTA states, "I see that at least half of you have drawn your pie of life with too little time for rest and relaxation. Why don't we spend some group time exploring some ways to add more relaxation and rest into your days? Let's each give one suggestion." This scenario is an example of a group functioning at the following level:

A. project group.
B. egocentric-cooperative group.
C. cooperative group.
D. mature group.

123. The COTA responds to an individual by paraphrasing in order to:

A. refocus or redirect the individual's comments.
B. show acceptance and understanding to the individual.
C. force the individual to make a choice.
D. elicit additional information from an individual.

124. A COTA using stress-management interventions is using which type of health promotion?

A. Primary prevention.
B. Secondary prevention.
C. Tertiary prevention.
D. Intermediate prevention.

125. The COTA is leading a reality-orientation group for nursing-home residents with dementia. The MOST important item for the COTA to focus on is:

A. the residents' plans for the future.
B. the name(s) of family members.
C. verbalization of the residents' thoughts and feelings.
D. remembering events from the past that would create a sense of well-being.

126. A Level II OTA student describes an individual she is working with to her fieldwork supervisor. The student comments that the individual is "one of her favorites," and that she frequently allows this individual to spend extra time in the craft area after group sessions are over. The fieldwork supervisor is most likely to wonder if the student's comments reflect:

A. self-disclosure.
B. over-involvement.
C. transference.
D. burnout.

127. The mental-health treatment environment that offers the least restrictive level of care is:
A. a quarterway house.
B. a halfway house.
C. a supervised apartment.
D. outpatient counseling.

128. The COTA is visiting a patient in the patient's home, working on a household budgeting activity. The patient, who is in her mid-60s, takes Tranxene, an anti-anxiety medication. The patient stands up from the kitchen table to get her eyeglasses, grabs the edge of the table, and says "I'm having a dizzy spell." Later, when she sits down to work with the COTA, the patient has difficulty telling the difference between the phone bill and the utility bill. The first thing the COTA should do is:
A. advise the individual to discontinue taking her anti-anxiety medication until the physician can be reached.
B. when she gets back to the clinic, read about the side effects of Tranxene in the Physician's Desk Reference.
C. ask the client how often she has these "spells," encourage her to sit back down until it passes, and stop working on the budget activity for today.
D. teach the client to get up slowly from seated and lying positions and to hold onto a stable surface until the dizzy feeling is over.

129. The COTA is working with an individual at risk for ingesting toxic substances. The craft material of greatest concern to the COTA is:
A. small mirror pieces.
B. white craft glue.
C. permanent markers.
D. leather dyes.

130. The COTA who uses pictures, music, and discussion questions with a group of elderly clients to encourage them to verbalize their thoughts and feelings about their first ride in a car is using:
A. remotivation
B. reality orientation
C. compensatory strategies
D. environmental modification

131. Ricky, an 18-year-old diagnosed with schizophrenia, takes a neuroleptic drug that caused him to feel extreme thirst. He is to continue taking the medication after discharge from the hospital. It is MOST important to remind Ricky to:
A. keep time in the sun as brief as possible.
B. drink coffee and caffeinated sodas whenever possible.
C. get up slowly from a standing, sitting, or lying position.
D. drink juices and caffeine-free colas when thirsty.

132. Tim has paranoia and prefers to stay away from the group, working alone at another table. The best action for the COTA to take is to:
A. encourage Tim to join the group.
B. tell Tim he is required to sit with the group.
C. tell Tim it is okay to work where he is until he feels comfortable joining the group.
D. stay with Tim until he is ready to join the group.

Questions 133–134 pertain to this case study:

Mr. R., a 54-year-old man, has been admitted with a diagnosis of reactive depression following an overdose of sleeping pills. Mr. R. was asked to take early retirement because of downsizing in the company that employed him for the past 30 years. His entire identity and self-concept revolved around his position as the Director of the public relations department. Mr. R. was referred to occupational therapy to increase his sense of competence and self-confidence and to encourage the development of enjoyable leisure activities.

133. When meeting Mr. R. for the first time it is MOST important for the COTA to introduce:
A. himself and provide the patient with a written schedule for his OT program.
B. himself and explain how OT activities will correlate with Mr. R.'s overall treatment plan.
C. himself and begin administering an interest checklist.
D. Mr. R. to the other patients in the OT clinic.

134. Based on Mr. R.'s OT goals, what is an appropriate FIRST activity to recommend for this patient?
A. pouring and glazing chess pieces.
B. designing and building a doll house.
C. copper tooling using a template.
D. learning how to play bridge.

135. The COTA changes a tile trivet activity by providing blue craft glue instead of white glue to clients who confuse the glue and the grout. The COTA is using:
A. activity analysis.
B. activity adaptation.
C. activity sequencing.
D. clinical reasoning.

Evaluating the Treatment Plan

136. The COTA is working with developmentally disabled clients in a sheltered workshop. She realizes that a worker is having difficulty learning the assembly sequence for a knife-fork-spoon package. The COTA decides to use backward chaining. In this case, backward chaining involves:
A. encouraging the individual to reverse the packaging sequence.

B. asking the client only to put the last piece into the package.
C. praising the client for close approximations (such as including a knife, fork, and two spoons).
D. demonstration and repetition by the COTA of the correct sequence before each of the worker's attempts.

137. After one session with a new patient in a psychosocial treatment setting, it has become apparent to the COTA that the woman is highly distractible and cannot complete a magazine collage when in a group. The best approach for the COTA to use is to:
A. speak slowly and softly to the patient.
B. coax and praise the patient until she completes the task.
C. ask the rest of the group members to stop talking.
D. position the patient so she is facing a blank wall.

Questions 138–141 pertain to this case study:

Shirley is a 65-year old, disheveled-looking woman with paranoid schizophrenia. She demonstrates poor eye contact, mumbles when she speaks to others, and is often belligerent. She frequently accuses men in her program of sexually abusing her. She refuses to walk without a walker, even though her hip fracture is well healed and she has no residual gait disorder. The COTA has been working with Shirley in a weekly beauty group and a daily current events group.

138. The COTA observes during beauty group that Shirley is more willing to allow the COTA to polish her nails than she was originally. What is the MOST likely reason for this change?
A. Shirley is experiencing less tactile defensiveness.
B. Shirley wants to make herself more attractive to men.
C. Shirley's self-esteem has increased.
D. Shirley is exhibiting improved social conduct.

139. The COTA observes Shirley arrive in current events group without her walker on three consecutive days. This is most likely indicative of:
A. improved social conduct.
B. improved balance.
C. forgetfulness.
D. improved interpersonal skills.

140. "Shirley arrived without her walker three out of three days this week." This statement belongs in which part of a SOAP note?
A. Subjective.
B. Objective.
C. Assessment.
D. Plan.

141. The statement that best substantiates a decrease in paranoid behavior is:
A. "Shirley is no longer as afraid of men."
B. "Shirley has not accused any men of attacking her this week."
C. "Shirley is participating more actively in beauty group."
D. "Shirley will tolerate sitting next to a man in group one time this week."

142. "Continue social skills training program and encourage client to attend one new after-school club activity, within the next week." This statement is an example of which part of a SOAP note?
A. Subjective.
B. Objective.
C. Assessment.
D. Plan.

143. The COTA is documenting a client's psychosocial responses to a stenciling activity. Which of the following is the most objective statement?
A. On 11-1-96, the client did not want to finish her stenciling activity.
B On 11-1-96, the client was hostile to another client in the activity group.
C. The client initiated working on the stenciling activity by selecting one of six available designs.
D. The client demonstrated an appropriate level of frustration tolerance during most of the activity.

Discharge Planning

144. The best work program for individuals who experience difficulty accepting supervision, difficulty relating to co-workers, and difficulty accepting the value of punctuality is:
A. competitive job placement.
B. working in a fast-food restaurant with a job coach.
C. supported employment.
D. work adjustment.

Questions 145–148 pertain to this case study:

The COTA is discussing discharge plans with Katrina, a 35-year-old homemaker who has identified her use of alcohol as a contributing factor to her depression. Katrina is scheduled for discharge the following week.

145. Katrina's discharge-planning group is likely to address all of the following issues except:
A. structuring her leisure time following discharge.
B. making living arrangements.
C. obtaining outpatient treatment .
D. relaxation and exercise.

146. Upon discharge, the most appropriate type of group to refer Katrina to is a(n):
A. advocacy group.
B. self-help group.

C. support group.
D. psychotherapy group.

147. Katrina asks the COTA for information about self-help groups. The COTA explains that the expectation for becoming a member of a self-help group for alcoholics is that members:
A. are encouraged to tell the other members their name and where they live and work.
B. share their experiences and struggles with alcohol use.
C. are required to attend a set number of meetings.
D. are encouraged to give advice to others.

148. The most appropriate self-help group to recommend to Katrina is:
A. Mothers Against Drunk Drivers (MADD).
B. Al-Anon.
C. Alcoholics Anonymous (AA).
D. Group Therapy.

149. The COTA is a member of a discharge team reviewing treatment options for a 70-year-old woman who no longer experiences the acute symptoms that necessitated admission but continues to require occupational therapy services to address her anxiety and isolation. The patient is functional in all daily living skills and will return to live with her sister, who works during the day. The best treatment environment for the patient to continue receiving occupational therapy services would be:
A. in her home, with services provided by a home health agency.
B. partial hospitalization.
C. adult day care.
D. day treatment.

150. The COTA is working with a group of individuals who are diagnosed with major depression. The group is focusing on issues related to being ready for discharge. The most helpful approach for the COTA to take would be to:
A. be upbeat, positive, and cheerful when encouraging the individuals to discuss their discharge plans.
B. allow more time for the individuals to respond to questions about discharge plans.
C. remain silent and still while the individuals are describing their feelings about discharge.
D. allow the individuals to structure the group discussion.

PROFESSIONAL PRACTICE QUESTIONS

Promote Professional Practice

151. A COTA faced with a dilemma concerning patient confidentiality should refer to which of the following documents?
A. Standards of Practice.
B. Uniform Terminology System for Reporting Occupational Therapy Services, 3rd Edition.
C. Her state's regulatory act.
D. Occupational Therapy Code of Ethics.

152. The primary purpose of licensure is to:
A. delineate the specific roles of and relations between occupational therapists and certified occupational therapy assistants.
B. protect consumers of occupational therapy.
C. ensure continued competency of therapists.
D. justify occupational therapy services for Medicare and Medicaid reimbursement.

153. Based on the service need, the role of the COTA may vary. A COTA who is called to give expert witness on behalf of a claimant in an Americans with Disability Act (ADA) lawsuit would be acting as a(n):
A. practitioner
B. consultant.
C. supervisor.
D. educator.

154. In which occupational therapy setting is a COTA most challenged to find creative alternatives for providing treatment equipment and overcoming professional isolation?
A. The acute-care hospital.
B. The nursing home.
C. Home care.
D. The rehabilitation hospitals.

155. The profession of occupational therapy is continually evolving and developing. As health care changes through the next century, the focus will move more toward health status and away from health care. In this context, the COTA's role in enhancing wellness through education, behavioral change, and cultural support is called:
A. occupational behavior.
B. intervention.
C. self-efficacy.
D. health promotion.

156. A COTA who has demonstrated service competency is about to apply paraffin to the hands of a client with arthritis. Before doing so, she explains the potential benefits and risks to the client. This explanation is required by the ethical concept of:
A. informed consent.
B. fidelity.
C. beneficence.
D. nonmaleficence.

157. A COTA working in a long-term care facility has her notes cosigned weekly by her supervising OTR. Which of the following is NOT a valid reason for this requirement?

A. The AOTA requires the cosignature of the supervising OTR.
B. Cosigning may be required for reimbursement.
C. The employer may require cosigning.
D. Cosigning may be required by the state regulatory act.

158. The COTA working with a 4-year-old child notices a bruise on the child's shoulder that looks like an adult hand- and fingerprint. Based on this observation, the COTA should:
A. discuss the bruises with family members who pick up the child.
B. wait until more injuries can be observed.
C. make a report to the appropriate authorities.
D. avoid getting involved in personal family matters.

159. A 1-year-old child with multiple disabilities is eligible to have which of the the following types of plan developed by an interdisciplinary team:
A. Individual education plan (IEP).
B. Least restrictive environment plan (LREP).
C. Individual family service plan (IFSP).
D. Early intervention program plan (EIPP).

160. A COTA practicing in a school-based setting is interested in training students in Level II fieldwork. Before accepting Level II students, the COTA should have at least:
A. 6 months experience.
B. 1 year experience.
C. 2 years experience.
D. 3 years experience.

161. Current trends in the field of occupational therapy reflect:
A. increased use of COTAs.
B. decreased use of COTAs.
C. increased use of OT resources in inpatient facilities.
D. decreased need for OTs in the community.

162. A COTA is providing treatment to two women, Jean and Liz, in the OT room. Jean observes Liz doing a cooking activity, which is not included in Jean's treatment plan; she asks if she can do a cooking activity, too. The COTA does not think that allowing Jean to do a cooking activity would be detrimental to her. What is the most appropriate action for the COTA to take?
A. Modify Jean's treatment plan.
B. Do not modify Jean's treatment plan and explain why not to Jean.
C. Notify the supervising OTR of Jean's interests so that the OTR may decide if it is a good idea to modify the treatment plan.
D. Discuss the occupational therapy program with the patient and her family and modify the program based on Jean's preferences.

163. A COTA is asked to provide paraffin treatments for a patient evaluated by the occupational therapist. At what minimal level may the COTA participate in this activity?
A. An entry-level COTA may perform the task unless state law prohibits it.
B. A COTA may perform the task following demonstration of service competency, unless state law prohibits this.
C. A COTA contributes to the process but does not complete the task independently, unless state law specifically allows the COTA to do so.
D. A COTA cannot perform the task.

164. Mrs. N. informs her COTA that she is concerned about returning home under her husband's care, indicating that he had been abusive to her before her stroke. What is the FIRST action the COTA should take?
A. Notify hospital security and limit the patient's husband to supervised visits.
B. Recommend alternative discharge plans.
C. Notify the supervising therapist of the situation.
D. Notify the hospital's protective services department.

165. The standard by which rightness or wrongness of choices and behaviors is determined for a professional group such as occupational therapy practitioners is called:
A. a policy or procedure.
B. regulations.
C. code of ethics.
D. protocol.

166. An entry-level COTA wants to know the extent of her liability when providing occupational therapy. Which of the following answers is MOST correct?
A. Only OTRs need to have liability insurance.
B. Only COTAs need to have liability insurance.
C. Both OTRs and COTAs should have liability insurance.
D. Neither OTR or the COTA need to have liability insurance.

167. A COTA working in outpatient rehabilitation teaches herself how to use paraffin by reading books on physical agent modalities (PAMs), carefully reading the instructions that came with the paraffin bath unit, and practicing on herself for several weeks. Is it now acceptable for this COTA to provide paraffin treatments?
A. No, COTAs may not administer PAMs.
B. No, it violates the Occupational Therapy Code of Ethics.
C. Yes, she has demonstrated service competency.
D. Yes, only when an OTR is on duty in the facility.

168. Before providing a paraffin bath to an individual with arthritis, the COTA must do all of the following EXCEPT:
A. demonstrate service competency in the use of paraffin.

B. inform the patient of the risks involved in using paraffin.
C. precede the paraffin bath with purposeful activity.
D. have the appropriate level of supervision from an OTR.

169. An OTR asks a COTA to lead a group in a quilting project during the upcoming holiday season. The most responsible action for the COTA to take is to:
A. ask his supervisor to teach him quilting.
B. change the activity to one in which he is competent and therefore able to accomplish the same goals.
C. refuse to lead a group activity that he is not competent in.
D. take a few days to teach himself the activity before leading the group.

170. A COTA's employer provides funding for only one person a year to attend continuing education. There are four OT practitioners in the department. The BEST way to ensure that the COTA achieves continuing education he or she needs is to:
A. wait for his or her turn to take employer-funded continuing education.
B. demand more funding for continuing education.
C. participate in the continuing-education workshops offered by the AOTA over the Internet.
D. schedule regular department inservices and take turns presenting.

171. All of the following are considered forms of continuing education except:
A. training fieldwork students.
B. reading professional journals.
C. providing continuous patient treatment.
D. attending a state occupational therapy conference.

172. A COTA witnesses a fellow employee charging a patient for services that were not provided and reports that practitioner to the Standards and Ethics Committee of the AOTA. After conducting a hearing, the Judicial Council decides upon its most severe form of disciplinary action—revocation. This action means that the practitioner:
A. loses his or her license to practice OT anywhere in the United States.
B. loses his or her license to practice OT in the state in which he or she was practicing.
C. permanently loses his or her membership in the AOTA.
D. loses his or her membership in AOTA for a specific period of time.

173. The primary diagnosis most frequently treated by COTAs is:
A. learning disabilities.
B. developmental delay.
C. CVA/hemiplegia.
D. fracture.

174. An OTR and COTA are hired to establish a department in a rural nursing home. As they develop the policies and procedures for documentation in the nursing home, the document they will MOST likely refer to is the:
A. Uniform Terminology, 3rd edition.
B. Occupational Therapy Code of Ethics.
C. Occupational Therapy Standards of Practice.
D. Occupational Therapy Roles.

175. A COTA has been assigned a patient who was diagnosed with lung cancer that has metastasized to his brain. The COTA spends 15 minutes reviewing the patient's chart and talking with his nurse, who indicates that the patient is preoccupied with finances. As the COTA enters the room, the man states that he does not want to be seen for occupational therapy because his insurance has run out and he cannot afford to pay for the treatment. What is the BEST response for the COTA?
A. Treat the patient according to the physician's order and notify the nurse that the man's preoccupation with finances continues.
B. Do not treat the patient, because of his refusal, and document the interaction in the chart.
C. Treat the patient but do not charge for or document the services.
D. Do not treat the patient but charge for the time spent completing the chart review.

176. A COTA is assigned to work with two new patients, Sam and Lou. Sam has a pleasant disposition and is a pleasure to work with. Lou is argumentative, swears a lot, and has not bathed in 3 weeks. Both men have extensive rehabilitation needs. The COTA works with Sam for a standard 45-minute session each day but shortens Lou's sessions to 30 minutes. Is the COTA violating the Occupational Therapy Code of Ethics?
A. Yes, by violating the concept of beneficence.
B. Yes, by violating the concept of competence.
C. Yes, by violating the concept of compliance with laws and regulations.
D. No, there is no ethical violation.

177. An OTA student completes a range-of-motion evaluation and asks her supervisor to retest the individual to check her results. This is an example of:
A. an appropriate request for supervision.
B. student incompetence.
C. interrater reliability.
D. a lack of self-confidence.

Support Service Management

178. The COTA is treating a middle-aged woman for carpal tunnel syndrome. The employer's industrial nurse indicated that the condition was a result

of repetitious fine-motor movement considered an essential job function. The payment program most likely to provide payment for occupational therapy services is:

A. Medicare.
B. Medicaid.
C. Workers' compensation.
D. Education for All Handicapped Children program.

179. The COTA is working with a patient on an acute-care floor when the patient's IV tube disengages and the COTA is splashed in the eye with medication and "backwash" fluid. The COTA's FIRST response should be to:

A. rub the eye and continue treatment.
B. rinse the eye with an eyewash or water immediately.
C. write an incident report.
D. cover the eye with a bandage and contact his or her immediate supervisor.

180. A COTA with several years of experience receives general supervision from an OTR supervisor. This COTA has contact with her supervisor:

A. once a day.
B. every 2 weeks.
C. once a month.
D. as needed.

181. Most of the clients of a COTA working in an outpatient setting are enrolled in HMOs. The term used to describe the preestablished rate of payment per diagnosis is:

A. fee for service.
B. capitation.
C. cost shifting.
D. cost control.

182. OT practitioners should wear gloves when working with:

A. individuals with open wounds who have been diagnosed with HIV.
B. individuals with third-degree burns.
C. individuals with open wounds who have been diagnosed with hepatitis.
D. all individuals with open wounds.

183. COTAs employed by home-health agencies primarily see patients who:

A. require a wheelchair for mobility.
B. are not able to drive to an outpatient treatment center.
C. are homebound.
D. require moderate assistance for ambulation.

184. One week after an experienced COTA begins a new job in a nursing home, her supervising OTR resigns. There is not another OTR on staff. The nursing home administrator advises the COTA to continue treating patients, and promises to hire an OTR within a week. The MOST acceptable action for the COTA to take is to:

A. refuse to provide OT services to patients until an OTR has been hired to supervise her.
B. agree to provide OT services to patients for the first week, but not beyond that.
C. provide OT services only to patients who will suffer if they don't receive OT services.
D. report the nursing home to the AOTA.

185. A referral for a woman s/p hip replacement is received in the OT department on a day when the only OTR is on vacation. The COTA observes that the patient is scheduled to be discharged before the OTR's return. The BEST action for the COTA to take is to:

A. obtain collaboration with or supervision from an OTR before beginning treatment.
B. perform an ADL evaluation.
C. provide the individual with the adaptive equipment she will need.
D. begin instruction in hip precautions.

186. Walking through the PT department, a COTA notices a man struggling to put on his shoes. Later that day, she observes the same individual attempting unsuccessfully to don a sweater. The most appropriate action for the COTA to take is to:

A. initiate a referral for OT.
B. begin instruction in upper- and lower-extremity dressing.
C. formally evaluate the man's dressing skills.
D. perform a full self-care evaluation.

187. OT practitioners working in a partial-hospitalization program are designing a quality assurance (QA) program. What is the LEAST appropriate area of practice for them to examine?

A. Patient satisfaction.
B. Medication effectiveness.
C. Progress toward goals.
D. Behavior ratings.

188. Once an occupational therapy department has received a referral, the role of the COTA may include:

A. responding to the referral.
B. determining information to be collected for the screening.
C. initiating the screening.
D. collecting screening data.

189. An entry-level COTA is working in a long-term care facility. Based on the COTA's level of experience, what form of supervision would be most effective?

A. Direct contact with supervisor, on site, daily.
B. Direct contact with supervisor, on site, once a week.
C. Indirect contact with supervisor once a day.
D. Indirect contact with supervisor once a week.

190. The COTA has been asked to write a patient-care quality-assurance monitor for the outpatient service area. The OT supervisor has stipulated that the results be measurable, reliable, valid, and within the OT scope of care. The monitor that best meets these criteria is:
A. family compliance with a home-exercise program.
B. appropriate physician referrals.
C. improvement in functional independence.
D. patient compliance with a home splinting schedule.

191. A COTA is supervising an occupational therapy aide. Duties that the COTA may assign to the aide include:
A. setting up or cleaning up treatment activities.
B. instructing a patient in an active range-of-motion exercise program.
C. completing ADL training with a patient.
D. selecting adaptive equipment from a catalog.

192. A COTA is involved in an emergency-response practice that is routinely done in the occupational therapy department. Which one of the following activities is the COTA most likely participating in?
A. A fire drill.
B. Electrical equipment inspection.
C. Maintenance check of fire extinguishers.
D. Clearing fire exits of equipment.

193. A COTA working in a school system has been asked by the OTR to perform most of the initial evaluation. She is concerned this goes beyond the scope of COTA practice, as well as beyond her own competence. The most responsible action for her to take is to:
A. resign from the job.
B. refuse to perform the evaluation.
C. discuss the problem with the OTR's administrative supervisor.
D. discuss her concerns with the OTR.

194. "All documentation is to be entered into the patient's permanent medical record by the end of the business day." This statement is an example of:
A. documentation.
B. a policy.
C. a procedure.
D. a job description.

195. Information about what to do in case of fire will most likely be found in the:
A. mission statement of the facility.
B. quality assurance report.
C. description of essential job requirements.
D. policy and procedure manual.

196. A COTA who needs to transfer an obese man is not confident she can manage the transfer alone. The best action for her to take is to:
A. use proper body mechanics.
B. ask someone from physical therapy to do the transfer.
C. ask another practitioner for help.
D. refrain from transferring the patient.

197. The activity that is most likely to involve toxic substances is:
A. wood burning.
B. copper tooling.
C. dough art.
D. papier mache.

198. A COTA is using a computer in the occupational therapy clinic for patient documentation. The COTA is most likely using a:
A. terminal program.
B. spreadsheet.
C. database manager.
D. word processing program.

199. Political trends in the United States suggest that:
A. government will pass legislation to make health insurance available to all American citizens.
B. government will pass legislation that will call for insurance company reform.
C. inpatient hospital care will increase.
D. managed healthcare systems will become extinct.

200. A COTA is completing a home assessment and making recommendations for equipment to be used in the home. He recommends a hospital bed, lightweight wheelchair, bedside commode, reachers, a long-handled sponge, a shower chair, and a handheld shower. The item(s) considered as durable medical equipment are:
A. lightweight wheelchair and reachers.
B. shower chair, long-handled sponge, and bedside commode.
C. hospital bed and shower chair with a handheld shower.
D. lightweight wheelchair and hospital bed.

ANSWERS FOR SIMULATION EXAMINATION 2

1. (B) decreased muscle tone. Decreased muscle tone is usually characterized by joints that are lax and hyperextensible. Low muscle tone and joint hyperextensibility are also frequent characteristics of Down syndrome. Answers A and C are incorrect because loss of range of motion resulting in contractures is characteristic of increased muscle tone. Clonus (answer D) refers to rapid, reflexive contraction of antagonistic muscles. See reference: Hopkins and Smith (eds): Simon, CJ, and Daub, MM: Human development across the life span.

2. (B) using a compensatory position to achieve stability. Answer B is correct because exclusive "W" sitting by a child with low muscle tone indicates that the child is probably not using side-, ring-, or long-sitting positions (all of which are developmentally appropriate). The child is compensating for an inability to achieve stability in a variety of positions that require dynamic postural control, depending on skeletal rather than neuromuscular structures for stability. Answers A and D are not correct because exclusive "W" sitting is not age-appropriate for a 5-year-old child, or a child at any age. Answer C is not correct because although exclusive "W" sitting is a compensatory position, it is used to achieve stability and in fact may limit mobility. See reference: Kramer and Hinojosa: Schoen, S, and Anderson, J: Neurodevelopmental frame of reference.

3. (C) has stated instructions for administration and scoring. Nonstandardized tests are subjective (answer A) and depend on the skill and judgment of the occupational therapy practitioner administering them (answers B and D). Entry-level COTAs are educationally prepared to administer some standardized tests. With experience and training, COTAs may become competent to administer additional standardized tests and some nonstandardized tests. See reference: Pedretti (ed): Pedretti: Occupational therapy evaluation and assessment of physical dysfunction.

4. (A) record attention span during classroom observation. "Cognitive integration is often assessed . . . through direct observation of the child during everyday tasks within the child's natural environments. An example of this is recording a child's attention span while the child is in the classroom (p. 167)." Answer A assesses psychosocial performance components, and answers C and D assess sensorimotor component. See reference: Case-Smith, Allen, and Pratt (eds): Stewart, KB: Occupational therapy assessment in pediatrics.

5. (A) Interview. Interviews provide an opportunity for the parents to identify their values and priorities in regard to the skills being assessed in occupational therapy. Open-ended questions are best for eliciting information about the family's feelings about the intervention. Answers B, C and D are structured observation methods, through which information on specific skills or functional levels is collected. See reference: Case-Smith, Allen, and Pratt (eds): Stewart, KB: Occupational therapy assessment in pediatrics.

6. (B) match picture dominoes. A game of matching dominoes involves visual form perception defined as "matching one design with another." Playing marbles (answer A) and assembling a puzzle (answer D) address spatial perception skills. Playing "Memory" (answer C) requires visual memory in addition to form-perception skills. See reference: Case-Smith, Allen, and Pratt (eds): Schneck, CM: Visual perception.

7. (C) the cultural context and family interaction patterns. Cultural expectations may determine behavior standards and the expression of family roles. Continued feeding of a young child with a handicap may be the expression of nurturing and caring. Such an expression may be viewed as more important than the promotion of independence and self-reliance. Answers A, B, and D may be valid issues as well but should be addressed after the COTA has familiarized himself or herself with the cultural and familial context of the skill. See reference: Case-Smith, Allen, and Pratt (eds): Shepherd, J, Procter, SA, and Coley, IL: Self care and adaptations for independent living. Also: Case-Smith, J, and Humphry, R: Feeding and oral motor skills.

8. (A) copying letters. The test administered consists of design-copying tasks that can yield information on the child's ability to translate a visual image into a motor output. Visual-motor integration is defined as "the ability to integrate the visual image of letters and shapes with the appropriate motor response necessary." Remembering (answer B), recognizing (answer C), and sequencing (answer D) are cognitive and perceptual skills, which do not require a motor response and therefore are not considered visual-motor skills. See reference: Case-Smith, Allen, and Pratt (eds): Schneck, CM: Visual perception.

9. (D) the presence of self-stimulatory behavior. Self-stimulatory behavior is often seen in autistic children and frequently interferes with function. The other answers are less relevant in terms of essential data for intervention planning; an autistic child may be normal in terms of ability to focus at close range (answer A), wrist flexibility (answer B), and hand preference (answer D) but will show poor adaptive behavior. See reference: Nelson DL: Typical strengths and weaknesses in children with pervasive disorders.

10. (A) a grand mal seizure. Grand mal seizures are the most commonly seen seizures (40–50% of all occurring seizures). The seizure may be preceded by an aura, and incontinence is common. The child may experience drowsiness or sleep for 1 to 2 hours following the seizure. Petit mal seizures (answer B) are accompanied by only a short loss of awareness. The only motor activity seen may be eye blinking or rolling. The seizure lasts only 5 to10 seconds, and there is no noted recovery period. In a psychomotor (answer C) or focal seizure the child may have auditory or olfactory sensations, may appear confused, and may demonstrate automatic movements such as lip smacking, chewing, or unbuttoning clothing. A seizure that lasts for 30 minutes or more is called status epilepticus (answer D). This is a serious condition requiring medical management. See reference: Case-Smith, Allen, and Pratt (eds): Gordon, CY, Schanzenbacher, KE, Case-Smith, J, and Carrasco, R: Diagnostic problems in pediatrics.

11. (D) all extremities. The word "quadriplegia" refers to involvement of all four extremities, and in cerebral palsy describes trunk, neck, and often oral motor involvement as well. Single-limb involvement (answer A) is called monoplegia and is very rare. The involvement of one body side (answer B) is called hemiplegia, which is why this answer is incorrect. Answer C assumes bilateral lower-extremity involvement, which is called paraplegia. See reference: Case-Smith, Allen, and Pratt (eds): Gordon, CY, Schanzenbacher, KE, Case-Smith, J, and Carrasco, R: Diagnostic problems in pediatrics.

12. (B) . forward and side-to-side movement with the child sitting on a ball. Answer B is correct because the position of the child requires the least resistance to gravity. By tilting the child in this position, the practitioner controls how much the child will work against gravitational pull. Answers A and D are incorrect, because they would require the child to lift her head directly against gravity. Answer C is also incorrect, because the head is positioned against gravity in the quadruped position, and a child with extremely poor head control probably could not hold a quadruped position. See reference: Hopkins and Smith (eds): Erhardt, RP: Cerebral palsy.

13. (A) 2 years. A powered wheelchair, which provides rapid mobility to the nonambulatory child, can be considered as early as 18 months. Because an 18-month-old child can direct his body through space safely, a nonambulatory child of the same age should also be able to direct a wheelchair. Answers B, C, and D are incorrect because the power wheelchair can first be considered at a much earlier age. See reference: Kramer and Hinojosa: Colangelo, CA: Biomechanical frame of reference.

14. (D) adapted teaching techniques. Answer D is correct, because a child with this type of disability will characteristically have learning problems that require such teaching methods as "chaining" or behavior modification. Answers A, B, and C are of secondary importance, because physical coordination may be impaired, or other physical limitations such as abnormal muscle tone or significant problems with balance could also be present. These additional problems may require adaptive equipment, clothing, or techniques. However, all aspects of dressing are dependent on the child's ability to learn procedures of dressing, and therefore it is necessary to consider task analysis and teaching approach first. See reference: Case-Smith, Allen, and Pratt (eds): Wright-Ott, C, and Egilson, S: Mobility.

15. (D) developing vocational skills. By adolescence, the focus in goal setting should be on functional skills that support maximal possible independence in community living. Answers A, B, and C are goals typically addressed in the younger child with MR. See reference: Case-Smith, Allen, and Pratt (eds): Gordon, CY, Schanzenbacher, KE, Case-Smith, J, and Carrasco, R: Diagnostic problems in pediatrics.

16. (A) Within 6 months, Billy will participate in classroom activities for 1 hour without disruptive outbursts, twice a day. A functional goal relates the skill to be developed to a child's environment or life tasks, therefore making it more meaningful to the child and the family. Answers B, C, and D are measurable but not functional goals, because they do not address the context in which the skill is applied. See reference: Case-Smith, Allen, and Pratt (eds): Case-Smith, J: Planning and implementing services.

17. (D) joint contractures. The functional ADL problems of children with arthrogryposis multiplex congenital disorder are caused by the presence of joint contractures from birth. Independent feeding is often an initial concern. Answer A is not correct, because obstetric paralysis refers to damage of the brachial plexus occurring at birth. Answer B is incorrect, because hip dislocation is not a usual feature of this disorder; when the lower extremities are involved, the characteristic problem is also joint contracture. Answer C is not correct, because joint inflammation is characteristic of juvenile rheumatoid arthritis, not arthrogryposis. See reference: Hopkins and Smith (eds): Atkins, J: Neural tube defect.

18. (A) play 'pat-a-cake' when prompted. Answer A is the only one that addresses the bilateral component of hand-skill development. Answers B and C deal with manipulation and finger isolation skills. Answer D addresses tolerance of tactile stimuli. See reference: Case-Smith, Allen, and Pratt (eds): Exner, CE: Development of hand skills.

19. (B) wide-base sitting on the floor while reaching for a suspended balloon. The child first practices skills in unsupported sitting on a stable surface using a wide base of support. As skills improve, the wide base is reduced to a more narrow one. Reaching activities are used to promote postural reactions, because they involve displacement of the center of gravity and weight shifting. Answers A, C, and D are activities involving unstable support surfaces, typical of more advanced skills. See reference: Case-Smith, Allen, and Pratt (eds): Nichols, DS: The development of postural control.

20. (B) Concentration. This game requires the player to remember visual cues. Answers A, C, and D require visual skills, but not memory. See reference: Case-Smith, Allen, and Pratt (eds): Schneck, CM: Visual perception.

21. (C) Rolling in a carpeted barrel. Answer C is the most appropriate initial activity for this child's treatment program. Because tactile defensiveness is an area of sensory integration treatment that should be approached cautiously, the child-controlled rolling on a textured surface would be less intrusive to her nervous system than the activity described in answer A, in which the practitioner provides sensory stimulation to the most sensitive areas of the body. In general, sensory integration therapy involves child-directed adaptive responses, and it is recommended by Dr. Ayres that occupational therapy practitioners consult with a sensory-integration therapist when applying direct sensory input. Answers B and D are not correct, because balancing and swinging activities generally do not address a problem of tactile defensiveness. See reference: Ayres: Developmental dyspraxia: A motor planning problem.

22. (B) overreactive to being touched. Tactile defensiveness is an overreaction or negative reaction to touch sensations. Touch sensations may be overwhelming probably due to a lack of central-nervous-system inhibitory influences. Light touch is particularly uncomfortable to the child with tactile defensiveness; therefore, answer D is also incorrect. See reference: Ayres: Tactile defensiveness.

23. (C) wedge-shaped seat insert that is higher in front. A wedge-shaped seat insert will increase hip flexion to more than 90 degrees, which is inhibitory to an extensor pattern. Answer A is incorrect, because lateral trunk supports will only prevent the trunk from falling to the side. Answer B is incorrect, because a seatbelt at the hips and ankle straps will hold a child in a chair but cannot inhibit an extension pattern. Answer D is incorrect, because although a lap board fastened to the arm rests may contribute to holding a child in a chair, it does not affect the angle of the hip joint, which is necessary to decrease extensor tone in sitting. See reference: Case-Smith, Allen, and Pratt (eds): Shepherd, J, Procter, SA, and Coley, IL: Self-care and adaptations for independent living.

24. (B) prone over the parent's thighs, then flex and abduct both legs. Answer B is correct, because it provides a position that is inhibitory to extensor patterns along with a reflex-inhibiting pattern (in opposition to abnormal pattern). Answer A is not the best method, because extension can predominate in supine position, making flexing of the hip and separation of the legs more difficult; however, the inhibitory pattern of flexion and abduction of the legs is correct. Answer A would be an appropriate choice if the child's neck were slightly flexed. Answer C is not the best position for a small child with undeveloped trunk balance but would be a good position as the child becomes larger and trunk balance develops; the inhibitory pattern is also incorrect (adduction is incorrect). Answer D is not correct, because although the positioning is optimal for decreasing extensor patterns the pattern of movement at the hip (extension and adduction) is not inhibitory. See reference: Case-Smith, Allen, and Pratt (eds): Hunter, JG: The neonatal intensive care unit.

25. (A) neurodevelopmental. Neurodevelopmental treatment emphasizes "the inhibition or restraint of abnormal reflex patterns through handling and sensory stimulation. The goal is to help the patient produce the desired normal movement pattern (p. 51)." Sensory integration (answer B) does not involve therapeutic handling; rather, it postulates that the provision of situations requiring an adaptive response can promote growth and change. Cognitive disabilities (answer C) addresses six levels of cognitive functioning as they relate to task performance. Answer D, the biomechanical frame of reference, focuses on increasing skill through practice (and the use of adaptive equipment for positioning) and does not address managing tone and movement through therapeutic handling. See reference: Ryan (ed): Madigan, MJ, and Ryan, SE: Theoretical frameworks and approaches. *The Certified Occupational Therapy Assistant.*

26. (D) held supine in feeder's arms. The supine position should be avoided, because in this position the infant has the least control over the food or liquid in his or her mouth. Positioning an infant with poor swallowing skills in supine position during feeding could lead to life-threatening conditions, such as choking. Answers A, B, and C describe positions that are well suited for a child with this problem. See reference: Case-Smith, Allen, and Pratt (eds): Case-Smith, J, and Humphry, R: Feeding and oral motor skills.

27. (A) single-pressure switch firmly mounted within easy reach. A child with fluctuating muscle tone lacks stability and demonstrates extraneous movement; therefore, deliberate motor action is most effectively executed on a securely mounted device using simple movement patterns. Answers B, C, and D involve devices that would respond to slight touch and would therefore not be effective for a person with extraneous movement and difficulty grading motor action. See reference: Case-Smith, Allen, and Pratt (eds): Struck, M: Augmentative communication and computer access.

28. (C) slow and predictable movement. The therapy ball provides slow, predictable, rhythmic movement for children with vestibular hypersensitivity. Answer A is not correct, because movement in any position or direction is used with children who have vestibular hyposensitivity. Answer B is not correct, because adaptation to movement will be an important goal for comfort in the child's life activities. Answer D is not correct, because it describes the type of movement most likely to be used in therapy when children are hyposensitive to movement. See reference: Hopkins and Smith: Kinnealey, M, and Miller, LJ: Sensory integration/learning disabilities.

29. (B) upright. For a child with increased tone, the upright position appears to give the best postural control. A forward (answer A) or backward tilt (answer C) increases the effect of gravity and thus adds to the difficulty of maintaining posture. At all times, the child should sit squarely with even weight distribution on both buttocks, never tilted asymmetrically (answer D). See reference: Case-Smith, Allen, and Pratt (eds): Wright-Ott, C, and Egilson, S: Mobility.

30. (C) raise it. Raising the feeding surface brings it higher relative to the child's trunk and helps with trunk stability. The higher tray also reduces the distance the arm has to travel to bring food to the mouth, thereby facilitating better control. By stabilizing the elbow on the tray, the child can also use a simpler pattern of elbow flexion and extension to feed himself. Answers A, B, and D would make feeding more difficult, either by increasing the distance the arm has to travel or by adding the challenge of stabilizing food on a tilted surface. See reference: Case-Smith, Allen, and Pratt (eds): Case-Smith, J, and Humphry, R: Feeding and oral motor skills.

31. (A) held supine in his mother's arms. Supine positioning is contraindicated, because food is most difficult to control in this position. The pull of gravity may cause bits of food to fall into the pharynx, causing aspiration of food; in addition, an effective protective cough is hard to achieve against gravity. The likely positioning of head and neck in extension may make a coordinated swallow difficult. Answers B, C, and D describe different forms of upright positioning, which are all acceptable depending on the level of trunk control Jason has achieved at this point. In upright position, food is easier to control and, combined with a slight chin tuck, a coordinated swallow is easier to accomplish. See reference: Case-Smith, Allen, and Pratt (eds): Case-Smith, J, and Humphry, R: Feeding and oral motor skills.

32. (D) wind-up toys. Wind-up toys give mostly visual stimulation and "do things" on their own, without requiring active exploratory play. Answers A and B lend themselves to active tactile exploration, and answer C provides auditory feedback, encouraging continued involvement. See reference: Logigian and Ward (eds): Logigian, MK: Physical disorders.

33. (D) be highly structured, to facilitate step-by-step learning. Therapeutic activities should be presented in an environment free from extraneous stimuli to help the child focus on the task. The activities should be carefully graded and presented in a sequence tailored to the sensory capacities and preferences of each child. Children with autism lack the imagination and self-direction needed to benefit from the environments described in answers A, B, and C. See reference: Logigian and Ward (eds): Ward, JD: Infantile autism.

34. (A) hard and firm. A firm seat or seat insert, often of a triangular shape, is best for providing a firm base of support for the child with postural difficulties. A softer, less stable surface (answers B, C, and D) adds the challenge of ongoing postural adjustments to the already difficult position of upright sitting. See reference: Logigian and Ward (eds): Logigian, MK: Cerebral palsy.

35. (C) gravitational insecurity. Gravitational insecurity, according to Clark et al, is described as "intense anxiety and distress in response to movement or to a change in head position." The child easily experiences a fear of falling and prefers to keep his or her feet firmly on the ground. Therefore, answer C is correct. Answer A, tactile defensiveness, is a term used to describe discomfort with various textures and with unexpected touch and therefore is not correct. Answer C (developmental dyspraxia) is not correct, because it is a term used to describe a problem with motor planning. Intolerance for motion (answer D) refers to a very similar and often related problem of inhibition of vestibular impulses, but one which is usually associated with sensory information received from the semicircular canals, whereas gravitational insecurity is associated with the utricle and saccule. Therefore, answer D is not correct. See reference: Case-Smith, Allen, and Pratt (eds): Parham, LD and Mailloux, Z: Sensory integration.

36. (B) treatment for this problem may be discontinued. The correct answer is B, because the child has developed the highest form of pencil grasp, which begins to appear at approximately 4 years of age. Answers A and C are incorrect, because these answers imply that further development of grasp can be achieved. Answer D is incorrect, because a dynamic tripod grasp of the pencil should be well-established by this age. See reference: Erhardt: Joanne.

37. (D) increased angle of flexion at the hip. The correct answer is D because increasing the angle of flexion of the hip will inhibit the extensor hypertonic pattern (or extensor reflex pattern). Answer A is not correct, because lengthening the back support will primarily aide in head and neck support and stability. Answer B is not correct, because a hip strap, although it may prevent thrusting out of the chair, primarily will stabilize the pelvis. Answer C is not correct, because a shoulder harness primarily prevents the child from falling forward. See reference: Kramer and Hinojosa: Colangelo, CA: Biomechanical frame of reference.

38. (B) a 3-inch screw-top jar. Since the goal was written as a functional behavioral objective, the COTA should reassess Luis for functional progress made in performance areas. Assessing his progress by measuring ROM with a goniometer (answer A), the strength of his grip using a dynamometer (answer C), or his degree of coordination using the Peabody Fine Motor Scale may provide useful information of individual performance components addressed; however, none of these will provide sufficient information to measure progress on his functionally written goal. See reference: Case-Smith, Allen, and Pratt (eds): Exner, CE: Development of hand skills.

39. (A) of the skin in the morning. Any sustained redness is an indicator that the splint needs to be refitted. To wait for skin breakdown (answer B) or signs of itching (answer C) in addition to the redness may prevent intervention at the time it is needed. Complaints of discomfort (answer D) in addition to redness may not occur, because Laurie may be limited cognitively or in her sensory perception. See reference: Case-Smith, Allen, and Pratt (eds): Exner, CE: Development of hand skills.

40. (B) verbal and gestural cues. The next least intrusive level of cues consists of the combination of verbal and gestural cues. Physical cues (answers C and D) are the most intrusive, and purely verbal ones (answer A) the least intrusive. See reference: Case-Smith, Allen, and Pratt (eds): Shepherd, J, Procter, SA, and Coley, IL: Self-care and adaptations for independent living.

41. (D) "When she can copy a triangle." Perception and reproduction of the oblique (or diagonal) angle represents the highest level of skill in the development of shape recognition and copying. Therefore, when Trinidad can copy triangles and diamonds—typically a 5-year-old's skill—she will be ready to begin to write letters, which involve a combination of right angles, diagonals, and circular lines. Scribbling and copying a circle (answer A) and imitating a cross (answer C) are earlier skills, typically achieved at 3 years of age, and do not indicate writing readiness. See reference: Case-Smith, Allen, and Pratt (eds): Dubois, SA: Preschool services.

42. (B) project group. The next level of group interaction is termed project group, since the group members are now able to share the completion of a group project; however, they still require strong group leadership to guide them. Following a project group, the next level of group interaction is the egocentric cooperative group (answer A), followed by the cooperative group (answer C), and the mature group (answer D), which is the most advanced. See reference: Ryan (ed): Blechert, TF, and Kari, N: Interpersonal communication skills and applied group dynamics. *The Certified Occupational Therapy Assistant.*

43. (D) Flushing, blanching, or perspiring. The most correct answer is D, because these responses are autonomic nervous system signs of sensory overload. Answers A, B, and C are not correct, because they do not describe autonomic response. See reference: Case-Smith, Allen, and Pratt (eds): Parham, LD and Mailloux, Z: Sensory integration.

44. (A) occupational therapy program works for the child. Answer A is correct, because parents need to see the success of the occupational therapy program in order to continue. A program that is too challenging (answer B) may be frustrating for both the child and parent. Answer C is incorrect, because parents will be more invested in the program if they have participated in goal setting. Answer D is incorrect, because incorporating a home program into the family's daily routine will make it easier in terms of time schedules as well as making the program more meaningful to both parent and child. See reference: Case-Smith, Allen, and Pratt (eds): Humphry, R, and Case-Smith, J: Working with families.

45. (A) index and middle fingers; place your thumb on the child's cheek." The correct position of the adult's hand for jaw control when feeding the child from the side is as described in answer A. Answers B and D are incorrect, because the thumb should be placed on the cheek to provide jaw stability. Answer C is incorrect, because controlling the child's jaw movement with the adult's whole hand provides less control of the child's jaw than the recommended method. Placing the adult's thumb on the ear (answer D) is also incorrect, because it would create discomfort for the child; in addition, thumb placement should be near the fulcrum of jaw movement (temporomandibular joint). When the child is fed from the front, the adult's thumb should be placed on the chin and the middle finger should be placed under the chin to control opening and closing of the jaw. The index finger then rests on the side of the child's face to provide stability. See reference: Case-Smith, Allen, and Pratt (eds): Parham, LD, and Mailloux, Z: Sensory integration.

46. (D) Praise her for what she does well; reinforce her independence. Since June has just achieved independence in spoon feeding, she may still need frequent reinforcement of the new skill. It is more effective to encourage her for what she does well than to point out her mistakes (answer B). To provide assistance either by using a hand-over-hand technique (answer A) or by feeding her as a reward appears to be counterproductive and may cause her to lose independence in this skill. See reference: Ryan (ed): McFadden, SA: The child with mental retardation. *Practice Issues in Occupational Therapy*.

47. (A) Whether the disability interferes with the child's education. Related services are defined as services needed to help a student benefit from education. If the student's disability no longer interferes with education, OT as a related service can be discontinued. Functional skills (answer B) and ADLs (answer C) may be ongoing goals in therapy as provided in a rehab setting or hospitals but would not be provided as a related service in the schools. Accessibility of the learning environment (answer D) is an important concern, but it would be covered in consultation with the school or teacher, not through direct service provision. See reference: Case-Smith, Allen, and Pratt (eds): Johnson, J: School-based occupational therapy.

48. (D) installation of a bidet with a spray wash and air-drying mechanism. Use of a bidet for hygiene after using the toilet eliminates any upper-extremity reach requirement. Answers A, B, and C describe adaptations appropriate for a child with poor postural control in need of external stability devices; these devices would not reduce reach requirements. See reference: Case-Smith, Allen, and Pratt (eds): Dudgeon, BJ: Pediatric rehabilitation.

49. (B) Boy Scouts. While answers A, C and D describe activities that may help build his sense of competence, only participation in Boy Scouts includes the necessary interaction with peers. Noncompetitive activities, a uniform to signify belonging, predictable routines, and exposure to role models are all elements of the Boy Scouts that can help him develop social competence. See reference: Case-Smith, Allen, and Pratt (eds): Davidson, DA: Programs and services for children with psychosocial dysfunction.

50. (A) large, easily interlocking pieces. For the child with fluctuating muscle tone, efforts should be made to provide a means of stabilizing toys and equipment. The interlocking quality of such toys as bristle blocks and magnets will provide some stability and assist with controlled release; the large size of the blocks will facilitate a more effective grasp. Small blocks (answer B) and lightweight ones (answer C) are more difficult to manipulate and are not recommended for constructive play for a child with coordination difficulties. Colorful blocks (answer D) may stimulate some interest but have no direct bearing on Luke's ability to engage in construction efforts. See reference: Case-Smith, Allen, and Pratt (eds): Morrison, CD, Metzger, P, and Pratt, PN: Play; and ibid., Dudgeon, BJ: Pediatric rehabilitation.

51. (A) apply the stimuli beginning at an area distal to the lesion progressing proximally. The general guidelines for sensation testing are that the person's vision should be occluded, the stimuli should be randomly applied with false stimuli intermingled (opposite of answer C), a practice trial should be performed before the test, and the unaffected side or area should be tested before the affected side or area (opposite of answer B). Also, the tested individual should be given a specified amount of time in which to respond; therefore, answer D is incorrect. See reference: Trombly (ed): Bentzel, K: Evaluation of sensation.

52. (B) pinch meter. A pinch meter is used to measure the strength of a three-jaw-chuck grasp pattern (also known as palmar pinch), as well as key (lateral) pinch and tip pinch. For each of these tests, the individual performs three trials, which the tester averages together; the result is compared to a standardized norm. An aesthesiometer (answer A) measures two-point discrimination. A dynamometer (answer C) measures grip strength, and a volumeter (answer D) measures edema in the hand. See reference: Trombly (ed): Evaluation of biomechanical and physiological aspects of motor performance.

53. (D) fair minus (3–). The grade of fair minus (3–) means the individual has the ability to move through less than full ROM when flexing against the pull of gravity or through complete ROM against slight resistance but with the pull of gravity eliminated. A grade of "good" (4) strength reflects the ability to move through full ROM against gravity and moderate resistance (answer A). A "fair" (3) grade (answer B) means the individual can move through full ROM, against gravity without any additional resistance. A grade of "poor plus" (2+) means the individual moves through full ROM, with gravity eliminated against minimal resistance, and suddenly relaxes (answer D). See reference: Trombly (ed): Evaluation of biomechanical and physiological aspects of motor performance.

54. (C) problems with initiation. Initiation, or the ability to begin a task, affects a person's spontaneity in performing activities and how much he or she is able to perform. An individual with initiation problems may be able to plan or carry out activities but unable to begin until prompted by another person. Problems with attention (answer A) or concentration (answer B), or apraxia (answer C) are evidenced by the incomplete or incorrect completion of an activity. See reference: Zoltan: Cognitive deficits.

55. (C) the Manual Muscle Test. The manual muscle test (answer C) is an example of a nonstandardized test. Although it includes instructions for the administration and scoring of the test, it lacks validity and reliability. The interpretation of a nonstandardized test often depends on the skill, judgment, and bias of the evaluator. A standardized test has instructions for the administration and scoring as well as information regarding the validity and reliability based on established norms from a specific population. The Motor Free Visual Perception Test (answer A), the Minnesota Rate of Manipulation Test (answer B) and the Purdue Pegboard Evaluation (answer D) all have information available regarding reliability and validity based on the established norms. See reference: Pedretti (ed): Kasch, M: Hand injuries.

56. (B) examining an analysis of the individual's job. The job analysis is a detailed description of the physical, sensory, and psychological demands of a job. Examples of performance requirements include tasks such as lifting, walking, sitting, standing, and reaching, as well as seeing and hearing and interpersonal skills. Interviewing the individual (answer B) is useful to obtain information about his or her perception of the injury, motivation for returning to work, and sense of responsibility for rehabilitation. However, the worker may not be able to give an objective, detailed, and concise analysis of the job. The Dictionary of Occupational Titles (answer C) provides generic job descriptions but does not contain as much specific information as a job analysis. A physician (answer D) is unlikely to have the depth of information necessary or the time available to provide the necessary information. See reference: Pedretti (ed): Burt, CM, and Smith, P: Work evaluation and work hardening.

57. (A) the ability to assess hand strength. The Purdue Pegboard Evaluation is a standardized assessment designed to measure fine-motor coordination.The COTA administering the evaluation must have the ability to measure fine motor coordination (answer D); knowledge of how to administer standardized evaluations in general (answer C) and in the Purdue Pegboard Evaluation specifically; and the observation skills (answer B) to observe the individual's performance and record the results. See reference: Hopkins and Smith (eds): Fess, EE: Hand rehabilitation.

58. (B) determine the roles the individual has performed in the past, is currently performing, and plans to perform in the future. In addition, the Role Checklist also addresses the value of each role to the individual concerned. Although is it possible to observe how well the individual follows direction (answer C) and to establish rapport with the individual (answer D) while administering the Role Checklist, these answers do not describe the purpose of the tool. The Occupational History Interview is a tool that addresses an individual's role performance and his perceptions of his strengths and weaknesses in regard to role performance (answer A). See reference: Early: Data gathering and evaluation.

59. (D) endurance. A deficit in endurance is demonstrated by his inability to sustain cardiac, pulmonary, and musculoskeletal exertion for the duration of the activity. Answer A, a deficit in postural control, would be correct if the client had been unable to maintain his balance while donning the shirt. A deficit in muscle tone (answer B) would have been evident if the client had demonstrated spasticity while donning the shirt. Inability to push his arms through the resistance created by the shirt sleeve would demonstrate a deficit in strength (answer C). See reference: AOTA: Uniform terminology for occupational therapy, 3rd edition.

60. (C) volumeter. A volumeter is a tool used to measure edema in the hand by measuring the amount of water displaced when the hand is placed into the container. A goniometer (answer A) is used to measure movement at a joint. An aesthesiometer (answer B) measures two-point discrimination by means of a movable point attached to a ruler that has a stationary point at one end. A dynamometer (answer D) measures grip strength through gross hand grasp. See reference: Trombly (ed): Zemke, R: Remediating biomechanical and physiological impairments of motor performance.

61. (C) trace newspaper headlines across the page with her right index finger from left to right. When tracing a headline across the page, the individual receives the same proprioceptive input and uses the same amount of space in the visual field as she would by writing on paper. This makes the transfer of skills easier when the time comes to attempt to write. A person who follows a line when wheeling a wheelchair (answer A) is focusing on midline positioning, not crossing the midline. Placing objects commonly used on the unaffected side (answer B) is a compensatory technique that does not involve crossing the midline. The individual with midline problems would need cueing not to start at midline when attempting to lay cards out from the left to the right side (answer D). Also, the person would have difficulty accurately completing a sequencing task on the neglected side, making it difficult to complete the midline crossing successfully. See reference: Zoltan: Body image and body scheme disorders.

62. (D) a cutting board with two nails in it. The potato is placed on the nails to hold it in place while working. The nonskid backing would only hold the cutting board in place, not the potato being cut. A plate guard would not be secured tightly enough to the plate to withstand the force of cutting the potato. A rocker knife is useful for one-handed cutting, but the potato would still need to be stabilized. See reference: Trombly (ed): Stewart, C: Retraining housekeeping and child care skills.

63. (D) an arm trough. An arm trough that slides onto the wheelchair armrest provides a stable surface that will keep Mrs. R.'s arm supported whether she is sitting straight or leaning to the right in order to push her wheelchair. Also, the arm trough supports the humeral head in the glenoid fossa at a natural angle. If edema in the hand is present, the COTA may place a foam wedge in the trough to elevate the hand and use a foam strap to keep the wedge and arm in place. A half laptray (answer A) would provide support, but could easily fall out of place if Mrs. R. leans to the side. The wheelchair armrest (answer B) would provide only a temporary means of support, because Mrs. R.'s arm would remain in place only until she shifted her weight, at which her arm will fall off the armrest. Although an arm sling (answer C) would provide support for the arm, it would immobilize the arm in adduction and internal rotation. The sling provides support for the shoulder when walking but should not be used when the individual is sitting, because the position of the arm in the sling in nonfunctional. See reference: Trombly (ed): Linden, CA, and Trombly, CA: Orthoses: Kinds and purposes.

64. (D) no, primarily because of her difficulty with position in space. The ability to determine how the ends of the strips relate spatially to themselves as well as the relationship of the loops to each other is critical in being able to glue the ends of the loops correctly and join the loops together. Deficits in sequencing would also limit Mrs. R's success with this activity. Even if methods to compensate for her one-handedness were provided (answer A), the activity would still have limited success because of the perceptual deficits. The fact that the activity is consistent with Mrs. R's interests (answer B) is worth noting, but that, too, is outweighed by her perceptual deficits. The contrast between the red and green strips makes this activity easier for individuals with a figure-ground deficit (answer C) who have difficulty differentiating between foreground and background forms and objects. See reference: AOTA: Uniform terminology for occupational therapy, 3rd edition.

65. (C) power mobility. An individual with paralysis of the left upper and lower extremities needs an arm trough and footrest for the involved side (answers A and B). One-arm drive (answer D) will enable him to propel the chair successfully using only his right arm. A motorized wheelchair is unnecessary for an individual with normal function on one side. See reference: Palmer and Toms: Wheelchairs, assistive devices and home modifications.

66. (D) to summarize the approach to managing the individual's condition. The treatment plan or plan of care is usually a multidisciplinary approach to an individual's treatment. Each member of the treatment team contributes to the plan, which may be documented on a specific form. Specific directions for the OT practitioner in treatment (answer A), measurements of the patient's progress (answer B), and organization of the patient's priorities (answer C) are all pieces of information included in the occupational therapy departmental documentation. See reference: Jacobs and Logigian (eds): Pagonis, J: Documentation.

67. (A) learning to type. Typing is the only compensatory strategy listed. Learning to type would allow the individual to communicate legibly in writing while avoiding the need to write by hand. Answers B, C, and D are all examples of remedial strategies that do not make handwriting unnecessary. See reference: Hopkins and Smith (eds): Culler, KH: Home and family management.

68. (D) swivel spoon. A swivel spoon allows the head of the spoon to rotate as the individual moves the handle into varying positions, thus compensating for poor supination. An individual who is unable to reach her mouth because of limitations in shoulder or elbow flexion would benefit from a spoon with an elongated handle (answer A). An individual who is unable to hold a spoon because of difficulty with grasp would benefit from a spoon with a built-up handle (answer C). A spork (answer B) is helpful for those who need to use one utensil as both fork and spoon. See reference: Hopkins and Smith (eds): Kohlmeyer, KM: Assistive and adaptive equipment.

69. (A) skin inspection. Visual inspection of an insensate area is essential for preventing pressure sores, which may develop when there are no sensory cues to alert a person to skin breakdown. Nail trimming (answer B) is an important issue to address with individuals with diabetes but is secondary to skin inspection in importance; moreover, the nursing staff may address this issue with the patient. Many individuals with diabetes have abnormalities in nail growth, and instead of trimming their own nails they have them trimmed by a podiatrist. Retirement planning (answer C) and returning to work (answer D) are issues that may be addressed when discussing discharge plans. See reference: Trombly (ed): Bentzel, K: Remediating sensory impairment.

70. (D) no adaptive equipment. A person with a spinal-cord injury at the C8 level will have full use of his or her upper extremities and should be able to perform self-feeding independently without adaptive equipment. An injury at the C4 or C5 level would allow scapular elevation, and the individual would be able to feed himself or herself independently using a mobile arm support (answer B). An injury at the C6 level would allow enough upper-extremity function for the individual to feed himself or herself independently using a universal cuff or built-up utensils (answers C and D). See reference: Trombly (ed): Hollar, LD: Spinal cord injury.

71. (D) "The patient will increase quadriceps strength to 5/5." Individuals with paraplegia are usually able to perform depression transfers independently. Strong triceps (answer A) are important for successful depression transfers, which involve pushing down with the scapular depressors and triceps while swinging the hips toward the desired surface. Independent manipulation of armrests, leg rests, and brakes (answer B), as well as adequate sitting balance (answer C) are also required. The quadriceps (a hip flexor) is nonfunctional in T8 paraplegia, therefore strengthening the quadriceps (answer D) is an inappropriate goal. See reference: Trombly (ed): Retraining basic and instrumental activities of daily living.

72. (B) wearing permanent press clothing. Using a wrinkle-resistant fabric eliminates or decreases the amount of ironing needed. The side-loading washer (answer A) is an example of household equipment adapted to eliminate excessive reaching from a wheelchair. An extended-handle dustpan (answer C) eliminates bending or stooping from a standing or sitting position. Neither the dustpan nor the washer, however, eliminates or reduces the amount of work needed for the tasks. Good body mechanics (answer D) are necessary to protect or maintain physical health, but they do not eliminate or reduce the amount of work either. See reference: Trombly (ed): Retraining basic and instrumental activities of daily living.

73. (A) prevent deforming stresses. It is very important to prevent deforming stresses and preserve joint integrity in the individual with arthritis by using adaptive equipment to avoid or reduce stresses on fragile joints. Adaptive equipment does not correct deformities (answer B), because deformities are corrected only by surgery or with orthotic devices that reposition the joints in correct alignment. Adaptive equipment allows activities to be completed but does not simplify work (answer C). Simplifying work involves eliminating steps in a task. Adaptive equipment is also used to increase independence (opposite of answer D). See reference: Pedretti (ed): Hittle, JM, Pedretti, LW, and Kasch, MC: Rheumatoid arthritis.

74. (D) compensation. Compensation techniques are used to work around a deficit by using alternative methods to accomplish the same task. An example of compensation is the use of elastic shoelaces or Velcro closures on shoes by persons unable to reach their feet or otherwise unable to tie their shoes. Retraining (answer B) and substitution (answer C) continue to use skills to accomplish the same task, whereas compensation techniques may include avoiding performance of the activity entirely. An individual uses problem solving (answer A), for instance, to organize information and reach a solution that would provide a method for handling memory problems. See reference: Zoltan: Body image and body scheme disorders.

75. (A) 10 degrees of neck flexion. Positioning the neck in 10 degrees of flexion ensures that the trachea is closed yet allows food to pass easily down the esophagus. Answers B and D both involve extension of the neck, which opens the trachea and may cause choking or aspiration. Extreme flexion of the neck (answer C) narrows the esophagus and causes a feeling of food sticking in the throat. See reference: Pedretti (ed): Nelson, KL: Dysphagia: Evaluation and treatment.

76. (B) (1) position shirt on lap; (2) place left hand into sleeve and pull up sleeve past elbow; (3) place right hand into sleeve and pull up sleeve; (4) pull shirt up over head. Answers A, C, and D are all examples of incorrect sequences that would result in failure to perform the activity. See reference: Pedretti (ed): Foti, D, Pedretti, LW, and Lillie, S: Activities of daily living.

77. (B) exercises using the uninvolved arm to move the involved arm across the midline. Exercises involving bilateral use of the arms to move the involved arm across the midline are one treatment for unilateral neglect. Other activities for treating unilateral neglect are: rubbing lotion on the takes limb (answer A) and participation in tasks that *do* require the individual to cross the midline (answer C). Tasks that focus on the uninvolved side of the body (answer D) only reinforce neglect of the involved side of the body. See reference: Zoltan: Body image and body scheme disorders.

78. (A) identify landmarks on the hand and arm to align the splint. Referring to landmarks on the hand and arm when donning the splint will facilitate proper placement of the splint. Incorrect placement could result in skin irritation and/or ineffectiveness. Redness occurs (answer B) when a splint does not fit properly or is not being properly positioned. The individual should return to the outpatient setting when the splint no longer fits properly. The patient must know the *specific* wearing schedule (answer C) in order for the splint to be worn appropriately and to receive maximum benefit. The patient needs to be able to remove and replace the splint (answer D) *independently* prior to discharge, since the OT practitioner will not be present to provide verbal cueing. See reference: Trombly (ed): Linden, CA and Trombly, CA: Orthosis: Kinds and purposes.

79. (D) place her left index finger through a belt loop, then stand and pull the slacks up past her hips. An individual with good balance prefers to stand to pull on slacks because it is easier than sitting to dress. Answers B and C are wrong because they involve remaining seated. Individuals who have difficulty bending benefit from using a dressing stick for distal activity such as bringing slacks or shoes near the feet, but using a dressing stick to pull slacks past the hips (answer A) would be very awkward. See reference: Pedretti (ed): Foti, D, Pedretti, LW, and Lillie, S: Activities of daily living.

80. (D) batting a balloon. An activity such as batting a balloon may be graded for increasing strength by adding resistance to the arm in the form of weights, and endurance may be improved by adding more repetitions of the movement. Passive range of motion (answer A) and Codman's exercises (answer B) both use passive movements of the upper extremities, which will not improve strength or endurance. A person who pops a balloon (answer C) would be able to increase the resistance needed for upper extremity performance by adding weight to the arms or using a balloon with thicker rubber. However, there would not be an appropriate method to increase the number of repetitions, since the repeated noise would be annoying. See reference: Pedretti (ed): Pedretti, LW, and Wade, IE: Therapeutic modalities.

81. (C) biomechanical. The biomechanical approach uses voluntary muscle control during performance of activities for people with deficits in strength, endurance, or range of motion. The biomechanical approach focuses on decreasing deficits in order to improve performance of daily activities. The neurophysiological approach (answer A) is applied to individuals with brain damage. Emphasis is on the nervous system and methods for eliciting desired responses. The neurodevelopmental approach (answer B) also focuses on the nervous system, but emphasizes eliciting responses in a developmental sequence. The rehabilitative approach (answer D) emphasizes teaching a person how to compensate for a deficit on either a temporary or permanent basis. See reference: Trombly (ed): Zemke, R: Remediating biomechanical and physiological impairments of motor performance.

82. (C) lordosis. Lordosis, a concave posterior curvature of the spine, is a result of excessive anterior pelvic tilt. Scoliosis (answer B) is a result of a lateral curve of the vertebral column and is unaffected by anterior pelvic tilt. Kyphosis (answer D), a concave anterior curvature of the spine, may develop in response to exaggerated lordosis. Stenosis (answer A) is a disease of the spine resulting in narrowing of the spinal column. See reference: Norkin and Levangie: The vertebral column.

83. (A) elevate the arm on pillows so it rests higher than the heart. Elevation, contrast baths, retrograde massage, pressure wraps, and active ROM are effective methods for managing edema. When massaging an edematous extremity, stroking should be performed from the distal area to the proximal, not the reverse (answer B). Active and passive ROM can both be *beneficial* to managing edema (answers C and D). See reference: Pedretti (ed): Kasch, MC: Hand injuries.

84. (A) ease the patient onto the floor, cushioning his fall. Proper body mechanics must be used when transferring patients. No one should "attempt a transfer that seems unmanageable because of the discrepancy between the patient's size and her own or because of the patient's level of dependency (p. 294)." Attempting to continue or reverse the transfer of an obese patient who has already begun to slip (answers B and C) is likely to result in injury to the COTA and perhaps to the patient as well. Once the patient has started to slip, the COTA should begin easing him to the floor immediately. Although calling for assistance is an appropriate action, the higher-priority action is to begin easing the patient to the floor to prevent injury to the individuals involved. See reference: Trombly (ed): Retraining basic and instrumental activities of daily living.

85. (A) slip a piece of cylindrical foam onto the fork handle. The criteria for selecting adaptive equipment include effectiveness, affordability, operability, and dependability. For this assessment, the COTA needs something fast and inexpensive; durability is not an issue because this is not a permanent piece of equipment. A cylindrical foam handle meets these criteria. Thermoplastic material (answer B) is easy to clean and durable, but it is expensive and takes more time to fabricate.

Adhesive-backed foam (answer C) is expensive and difficult to clean, and once it is attached to a fork it is difficult to remove. It is not a good idea to use plastic forks (answer D) for feeding evaluations because they are easily broken, although wrapping a washcloth around a fork handle is quick and inexpensive, easily washable, and appropriate for a temporary need. See reference: Hopkins and Smith (eds): Kohlmeyer, KM: Assistive and adaptive equipment.

86. (B) reposition him in the wheelchair to allow optimal range of motion. When a person who uses a wheelchair and an augmentative communication device suddenly begins making errors, it is necessary first to check his positioning. Improper positioning can result in inability to access his communication device because of restricted ROM or interference from the wheelchair. If the COTA notices other changes that may be indicative of changing medical status, a referral to a physician (answer A) would be in order. However, it is best for the COTA to seek a solution to the problem if there is no reason to suspect a new medical problem. The COTA would reassess communication abilities (answer C) only if after repositioning the client to the best possible position in the wheelchair the client continues to make the errors. Replacing a communication device (answer D) would be indicated only if the device did not work and could not be fixed. See reference: Church and Glennen (eds): Harryman, S, and Warren, L: Positioning and power mobility.

87. (D) the same method used initially. Tissues, cotton balls, and monofilaments (answers A and C) are all acceptable methods to use for testing light-touch sensation. When retesting, however, it is important to use the same method used initially in order to make an accurate comparison of status before and after treatment. In addition, evaluation results are more consistent when the individual who performed the initial evaluation performs subsequent reevaluations. An aesthesiometer (answer B) is used to measure two-point discrimination, not light touch. See reference: Pedretti (ed): Evaluation of sensation and treatment of sensory dysfunction.

88. (C) To teach the caregiver how to lift and turn the client safely. Individuals unable to move themselves and those with sensory loss are susceptible to the development of decubiti. Skin damage results from pressure on the skin over a prolonged period of time. The skin over bony prominences is particularly prone to the development of decubitous ulcers. Frequent position changes are essential for these individuals to prevent skin breakdown and the risk of serious infection. If the patient were already involved in a strengthening program (answer A), it may be appropriate to change it to a maintenance program at this point. A bed-mobility program (answer B) and an environmental control unit (answer D) would be appropriate if the individual has potential in these areas, but instructing the care giver in how to reposition the patient is the highest priority modification. See reference: Trombly (ed): Bentzel, K: Remediating sensory impairment.

89. (B) treatment planning. The COTA recognized a change in the patient's status that necessitates a change in the treatment plan. Before implementing any change (answer C), the COTA must notify the supervising OTR of change in the patient's status and recommend the modification to the treatment plan. The COTA has already evaluated (answer A) by palpating the glenohumeral joint. A new referral (answer D) is not necessary following a change in the treatment plan. See reference: Ryan (ed): The therapeutic intervention process. *Practice Issues in Occupational Therapy.*

90. (B) information about the effect the individual's illness will have on role performance. The purpose of involving the family in the treatment process is to "reduce the incidence of family disorders and breakdown." The role of the OTR or COTA is to provide the family with information about how the illness or injury affects the individual's ability to carry out occupational roles. The OT practitioners also involve family members in the goal-setting process. Information about the prognosis for the patient's condition (answer A) should come from the physician. Options concerning discharge (answer C) are usually presented by the social worker. If the anticipated length of stay is short, the COTA might present anticipated equipment needs (answer D) at the first meeting, but this step does not have the priority that answer B has. See reference: Hopkins and Smith (eds): Versluys, HP: Family influences.

91. (C) "You sound like things are looking pretty bad to you right now." This is an example of paraphrasing the patient's comment. This type of response conveys to the patient that you understood what he says and that you are listening to him. Answers A, B, and D are examples of well-meaning but poorly designed responses. Answer A may give him false hope. Answer B may imply his concerns are trivial and can be soothed away with idle chit-chat. Answer D may imply that the COTA knows more than the patient does about the types of things that will make his life meaningful. See reference: Denton, PL: Effective communication.

92. (B) "Pt. will draw for 1 hour, taking stretch breaks every 20 minutes." Goals should be functional, measurable, and objective. This answer meets those criteria. Answer A is not measurable. "Goals need to be written to show what the patient will accomplish, not what the [OT practitioner] will do (p. 94)." Answers C and D describe what the OT practitioner will do. See reference: AOTA: Writing functional goals. *Effective Documentation for Occupational Therapy.*

93. (D) resumption of the homemaker role. The Commission on Accreditation of Rehabilitation Facilities defines work hardening as "a highly structured, goal oriented, individualized treatment program designed to maximize a person's ability to return to work." A homemaker's job is working in the home. A work-hardening program would not focus on obtaining employment outside the home for this individual (answers A and B). Although a work-hardening program may help to reduce pain levels, the emphasis is on a return to work. See reference: Pedretti (ed): Burt, CM, and Smith, P: Work evaluation and work hardening.

94. (A) an electric razor. An electric razor is the safest shaving tool, because a rotary head or foil is in contact with the skin instead of a blade. The patient should be instructed not to shave over or near the incision until the incision is healed. The other razors have blades that could nick or cut the skin, and cuts must be avoided until the patient is no longer taking blood thinners and normal blood coagulation can occur. See reference: Trombly (ed): Retraining basic and instrumental activities of daily living.

95. (A) remove all throw or scatter rugs. Whether an individual with instability during walking uses a walker, cane, or no equipment, the floor should be cleared of any obstacles that may cause slipping or tripping. Scatter or throw rugs may catch on a person's foot or the tip of an assistive device, resulting in a fall. Alternatively, rugs can be firmly taped down or secured with nonskid backing. Installing lever handles, a ramp, or a handheld shower (answers B, C, and D) would make certain tasks easier for this individual but would not be necessary for safety. See reference: Ryan (ed): Gower, D, and Bowker, M: The elderly with a hip arthroplasty. *Practice Issues in Occupational Therapy.*

96. (D) A bath using lukewarm water. A person with COPD would have difficulty breathing in hot, humid environments, such as those produced by the methods in answers A and B. Showers (answer C) result in high levels of evaporation, which also makes breathing more difficult. A lukewarm tub bath would provide the lowest humidity by using the coolest water temperature combined with the method of dispensing water that keeps evaporation at a minimum. See reference: Trombly (ed): Atchison, B: Cardiopulmonary disease.

97. (B) outpatient OT. "It is no longer expected that patients discharged to home will be totally independent. . . These patients are frequently capable of achieving further gains and could appropriately be followed . . . in an outpatient setting." A patient with such high levels of function is not an appropriate candidate for a home health referral (answer A). Work-hardening programs (answer C) are for individuals who are severely deconditioned as a result of disease or injury or those who have significant discrepancies between their symptoms and objective findings. If Sam has potential for further functional improvement, continuation—not discontinuation (answer D)—of services is indicated. See reference: Trombly (ed): Woodson, AM: Stroke.

98. (A) instructing Mrs. Z. in joint-protection techniques. "Among other tasks, the COTA may assist in [the discharge planning] process by providing specific information on progress. . . The COTA may also provide instructions for a home-based program, identify community resources and personnel, or recommend environmental adaptations that may assist the patient after discharge." Answers B, C, and D match these criteria. Although instruction in joint-protection techniques is a critical part of Mrs. Z.'s program, it would be considered a part of treatment implementation, not discharge planning. See reference: Ryan (ed): Therapeutic intervention process. *Practice Issues in Occupational Therapy.*

99. (C) marking the end of each step with high-contrast tape. Difficulty in seeing contrast and color are two forms of decreased visual acuity that cannot be addressed by corrective lenses. Two effective environmental adaptations to these deficits are increasing background contrast and increasing illumination. Using tape or paint to make the edge of each step contrast sharply with the rest of the step is an inexpensive way to adapt the environment for Rita. Installing a stair glide or installing handrails (answers A and B) are more costly adaptations that do not address the problems of decreased visual acuity. Instructing Rita to take only one step at a time when going up or down may cause her to be unnecessarily slow and does not address the problems of decreased visual acuity. See reference: Pedretti (ed): Warren, M: Evaluation and treatment of visual deficits.

100. (C) doughnut shop. The Rehabilitation Act of 1973 required only institutions receiving federal funding, such as post offices (answer A) and libraries (answer B), to be wheelchair accessible. The Americans with Disabilities Act (ADA) requires that new structures (answer D) and the facilities within them be accessible to individuals using wheelchairs. Therefore, municipal buildings and new construction are more likely to be wheelchair accessible than small, private businesses. See reference: Hopkins and Smith (eds): Reed, K: The beginnings of occupational therapy.

101. (C) Comprehensive Occupational Therapy Evaluation (COTE) Scale. All the instruments listed include observation of behaviors. The COTE scale guides the COTA in rating behaviors in the categories of general behaviors, interpersonal behaviors, and task behaviors. The Milwaukee Evaluation of Daily Living Skills (MEDLS) (answer A) assesses 21 daily living skills. The Kohlman Evaluation of Living Skills (KELS) (answer B) assesses self-care, safety and health, money management, transportation and telephone, and work and leisure. The Allen Cognitive Level (answer D) assesses levels of cognitive disability. See reference: Early: Data gathering and evaluation.

102. (C) tardive dyskinesia. Long-term use of antipsychotic medications results in tardive dyskinesia in approximately 15% of individuals taking these medications. Because the side effects can seriously affect an individual's ability to perform skills of daily living as well as his or her self-concept, it is the COTA's responsibility to know about the side effects during assessment, treatment planning, and implementation. Tremors, muscular weakness, and rigid gait, signs associated with Parkinsonian syndrome (answer A), are sometimes seen as side effects of antipsychotic medications. Overdose symptoms (answer B), would vary according to the specific antipsychotic medication ingested. Lithium toxicity (answer D) is linked to antimanic medications. See reference: Early: Psychotropic medications and somatic treatments.

103. (A) has a dual diagnosis. Examples of dual diagnostic categories are Mental Health/Mental Retardation and Mental Health/Substance Abuse. A person who is described as multiply handicapped (answer B) has at the same time both physical and mental health problems. Answers C and D are not terms commonly used in health care. See reference: Hopkins and Smith (eds): Humphry, R, and Jacobs, K: Mental retardation.

104. (D) psychological. Psychological performance components include values, interests, and self-concept. Social components (answer C) involve interactions with others. Sensory-perceptual and cognitive components (answers A and B) involve an awareness and processing of incoming information. See reference: Early: Treatment planning.

105. (A) allows the COTA to obtain facts. Fact gathering is the primary advantage to closed questions. The COTA should be aware that posing mostly closed questions can lead to biased information gathering, as with answer B and D. Although one can generally ask more closed questions in a short amount of time (answer C), this is generally not a patient-focused goal. See reference: Denton: Effective communication.

106. (A) the Magazine Picture Collage. These are projective methods, and the only instrument with protocol developed by and for occupational therapy practitioners is the Magazine Picture Collage. The Rorschach and H-T-P (answers B and D) are typically administered by psychologists. Proverb interpretation (answer C) is part of the mental status examination typically carried out by the psychiatrist. See reference: Early: Data gathering and evaluation.

107. (B) introduce herself, briefly describe what the patient might gain from occupational therapy, and set a time for the next meeting. Providing an overview of and a schedule for occupational therapy helps to promote trust and to orient the patient to the occupational therapy process. Answers C and D might be overwhelming to the patient. Answer C implies that the patient has an understanding of the occupational therapy process and answer D might be overstimulating to a new patient. Presenting the patient with personal information (answer A) on the first visit is inappropriate and not useful. See reference: Early: Therapeutic use of self.

108. (C) "The OTR and I will review the information you have given me and meet with you tomorrow afternoon to plan an activity program that best meets your needs." It is important to inform the patient of when and with whom the next session will take place and to explain in general what will take place. The OTR is responsible for analyzing data (answer B). Answer D is too vague. Answer A does not include input from the patient on his or her interests or goals, and it is not appropriate for the COTA to analyze the conversation. See reference: Early: Data gathering and evaluation.

109. (C) provide a summary of observations of the patient's behavior, including what the patient said and did during the interview. An observation summary should present a concise and accurate picture of what happened so that the OTR can understand almost as well as if she were present during the interview. It is a summary and should not include extensive descriptions (answer A) or interpretations of the interview (answer D). A treatment plan (answer B) should be developed collaboratively with the OTR. See reference: Early: Data gathering and evaluation.

110. (B) "Patient demonstrates possible cognitive disability, indicated by numerous errors in task execution." This statement presents a concise example to support the observation of a problem connected to problems that might affect the individual's ability to function. It supports the need for further assessment in this area. Answer A not only uses a personal pronoun ("I think . . .") but expresses an opinion. Answers C and D do not offer an accurate description of the problem. See reference: Early: Medical records and documentation.

111. (B) The COTA asks members of a small group to draw pictures of themselves on a piece of paper. The COTA then leads a discussion about body-image concerns and links the discussion to the group members' drawings. Adapting the activity procedures allows the COTA to use one activity to address different treatment goals. Selecting an activity appropriate for eating disorders is based on a primary problem focus for this population—body image distortions. Only answer B focuses on this problem area. Answer A focuses on cognitive deficits; answer C focuses on family dynamics; and answer D is an assessment task from the BAFPE. See reference: Denton: Treatment planning and implementation.

112. (A) A group consisting of fewer than five members. Group size strongly influences how members relate to one another. In general, a group of between 7 and 10 members (answer C) is likely to have the most interaction among members. In groups with fewer than five members (answer A), the focus of interactions is more likely to be on the group leader. Groups whose members have similar goals (answer D) tend to be more cohesive and to have fewer interactions. Variety in member ages (answer B) has not been shown to have an affect on the number of interactions. See reference: Howe and Schwartzberg: The group.

113. (A) playing "Whisper Down the Lane." When working with the individual with paranoid ideation, it is important to select structured activities that use "controllable" materials. Answers B, C, and D all meet this criterion. The game "Whisper Down the Lane" involves whispering, and the paranoid individual is likely to believe the other players are talking, or whispering, about her. See reference: Early: Responding to symptoms and behaviors.

114. (B) whether the program allows the "teacher," i.e., the COTA, to adjust the number, type, and frequency of attempts the individual can make to use the program. The use of computer applications within psychosocial settings should be linked to the overall goals of treatment. In the treatment of behavioral disorders, behavior management and reinforcement are overall goals. Answer B includes the software features that best enable the COTA to grade and adapt reinforcement. Answers A and C are criteria that are important for individuals with social-skill deficits. Noncompetitive games (answer D) are appropriate for individuals with paranoia. See reference: Hopkins and Smith (eds): Simon, CJ: Use of activity and activity analysis.

115. (B) provide enough chairs around a round table. Circular seating arrangements generally facilitate the most communication among members. Rectangular tables (answer A) can contribute to unbalanced communications. Difficulties in maintaining comfort and attention are problems related to floor seating arrangements (answer C). Using available chairs and couches (answer D) may result in group members sitting in rectangular or square arrangements, which frequently results in group members sitting at different seating heights. See reference: Posthuma: Group dimensions.

116. (B) the client will use facial expressions and gestures that are consistent with stated emotions during assertive, passive, and aggressive role-playing situations. Self-expression is the use of a variety of styles and skills to express thoughts, feelings, and needs. It is also the ability to vary one's expressions, thoughts, feelings, and needs. Being able to vary one's expression during three types of role-playing is an example of this. Identifying pleasurable activities (answer A) is an example of interest identification. Recognition of one's behaviors and consequences (answer C) promotes development of self-control. Identifying one's own assets and limitations (answer D) promotes development of self-concept. See reference: AOTA: Uniform terminology for occupational therapy, 3rd edition.

117. (B) relevant to the patient's needs and values. It is essential that goals for treatment be relevant to the patient's needs and realistic for the patient. Treatment goals may be written by the OTR or the supervised COTA (answer A) but should involve the patient to the extent of the patient's cognitive ability (answer C). See reference: Early: Treatment planning.

118. (A) a mosaic tile project. A simple mosaic project is a good choice for this patient, because the activity characteristics have a definite sequence and can be done in short intervals. The activities listed in answers B, C, and D are not appropriate for this patient because they all require a higher level of concentration and attention to detail. See reference: Early: Responding to symptoms and behaviors.

119. (C) oil painting on a large canvas. The manic patient usually has a high energy level, is easily distracted, and has a poor frustration tolerance. It is important to provide activities that are structured (answers A and D) and include opportunities for the patient to move around (answer B). Unstructured activities, such as oil painting on a large canvas, require decision making and are unfocused. These activities would be inappropriate for individuals with manic behavior. See reference: Early: Responding to symptoms and behaviors.

120. (C) games of chance. Because winning a game of chance depends essentially on luck, players at various functional levels have equal opportunities at winning. Hobbies (answer B) is not considered a category of games. Puzzles and strategy games (answers A and D) require specific skills to succeed. See reference: Early: Leisure skills.

121. (A) punctuality, accepting responsibility for oneself, accepting directions from a supervisor, and appropriately interacting with peer co-workers. Psychosocial components include time management, social conduct, and self-control. Punctuality, accepting responsibility, and accepting feedback are important prevocational skills that call upon these psychosocial performance components. Memory, decision making, and sequencing (answer B) are considered to be cognitive components. Standing tolerance, endurance, and eye-hand coordination (answer C) are categorized as sensory motor components. Grooming and adhering to safety precautions (answer D) are work-performance areas and not psychosocial performance components. See reference: AOTA: Uniform terminology for occupational therapy, 3rd edition.

122. (B) egocentric-cooperative group. Structured learning activities that focus on beginning to use group roles or encourage additional group roles (asking all to contribute briefly as experts), combined with the COTA's giving and asking for feedback are consistent with an egocentric-cooperative developmental group. The COTA makes activity-based suggestions, if needed, in project groups (answer A). The COTA is an advisor in cooperative groups (answer C) and a group member in a mature group (answer D). See reference: Early: Group concepts and techniques.

123. (B) show acceptance and understanding to the individual. Paraphrasing is used to clarify and relay acceptance of what an individual has communicated. The COTA paraphrases by repeating in her or his own words what the client has said. Redirection (answer A) is used to promote healthier thoughts and behaviors. Forcing the individual to make a choice (answer C) may be accomplished by providing a question that includes two possible choices. The COTA encourages a client to provide additional information (answer D) by asking open-ended questions. See reference: Denton: Treatment planning and implementation.

124. (A) primary prevention. Primary prevention strategies are designed to prevent occurrences before symptoms occur. Secondary and tertiary (answers B and C) prevention strategies focus on interventions for emerging and existing symptoms. Intermediate prevention (answer D) is not a type of prevention. See reference: Hopkins and Smith (eds): Levy, LL: The health care delivery system today.

125. (B) the name(s) of family members. Reality orientation is used with confused individuals. The emphasis is on awareness of personal identity, names, places, events, and time. Remotivation is a group-discussion technique used to help depressed and confused individuals verbalize their thoughts and feelings. It often focuses on objects and memories from an individual's distant past (answers C and D). Discussing plans for the future (answer A) could be useful in planning for an upcoming activity but is not generally a component of reality orientation. See reference: Early: Cognitive and sensorimotor activities.

126. (B) over-involvement. The conscious use of self is an area that should be addressed in supervision. There are some practitioner-patient interactions that can stall or interfere with treatment goals. One of these problematic interactions is over-involvement. One behavior that may be a signal of over-involvement is making extra time for an individual at the expense of others. Long-term over-involvement can lead to burnout (answer D). Self-disclosure (answer A) is the use of personal comments by the COTA to an individual to emphasize a point made by the individual. Transference (answer C) occurs when one individual unconsciously relates to another as if that person were someone else. See reference: Hopkins and Smith (eds): Schwartzberg, SL: Tools of practice - Therapeutic use of self.

127. (D) outpatient counseling. Transitional programs after hospitalization offer a range or continuum of support to mental-health consumers. Outpatient counseling is the least restrictive situation; it provides support through counseling but does not require any residential treatment. Answers A, B, and C are all residential programs with varying amounts of supervision. See reference: Hopkins and Smith (eds): Gibson, D, and Richert GZ: The therapeutic process.

128. (C) ask the individual how often she has these "spells," encourage her to sit back down until it passes, and stop working on the budget activity for today. Advising the discontinuation of prescribed medications (answer A) is outside the domain of occupational therapy. The COTA should already have a general understanding of possible adverse reactions to common anti-anxiety medications (answer B). Frequent adverse reactions are dizziness and confusion. Although the ultimate responsibility of the COTA is to report the individual's reactions to the OTR supervisor as soon as possible, additional information from the individual as well as recommending immediate safety precautions is necessary. Answer D is the safety precaution for orthostatic hypotension, not dizziness. See reference: Hopkins and Smith (eds): Gibson, D, and Richert GZ: The therapeutic process.

129. (D) leather dyes. Leather dyes are toxic when swallowed or ingested. Small mirror pieces (answer A) could present a risk to individuals who are suicidal or violent toward others, because of the sharp edges when shattered. White glue (answer B) is nontoxic. The precaution associated with permanent magic markers (answer C) is inhaling fumes with extended use. See reference: Early: Safety techniques.

130. (A) remotivation. Remotivation approaches are used to encourage the expression of thoughts and feelings related to intact long-term memories. The topic should be linked to past experiences that are easy to understand. Reality orientation (answer B) is designed to maintain or improve awareness of time, situation, and place. Compensatory strategies (answer C) are appropriate when cognitive impairment is not expected to improve. Environmental modification (answer D) is a type of compensatory strategy. See reference: Early: Cognitive and sensorimotor activities.

131. (D) drink juices and caffeine-free colas when thirsty. Continual dry-mouth and thirst are common side effects of many drugs and can be intensified by the dehydrating effects of caffeinated drinks and alcohol (answer B). Therefore, juices and caffeine-free drinks are preferable Photosensitivity, an increased sensitivity to the sun, is another side effect often associated with neuroleptic medications that can be addressed by limiting sun exposure (answer A). Answer C is a strategy that can be used to avoid postural hypotension, a sudden drop in blood pressure resulting in feeling faint or loss of consciousness when moving from lying or sitting to standing. All of the answers are strategies for possible side effects of neuroleptic medications, but answer D is most important because it addresses the only side effect Ricky has experienced. See reference: Early: Psychotropic medications and somatic treatments.

132. (C) tell Tim it is okay to work where he is until he feels comfortable joining the group. The paranoid patient frequently isolates himself or herself from the rest of the group as a self-protective measure. Such a patient should be allowed to do this until he or she feels comfortable joining the group. Although it is a good idea to encourage Tim to join the group (answer A), the COTA should not insist when Tim is uncomfortable (answer B). The paranoid patient may attempt to take control of an uncomfortable group situation by demanding the COTA stay with him, away from the group (answer D). In this instance it is important for the COTA to be supportive of the patient's need but to remain with the group. See reference: Early: Responding to symptoms and behaviors.

133. (B) himself and explain how OT activities will correlate with Mr. R.'s overall treatment plan. Although it may be desirable to provide the patient with a written schedule, administer an interest checklist, and introduce him to other patients (answers A, C, and D), when first meeting the patient it is most important for the COTA to explain the function of occupational therapy in the patient's overall treatment program. See reference: Early: Therapeutic use of self.

134. (C) copper tooling using a template. When choosing activities to address self-competence and self-confidence, it is important first to choose activities that are relatively simple, structured, of short duration, and guaranteed to provide a successful experience to the patient. Answers A and B are fairly complex projects that require decision-making and several sessions to complete and have the potential for problems in any of the many stages of construction. Although they may be appropriate later, they are contraindicated at the beginning of treatment. Learning to play bridge (answer D) may be a good choice when addressing development of leisure activities, but it also involves learning a series of steps and interacting with others, requirements that are inappropriate at this stage in treatment. See reference: Early: Responding to symptoms and behaviors.

135. (B) activity adaptation. Modifying the materials being used is one way to adapt activities. Activity adaptations enable the individual to become more functional in task performance. Activity analysis (answer A) is the process of identifying the aspects, steps, and materials used in performing the activity. Activity sequencing (answer C) is one method of grading activities. Clinical reasoning (answer D) is the problem-solving process that occupational therapy practitioners use in thinking about a client's treatment. See reference: Early: Analyzing, adapting, and grading activities.

136. (B) asking the client only to put the last piece into the package. "Working backwards" from the last (successful) step of a sequence is known as backward chaining. Answer A is the *opposite* of what backward chaining means. Answer C is more descriptive of shaping behaviors, and answer D is more descriptive of modeling behaviors. See reference: Early: Models of mental health and illness.

137. (D) position the patient so she is facing a blank wall. One way to modify the environment for an individual who is easily distracted is to position him or her facing a blank wall (answer D), thereby lessening possible distracters. It may also be necessary to speak loudly in order to get the patient's attention, which is why answer A is not recommended. If the patient is unable to participate in the activity successfully, the COTA should direct her to a simpler activity. Coaxing and praising (answer B) will not increase the patient's skill level. Asking the rest of the group members to stop talking (answer C) would probably interfere with the goals of the rest of the group. See reference: Early: Responding to symptoms and behaviors.

138. (C) Shirley's self-esteem has increased. Low self-esteem is a common characteristic of individuals with paranoia, and Shirley's disheveled appearance and poor eye contact are indicative of low self-esteem. There was no information in the case study to indicate that tactile defensiveness (answer A) is an issue for Shirley. Given her distrust of men, Shirley is unlikely to want to increase her attractiveness to men (answer B). Improved social conduct (answer D) would be better demonstrated though increased eye contact and improved verbalization. See reference: Early: Responding to symptoms and behaviors.

139. (D) improved interpersonal skills. Using the walker although she didn't need it was Shirley's nonverbal way of indicating distrust and discomfort in the presence of others. By relinquishing the walker, Shirley indicated she was prepared to interact more closely with others. She did not require the walker for a deficit in balance (answer B). Arriving without the walker one day might have been the result of forgetfulness (answer C), but doing so on three consecutive days indicates that Shirley has made a decision. Improved social conduct (answer A) would have been better demonstrated by improved eye contact and/or decreased belligerence. See reference: AOTA: Uniform terminology for occupational therapy, 3rd edition.

140. (B) objective. Measured results based on an individual's performance are included in the objective section. The subjective portion (answer A) of the SOAP note contains information provided by the patient or family. Analysis of the measurements is recorded in the assessment area (answer C) of the SOAP note. Plans for future sessions are included in the plan section (answer D). See reference: Early: Medical records and documentation.

141. (B) "Shirley has not accused any men of attacking her this week." The number of times Shirley demonstrates one aspect of paranoid behavior (fear of men) is objectively stated in the correct answer. Answer A indicates improvement, but does not provide substantiation for the statement. Answer C may be indicative of improved interpersonal skills and self-esteem but does not reflect decreased paranoid behavior. Answer D is a statement of a goal, not of improvement. See reference: Early: Medical records and documentation.

142. (D) plan. The plan section of a SOAP note includes statements related to continuing treatment; the frequency and duration of the treatment; suggestions for additional activities or treatment techniques; the need for further evaluations; and, when needed, recommendations for new goals. The subjective portion of a SOAP note (answer A) refers to what the patient reports or comments about the treatment. The objective portion of the SOAP note (answer B) focuses on measurable and/or observable data obtained by the OT practitioner through specific evaluations, observations, or use of therapeutic activities. The assessment part of a SOAP note refers to the effectiveness of treatment and any changes needed, the status of the goals, and justification for continuing occupational therapy treatment. See reference: Ryan (ed): Backhaus, H: Documentation. *Practice Issues in Occupational Therapy.*

143. (C) The client initiated working on the stenciling activity by selecting one of six available designs. The notation of the client's response to treatment that contains the most objective information is C. The notations that address the client's "wanting" and "hostility" (answers A and B) are interpretations of behavior, not reports of directly observable responses. The words "appropriate" and "most" (answer D) are vague, generalized terms. See reference: Early: Medical records and documentation.

144. (D) work adjustment. Work adjustment programs are designed to address problems with valuing work and with interpersonal skills in the workplace. Competitive job placement (answer A) is rarely done by COTAs. Job coaching (answer B) is specific to one job setting and may not address interpersonal concerns. Supported employment (answer C) is for noncompetitive skills. See reference: Hopkins and Smith (eds): Jacobs, K: Work assessment and programming.

145. (D) relaxation and exercise. Stress-management groups typically include sessions on recognizing stressors and the effects of stress; self-awareness and communication skills; time management; nutrition, relaxation, and exercise; and goal development and implementation. Discharge-planning groups facilitate the transition from inpatient to outpatient. They usually include mutual problem solving for issues involving daily and leisure time structure (answer A), educational and financial planning, planning living arrangements (answer B) and transportation, outpatient treatment (answer C), and relationships. See reference: Hopkins and Smith (eds): Richert, GZ: Program planning, development, and implementation.

146. (B) self-help group. Self-help groups are supportive and educational and focus on personal growth around one major, life-disrupting problem. Support groups (answer C) focus on assisting members who are in crises until the crisis is past. Advocacy groups (answer A) focus on changing others or changing the system rather than on changing one's self. Psychotherapy groups (answer D) focus on understanding the influence of past experiences on present conflicts. See reference: Early: Special populations.

147. (B) share their experiences and struggles with alcohol use. Shared experiences can build feelings of understanding, hope, and acceptance among the members of a self-help group. Answers A, C, and D are all examples of member roles that are *not* encouraged in self-help groups. See reference: Early: Special populations.

148. (C) Alcoholics Anonymous (AA). Self-help groups focus on personal growth. Leadership comes from the group members. AA is an example of such a group. MADD (answer A) is an advocacy group focusing on changing the legal system. Group therapy (answer D) involves leadership and expertise from outside the group itself. Al-Anon (answer B) is a combination of support group and self-help group for family members of alcoholics. See reference: Early: Special populations.

149. (C) adult day care. Adult day care is long-term care that provides structured daily activities for older individuals to enable them to maintain current levels of functioning. Usually, occupational therapy services are provided in the home (answer A) only if the client has another, nonpsychiatric diagnosis. Partial hospitalization (answer B) is appropriate for individuals who are experiencing acute psychiatric symptoms and who have a place to stay at night. This patient does not, at this time, present with acute symptoms. Day treatment (answer D) focuses on assisting individuals to adapt to their illness and develop daily living skills at the program site. See reference: Early: Treatment settings.

150. (B) allow more time for the individuals to respond to questions about discharge plans. Depression slows patients' responses, so allowing them more time to respond is important. Both silence and a cheerful approach (answers A and C) can be perceived as unaccepting or insincere. The COTA needs to structure the discussion (and therefore answer D is wrong), because initiating and maintaining is often difficult for depressed individuals. See reference: Early: Responding to symptoms and behaviors.

151. (D) Occupational Therapy Code of Ethics. This document, which states the underlying values and basic moral beliefs underlying occupational therapy practice, was adopted by the AOTA in April, 1977, and was most recently revised in 1994. The Standards of Practice (answer A) were designed as a guideline for the provision of occupational therapy services. Six sets of standards exist, one of which is a general standard of practice for all patients; each of the remaining five was written to cover patients with physical disabilities, patients with developmental disabilities; and patients in mental-health programs, home-health programs, and schools. The Uniform Terminology System for Reporting Occupational Therapy Services, 3rd Edition (answer B) defines areas of practice and descriptors of services. Regulatory acts (answer C) define state practice standards and often include codes of ethics. See reference: Jacobs and Logigian (eds): Bloom, G: Ethics.

152. (B) protect consumers of occupational therapy. The purpose of licensure is to protect consumers of occupational therapy services and to improve the status of occupational therapy, thereby increasing coverage of service. Although licensure guidelines cover in a general way the roles of OTRs and COTAs, they do not clearly delineate the roles (answer A). Ensuring the continued competency of OT practitioners (answer C) is not the primary purpose of licensure boards. Although some states require evidence of continuing education to maintain licensure, many do not. And although the existence of licensure may contribute to the willingness of Medicare, Medicaid, and other third-party payers to cover OT services (answer D), this is not the primary reason for licensure. See reference: Hopkins and Smith (eds): Hopkins, HL: Scope of occupational therapy.

153. (B) consultant. A consultant provides information based on his or her skill and knowledge base. A COTA acting as a practitioner (answer A) provides services to assigned individuals under the supervision of an OTR. A COTA acting as a supervisor (answer C) manages other OT personnel. A COTA acting as an educator (answer D) provides training to consumers, peers, and layperson or community groups. See reference: AOTA: Occupational therapy roles.

154. (C) home care. Working in home care environment requires, the COTA to transport equipment to the home or use what is available for a therapeutic result. This limitation in equipment resources requires the COTA to find creative alternatives for treatment. Acute-care hospitals, nursing homes, and rehabilitation hospitals (answers A, B, and D) usually provide equipment that the COTA may draw upon in treatment planning. See reference: Hopkins and Smith (eds): Levine, RE, Corcoran, MA, and Gitlin, L: Home care and private practice.

155. (D) health promotion. Health promotion is encouraging healthy lifestyles through education, behavioral change, and cultural support. Occupational behavior (answer A) is the developmental continuum of play to work. Intervention (answer B) is the provision of treatment to enhance performance in well or involved individuals. Self-efficacy (answer C) would be promoting the positive effects of occupational therapy services. See reference: Hopkins and Smith (eds): Levy, LL: The health care delivery system today.

156. (A) informed consent. This concept refers to the rights of individuals to be provided with information concerning potential risks of an intervention, as well as the right to decide if they want to participate in the intervention. Fidelity (answer B) involves remaining faithful to the patient's best interests and observing confidentiality. Beneficence (answer C) is the duty to do what is best for the patient or client. Nonmaleficence (answer D) is defined as the obligation of the provider to avoid causing harm or injury to a patient. See reference: Hopkins and Smith (eds): Hansen, RA: Ethics in occupational therapy.

157. (A) The AOTA requires the cosignature of the supervising OTR. The AOTA does *not* require that a COTA's notes be cosigned by an OTR, unless required by the employer or legislation. It is not uncommon for insurance carriers and licensure acts to require cosignature. Cosignature indicates that an OTR has read, sanctioned, and assumed responsibility for the documentation. It is also one method of demonstrating that the OTR is supervising the COTA. See reference: Jacobs and Logigian (eds): Pagonis, J: Documentation in health care.

158. (C) make a report to the appropriate authorities. In many states, the occupational therapy practitioner, as a health professional, is a "mandated reporter," who must make a report if there is reason to believe a child has been abused. A report of the injury should be made to appropriate authorities. Answers A, B, and D delay or prevent the provision of proper assistance to a family involved in child abuse and therefore are wrong answers. All agencies serving children have policies and procedures for reporting injury in these situations. See reference: Hopkins and Smith (eds): Simon, CJ: Child abuse and neglect.

159. (C) Individual family service plan (IFSP). Answer C is correct, because the service plan mandated by federal law (PL 99-457, part H) and provided through early intervention programs is called an "Individual Family Service Plan." Answer A is not correct, because the IEP is a service plan provided for children of school age. Answer B is not correct because there is no service plan called the "least restrictive environment plan." Answer D is not correct because there is no such service plan as the "Early Intervention Service Plan" covered by any federal law. See reference: Case-Smith, Allen, and Pratt (eds): Stephens, LC, and Tauber, SK: Early intervention.

160. (B) 1 year experience. Fieldwork educators, or supervisors, may be COTAs or OTRs with a minimum of 1 year of experience. These individuals should be competent and knowledgeable and able to function as good role models. There is no guideline indicating the amount of experience needed to supervise Level I students. See reference: Hopkins and Smith (eds): Cohn, EN: Fieldwork education: Professional socialization. Also AOTA: Essentials and guidelines for an accredited educational program for the occupational therapy assistant.

161. (A) increased use of COTAs. A continuing trend in occupational therapy service is the strong emphasis on providing optimal care at the lowest rate. This practice trend is increasing the roles of COTAs and OT aides and at the same time increasing the supervision responsibilities of the OTR. In addition, resources are shifting from inpatient areas to home health and/or outpatient care. Occupational therapy practitioners continue to be in high demand. See reference: AOTA: 1996 Member data survey.

162. (C) notify the supervising OTR of Jean's interests so that the OTR may decide if it is a good idea to modify the treatment plan. It is the COTA's responsibility to notify the supervising OTR of any changes in the patient's status. Changes may include an improvement in function, a decline in status, or altered patient or family goals. Working together, the OTR and COTA may update the individual's treatment plan as appropriate based on the new information. Answers A and D are incorrect, because the COTA should not modify the treatment plan without first consulting the OTR. Although it is desirable to honor patient interests (answer B), the activity provided must provide a positive benefit. See reference: Ryan (ED): Backhaus, H: Arts and crafts. *The Certified Occupational Therapy Assistant.*

163. (B) a COTA may perform the task following demonstration of service competency, unless state law prohibits this. Providing paraffin treatments requires advanced knowledge and skills that are not considered entry-level practice. In addition, this treatment requires ongoing interpretation of the patient's response. The practitioner providing the treatment must be able to interpret the patient's responses so as to identify patient sensitivity to the application of heat or the resulting increase in circulation and modify the treatment as needed. Therefore, it is necessary for OT practitioners to establish service competency in this area in order to ensure patient safety and achieve the desired results. Answer A does not take into account the additional skill required. Answers C and D are not correct, because this activity may be completed independently by a COTA once service competency has been established. State laws concerning the use of physical agent modalities by OT practitioners supersede AOTA policies. See reference: AOTA: Occupational therapy roles.

164. (C) notify the supervising therapist of the situation. The COTA is responsible for communicating information on the patient's status or change in status to the supervising OTR. In complicated situations such as this one, the occupational therapy team may have to consult the facility's ethics board to help determine how to safely and effectively manage the case. Answers A, B, and D are all possible results of such determinations. See reference: AOTA: Occupational therapy code of ethics.

165. (C) code of ethics. These are the moral guidelines used by members of a professional group to direct their behavior. Policies and procedures (answer A) are the facility guidelines for performing activities and tasks when working for the facility. The federal and state governments issue regulations (answer B) to define the rules for conduct of a professional group. Protocols (answer D) are the standard approaches to a problem that a professional may use in practice. See reference: Ryan (ed): Cummings, G: Principles of occupational therapy ethics. *Practice Issues in Occupational Therapy.*

166. (C) both OTRs and COTAs should have liability insurance. Liability insurance protects occupational therapy practitioners from financial damage when they are sued for negligence or misconduct. Most facilities maintain coverage for licensed professionals, but the level of coverage may not be sufficient to cover the amount sought for by the claimant. Therefore, occupational therapy practitioners may chose to insure themselves at a higher level. See reference: Ryan (ed): Jones, RA: Service operations. *Practice Issues in Occupational Therapy.*

167. (B) no, it violates the Occupational Therapy Code of Ethics. Despite the level of training she has achieved, according to the code it is still necessary for the COTA to demonstrate service competency in order to administer physical agent modalities. "Physical agent modalities may be used by occupational therapy practitioners when used as an adjunct to or in preparation for purposeful activity by a practitioner who has demonstrated service competency." Service competency in this area includes the theoretical background and technical skills for the safe and effective use of the modality. Although study and practice are necessary to establish service competency, they are not by themselves sufficient; an OTR must determine that the COTA is competent before the COTA can administer PAMs (answers A and C). Having an OTR on duty in the facility (answer D) does not make it acceptable for a COTA to administer a modality if the COTA has not demonstrated service competency. See reference: AOTA: Policy: Registered occupational therapists and certified occupational therapy assistants and modalities.

168. (C) precede the paraffin bath with purposeful activity. Purposeful activity should follow, not precede, a paraffin bath. "Physical agent modalities may be used by occupational therapy practitioners when used as an adjunct to or in preparation for purposeful activity by a practitioner who has demonstrated service competency" (answer A). An appropriate level of supervision is required (answer D). The OT Code of Ethics requires that the patient be informed of the risks involved with any intervention (answer B). See reference: AOTA: Occupational Therapy Code of Ethics. Also AOTA: Policy: Registered occupational therapists and certified occupational therapy assistants and modalities.

169. (D) take a few days to teach himself the activity before leading the group. This action demonstrates such important professional behaviors as initiative, problem solving, and respect for his supervisor's time. Answer A requires the supervisor to take time out of his or her schedule. Answer B could be an appropriate action, but the COTA would need to discuss the change in treatment plan with the OTR before implementing it. In addition, taking the initiative to learn a new intervention and add to his repertoire is an example of professional behavior. *No* COTA should engage in an activity that he or she is not competent in, but refusing to lead the quilting group (answer D) is the least professional way of responding. The other answers are better alternatives. See reference: Early: Supervision.

170. (D) schedule regular department inservices and take turns presenting. The OT Code of Ethics requires OT practitioners to maintain high standards of competence by participating in professional development and continuing education. Some state licensure acts also require evidence of continuing education. There are many ways to participate in professional development and continuing education that do not require funding, e.g., reading professional journals, attending local (often free or inexpensive) occupational therapy meetings, taking in-service training, training fieldwork students, and participating in professional organizations. Waiting up to 4 years for a continuing education opportunity is too long (answer A). Demanding something (answer B) is usually not effective. Participating in on-line workshops (answer C) is expensive. See reference: Ryan (ed): Blechert, TF, and Christiansen, MF: Intraprofessional relationships and socialization. *Practice Issues in Occupational Therapy.*

171. (C) providing continuous patient treatment. Although engaging in patient treatment is important to maintaining professional skills, it is not a form of continuing education. Answers A, B, and D are all examples of continuing education. Additional methods include attending in-services, workshops, seminars, and conferences and using programmed learning packets and audiovisual materials. See reference: Ryan (ed): Blechert, TF, and Christiansen, MF: Intraprofessional relationships and socialization. *Practice Issues in Occupational Therapy.*

172. (C) permanently loses his or her membership in the AOTA. The Commission of Standards and Ethics (SEC) of the AOTA has jurisdiction over all members of AOTA. Disciplinary actions the SEC may impose include reprimand, a private, written expression of disapproval; censure, a formal, public expression of disapproval; suspension, a loss of AOTA membership for a specific period of time (answer D); and revocation, a permanent loss of AOTA membership. Revocation of licensure (answers A and B) can only be imposed by state regulatory bodies. See reference: AOTA: Enforcement procedure for the Occupational Therapy Code of Ethics.

173. (C) CVA/hemiplegia. A 1996 study completed by the American Occupational Therapy Association revealed that the diagnosis most frequently being treated by COTAs was CVA/hemiplegia. The second most commonly seen diagnosis was fractures (11.6%). This was followed by developmental delay (8.6%) and learning disabilities at (4.7%). See reference: AOTA: 1996 Member data survey.

174. (C) Occupational Therapy Standards of Practice. Guidelines for documentation that may be used for reimbursement, research, and education or to provide legal information are included in the Occupational Therapy Standards of Practice. This document was originally published in 1978 and was revised in 1992. Uniform Terminology, 3rd edition (answer A), defines occupational therapy in relationship to performance areas and performance components. This document is used throughout the practice of occupational therapy so that there may be uniform use of the definitions provided. The Code of Ethics (answer B) outlines the standard for the conduct expected of an occupational therapy practitioner. The Occupational Therapy Roles document (answer D) defines the various educational and skill levels of occupational therapy practitioners. See reference: AOTA: Standards of practice for occupational therapy.

175. (B) do not treat the patient, because of his refusal, and document the interaction in the chart. As stated in the Code of Ethics (principle 2), "Occupational therapy personnel shall respect the individual's right to refuse professional services." Answers A and C are incorrect, because the COTA disregards the patient's refusal and proceeds to treat the patient. Answer D is incorrect, because it does not conform to Principle 4 of the Code of Ethics, "Occupational therapy personnel shall accurately record and report information related to professional activities." See reference: AOTA: Occupational Therapy Code of Ethics.

176. (A) yes, by violating the concept of beneficence. "Occupational therapy personnel shall provide services in an equitable manner for all individuals." Beneficence is the concern that the OT practitioner must demonstrate toward patients. This includes providing services without discrimination, providing appropriate information to patients regarding the practitioner's education and research experience, and involving the patient in treatment planning. Competence (answer B) concerns the requirement that the practitioner's credentials and competence match the requirements of the practitioner's job description. The OT Code of Ethics requires practitioners to refer patients to other service areas when the skills required do not fall within their expertise. Compliance with laws and regulations (answer C) means adherence to state, local, and federal laws in addition to the guidelines of the facility and the requirements for accreditation. See reference: AOTA: Occupational Therapy Code of Ethics.

177. (C) interrater reliability. Interrater reliability is a measure of the variation among various observers' perceptions of a subject's performance or some other characteristic. Although the need for supervisory feedback (answer A), an inability to competently administer the evaluation (answer B), and a lack of confidence may also be reasons for a student to ask the supervisor to check her results, there is nothing in the question indicating that these were issues for this student. See reference: Bailey: Collecting and analyzing qualitative data.

178. (C) worker's compensation. Worker's compensation is a state program funded in part or whole by employers' contributions. Beneficiaries receive coverage for services covered by their respective state programs. Medicare (answer A) is a federal program for health coverage for individuals 65 years old or older, disabled individuals, and people in end stage renal disease. Medicaid (answer B) is a joint state and federal program that provides coverage for the poor and medically indigent. The Education for All Handicapped Children program (answer D) is funded by state and federal grants. See reference: Bair and Gray (eds): Scott, S, and Somers, FP: Payment for occupational therapy services.

179. (B) rinse the eye with an eyewash or water immediately. The exposed area must be washed immediately with warm water or normal saline because the "backwash" fluid in the IV is unidentifiable body fluid and universal precautions should be followed. Therefore, answers A, C, and D are incorrect. Following the cleansing of the eye, the COTA should contact his or her immediate supervisor and report the exposure through the facility reporting system. See reference: Occupational Safety and Health Administration.

180. (C) once a month. Levels of supervision vary depending on the expertise of the supervisee. The description of general supervision given by the AOTA includes a minimum of monthly direct contact with supervision available as needed by phone or other forms of communication. Answer A describes close supervision with direct contact occurring daily. Answer B refers to routine supervision or direct contact occurring a minimum of every 2 weeks. Answer D is minimal supervision that occurs as needed. COTAs at all levels are required to have at least general supervision from an OTR. See reference: AOTA: Occupational therapy roles.

181. (B) capitation. Capitation is a uniform payment or fee per diagnosis. This form of reimbursement has evolved with healthcare reform. Fee for service (answer A) is an outdated model, in which health care providers were paid what they billed. This type of system allowed for various forms of abuse in the healthcare system. Cost shifting (answer C) occurs when a facility increases prices for all individuals who need service to cover the shortfalls in reimbursement by some of the carriers. Cost control (answer D) is the strategy that focuses on keeping the expenses below the revenue generated. See reference: Bair and Gray (eds): Scott, SJ and Somers, FP: Payment for occupational therapy services.

182. (D) all individuals with open wounds. Treating blood and body substances of all individuals as though they are contaminated is the concept of universal precautions. There are several strategies to protect employees from potential exposure. Engineering controls modify the work environment to reduce risk of exposure; for example, using sharps containers, eyewash stations, and biohazard waste containers. Work practice controls are policies that require a procedure be performed a certain way so that potential for exposure is minimized. Examples of work practice controls include the technique for disposal of sharps using only one hand and frequent hand washing during and after patient contact. Personal protective equipment, another strategy, is wearing appropriate gear to prevent contact with blood or identified bodily substances. Equipment may include goggles, masks, gowns, and gloves. Answers A, B, and C are all examples of individuals with open wounds, where exposure to blood is likely. Both the healthcare provider and the patient could be placed at risk unless gloves are worn. See reference: Occupational Safety and Health Administration.

183. (C) are homebound. Homebound patients are physically unable to leave their homes with or without assistance. Homecare services are not covered if the patient merely requires a wheelchair or assistance for mobility (answers A and D). If a patient is unable to drive to an outpatient center (answer B), community transportation services can usually be arranged. See reference: Hopkins and Smith (eds): Levine, RE, Corcoran, MA, and Gitlin, L: Home care and private practice.

184. (A) refuse to provide OT services to patients until an OTR has been hired to supervise her. A COTA cannot provide OT services without supervision from an OTR. Doing so could result in disciplinary action. Providing services for a limited period of time and treating only a few select patients (answers B and C) are both violations of certification, state licensure, the Code of Ethics, and the Standards of Practice. Answer D is incorrect, because the AOTA has no authority over nursing homes. In addition, no laws or regulations would be broken unless the COTA proceeded to provide OT services without supervision. See reference: Ryan (ed): Ryan, SE: COTA supervision. *Practice Issues in Occupational Therapy.*

185. (A) obtain collaboration with or supervision from an OTR before beginning treatment. According to the AOTA Statement of Occupational Therapy Referral, a COTA may identify or screen individuals for potential referral but may not accept or enter a case without the supervision or collaboration of an OTR. Answers B, C, and D are all actions the COTA would take after accepting the case. See reference: AOTA: Statement of occupational therapy referral.

186. (A) initiate a referral for OT. Because COTA education emphasizes activities of daily living the COTA is able to initiate referral for individuals with deficits in these areas. Answers B, C, and D are all examples of evaluation or intervention, which can only begin following acceptance of the case by the OTR. See reference: AOTA: Statement of occupational therapy referral.

187. (B) medication effectiveness. "Three major areas that should be assessed in quality assurance programs for mental health occupational therapy [include]: progress toward goals, patient satisfaction with care, and behavior rating scores" (p. 288). Medication is considered a medical intervention and is not an appropriate subject for an occupational therapy department's QA program. See reference: Early: Treatment planning.

188. (D) collect screening data. Screening is the process in which occupational therapy practitioners review the status of the patient and, if warranted, identify appropriate interventions. Once service competency has been established, the COTA may participate in collecting the screening data. See reference: Ryan (ed): Ryan, SE: Therapeutic intervention process. *Practice Issues in Occupational Therapy.*

189. (A) direct contact with supervisor, on site, daily. This level of supervision allows the entry-level COTA to collaborate and practice problem solving with the supervisor daily. This form of supervision is necessary to establish service competency and develop clinical skills. Answers B, C, and D do not provide the frequency of consultation required for skill development. See reference: Ryan (ed): Ryan, SE: COTA supervision. *Practice Issues in Occupational Therapy.*

190. (C) improvement in functional independence. Increased functional independence is an area that may easily be monitored by comparing a patient's function upon admission to his or her function at discharge. There are many programs that allow the OT practitioner to quantify improvement. Because occupational therapy practitioners provide the information for this monitor, the results will have a higher rate of reliability and validity than other answers provided. Answers A and D are difficult for the OT practitioner to monitor and control. Information provided by family members may not always be accurate, resulting in decreased reliability and validity. Answer B is outside the OT scope of care in that referrals are written by physicians. See reference: Early: Treatment planning.

191. (A) setting up or cleaning up treatment activities. Aides are noncredentialed personnel who are delegated routine nonskilled tasks. Answers B, C, and D require skill and judgment to complete the task. See reference: Ryan (ed): Ryan, SE: COTA supervision. *Practice Issues in Occupational Therapy*.

192. (A) a fire drill. Emergency plans typically include fire drills, code blue or patient emergencies, weather emergencies, local disaster emergencies, and behavioral emergencies. COTAs should be familiar with facility policy for the appropriate response in each emergency. Inspection of electrical equipment and fire extinguishers (answers B and C) is usually carried out by engineering or service personnel. Answers B, C, and D are all ongoing activities that are performed in preparation of an emergency situation. See reference: Ryan (ed): Jones, RA: Service operations. *Practice Issues in Occupational Therapy*.

193. (D) discuss her concerns with the OTR. Bringing concerns to a supervisor for discussion and problem-solving is an important way of participating in a collaborative supervisory relationship. Answers A, B, and C all avoid discussion of the issue with the supervisor, which can limit professional growth and damage a supervisory relationship. See reference: Early: Supervision.

194. (B) a policy. "A policy is a general statement that outlines an expected course." A procedure is a stepwise description of how a desired act is performed. (answer C). Documentation (answer A) is the preparation of written reports concerning evaluation and treatment. A job description (answer D) includes the job title, organizational relationship, and required skills and functions. See reference: Jacobs and Logigian (eds): Pagonis, J: Documentation in health care.

195. (D) policy and procedure manual. The policy and procedure manual is a set of guidelines unique to each facility that defines what personnel are expected to do and how they are expected to do it. A mission statement (answer A) reflects the philosophy of the facility. A quality assurance report (answer B) provides the results of a quality assurance program. Essential job requirements (answer C) are usually included in a job description. See reference: Hopkins and Smith (eds): Perinchief, JM: Service management.

196. (C) ask another OT practitioner for help. Trying to attempt this transfer alone could result in injury to the patient and/or the COTA, even if she uses proper body mechanics (answer A). It is often necessary to get assistance when transferring obese individuals. Asking someone else to do a difficult task for you (answer B) is not professional. If the patient needs to be transferred, not transferring him (answer D) is not an option. See reference: Pedretti (ed): Adler, C, and Tipton-Burton, M: Wheelchair assessment and transfers.

197. (B) copper tooling. Liver of sulfate, used to antique the copper design, is toxic. Wood burning (answer A) may create smoke and odor noxious to individuals with respiratory disease. Dough art (answer C) contains salt and is very drying to the skin. Papier mache (answer D) is very messy but uses flour and water, which are nontoxic. See reference: Johnson, C, Lobdell, K, Nesbitt, J, and Clare, M: Therapeutic crafts.

198. (D) word processing program. Word processing programs allow the user to input and edit necessary patient data. Many systems are now designed with evaluation and update status forms formatted into the word processor so that the clinician does not need to input repetitive data or formats. A terminal program (answer A) is a system that allows individuals in different computer systems to "talk" to each other through telephone lines. A common example of this would be the E-mail system. A spreadsheet (answer B) is typically used to manage numerical data such as productivity or budgetary information. A database manager (answer C) coordinates all of the facility's patient data regarding diagnoses, insurance, and demographics as designed by the program. See reference: Ryan (ed): Ryan, SE, Ryan, BJ, and Walker, JE: Computers. *The Certified Occupational Therapy Assistant*.

199. (A) government will pass legislation to make health insurance available to all American citizens. State and national governments have been debating the healthcare reform issue since the early 1990s. Although legislation mandating availability of insurance has not yet been passed, many states have written their own healthcare plans. Answers B, C, and D are incorrect. Government has not called for insurance-company reform, the use of inpatient hospital care is expected to decline, and managed healthcare systems are now booming. It is expected that by the year 2000, 50% of all patients treated will be in a managed care system.

200. (D) lightweight wheelchair and hospital bed. Durable medical equipment is defined by Medicare as "that which can withstand repeated use, is primarily and customarily used to serve a medical purpose, and generally is not useful to a person in the absence of illness or injury." Answers A, B, and C are incorrect because they include items such as reachers, shower chair, handheld shower and long-handled sponge, which are not considered as serving a "medical purpose." Depending on the patient's medical condition, a bedside commode may be covered. See reference: Bair and Gray (eds): Scott, S, and Somers, FP: Payment for occupational therapy services.

SIMULATION EXAMINATION 3

Directions: Circle the correct answer to the following questions. When you have completed this examination, check your answers against the answer key that follows. As you will see, an explanation is given for each answer along with a reference for further study. The book author is listed as well as the chapter author. See the bibliography for complete references. Study the areas in which your comprehension was low, then test yourself again by taking Simulation Examination 4.

PEDIATRIC QUESTIONS

Data Collection

1. A 7 year old child with a visual perceptual problem is lacing a series of geometric beads based on a stimulus card. She is unable to identify a triangle shape when the lacing bead is turned sideways on the table. This problem is BEST described as a deficit in:
A. figure-ground perception.
B. form constancy perception.
C. visual memory.
D. visual sequencing.

2. While observing a child for the first time, the COTA notes that the child responds to a loud noise by abducting and extending her arms. The reflex, or reaction, observed in this child is called:
A. rooting.
B. Moro.
C. flexor withdrawal.
D. neck righting.

3. The following procedure should be followed when administering standardized tests to young children:
A. test in a stimulating environment.
B. follow test manual directions.
C. remove all test materials before presenting the next item.
D. carry on a conversation with the child.

4. A 12-year-old girl is hospitalized with anorexia nervosa. The COTA has been assigned to collect data on her family background, education, and habits via chart review. The COTA would find this information in the :
A. nurse's notes.
B. doctor's notes.
C. social worker's notes.
D. admitting note.

5. A 3-year-old child with a diagnosis of spina bifida has been referred for an assessment. As directed by the OTR, the COTA is collecting initial data by interviewing the child's mother. The COTA should primarily focus on:
A. the mother's concerns and goals for her child.
B. medical management.
C. equipment needs.
D. the physical lay-out of the home.

6. To do a naturalistic observation of dressing skills in 6-year-old boy with a diagnosis of developmental delay, the COTA:
A. provides oversized clothing to ensure success.
B. has the child dress and undress in a distraction-free corner of the clinic.
C. provides assistance as needed to minimize frustration.
D. observes the child as he enters the clinic and takes off his coat and shoes.

7. By using an interest checklist that includes a report of both interests and actual participation in activities, a COTA may collect information on a client's:
A. use of time.
B. developmental level.
C. mood and affect.
D. communication skills.

8. During the administration of a standardized test, the child becomes uncooperative and complains that the test is "too hard". The COTA's MOST appropriate response is to:
A. switch to easier items to improve the child's self esteem.
B. terminate the session and reschedule for the remainder of the test.

C. follow administration instructions and note changes in behavior.
D. adapt the remaining test items to ensure success.

9. A COTA witnesses a seizure in his 6-year-old client with hydrocephalus. The MOST relevant information to document and report to the supervising therapist is:
A. the child's positioning during the seizure.
B. objective signs and duration of the seizure.
C. responsiveness during the seizure.
D. facial expression during and after the seizure.

10. During a coloring activity, the COTA observes a preschooler stabilizing his crayon between thumb and fingertips. The COTA documents this grasp correctly as:
A. pincer grasp.
B. radial-digital grasp.
C. palmar grasp.
D. lateral pinch.

Treatment Planning

11. The *BEST* activity to develop "position in space" skills in a 6-year-old child is:
A. identifying letters on a distracting page.
B. finding geometric shapes scattered in a box.
C. following directions about objects located in front, back, and to the side.
D. making judgments about moving through space.

12. A 12-year-old child with Duchenne's muscular dystrophy is able to independently use a manual wheelchair to get from one class to another, but she is tired upon arrival. The OTR and COTA are collaborating with a team to recommend the MOST appropriate wheelchair for this child. The BEST recommendation would be to:
A. retain the manual chair to build up strength.
B. change to an ultralight sports model since it requires less strength.
C. change to a power wheelchair to eliminate effort.
D. encourage walking with a walker to alternate mobility methods.

13. A child with a poor postural stability is developmentally ready for toileting. The element of the treatment plan that should be considered FIRST is:
A. training in management of fasteners.
B. provision of foot support.
C. provision of a seatbelt.
D. training in climbing onto the toilet.

14. The treatment plan for a child with a visual discrimination problem should include the following adaptation of visual materials:
A. low contrast and defined borders.
B. high contrast and defined borders.
C. high contrast and ambiguous borders.
D. low contrast and ambiguous borders

15. The COTA and the speech therapist collaborate on a communications goal for a 6-year-old child with multiple handicaps. The COTA focuses on positioning for function and the speech therapist on the development of a communications system. This is an example of what type of approach?
A. unidisciplinary.
B. multidisciplinary.
C. interdisciplinary.
D. transdisciplinary.

16. To promote play skills and self expression in a 7-year-old withdrawn child, the COTA should FIRST select activities that:
A. promote open-ended symbolic play, such as action figures, puppets, dolls.
B. provide a defined structure, such as simple craft activities with instructions.
C. promote social interaction, such as a game of tag with peers.
D. provide a means of tension release, such as leather tooling or wedging clay.

17. When developing play activities for a 10-year-old child with acute juvenile rheumatoid arthritis, the COTA should keep in mind the following precaution:
A. avoid light touch.
B. avoid rapid vestibular stimulation.
C. avoid resistive materials.
D. avoid elevated temperatures.

18. The COTA is helping a preschooler develop letter recognition skills. The BEST activity would be:
A. forming letters out of clay.
B. flash cards.
C. matching cut-out letters to a sample.
D. coloring in large letter outlines.

19. Angela's long-term goal is to increase fine motor skills. A deficit in tactile discrimination, specifically stereognosis, was identified. A relevant short-term goal would be: "Within two weeks, Angela will identify, with vision occluded:
A. five out of five fingers touched, when given tactile stimulus"
B. five out of five shapes drawn on the dorsum of the hand."
C. five out of five matching textures."
D. five out of five common objects, by feel only."

20. An 8-year-old child has low muscle tone, resulting in problems in the following printing/handwriting subskill areas: 1) postural stability, 2) shoulder stability, 3) immature grasp of the pencil. Treatment of her problems should proceed in the following order if the COTA follows a proximal-to-distal approach to development:

A. improve posture, then improve shoulder stability, then improve grasp.
B. improve shoulder stability, then improve posture, then improve grasp.
C. improve grasp, then improve posture, then improve shoulder stability.
D. improve shoulder stability, then improve posture, then improve grasp.

21. Haruka has poor sitting balance, which interferes with her school work, especially desk top activities. In order to promote the development of ongoing postural adjustments in sitting, the use of the following is recommended:
A. a sturdy chair with lateral trunk supports.
B. a corner floor seat with built in desk surface.
C. a bolster for back support.
D. a therapy ball to sit on during desk work.

22. Dorothy is easily aroused due to a sensory processing disorder. What environmental adaptation would be MOST effective in helping her go to sleep?
A. Mini-trampoline in the bedroom to tire her out before going to bed.
B. Use of a noise machine producing white noise at bedtime.
C. Lightweight, fuzzy blanket providing light touch.
D. Shutters on the windows to produce total darkness.

Treatment Implementation

23. A child with mental retardation who is in the moderate (trainable) range of intellectual ability probably functions in the following manner:
A. requires nursing care for basic survival skills.
B. can usually handle routine daily functions.
C. requires supervision to accomplish most tasks.
D. is able to learn academic skills at the 3rd to 7th grade level.

24. When dressing a child with strong extensor tone in the lower extremities, which position would make donning shoes and socks easier?
A. Extend the child's hips and knees.
B. Flex the child's hips and knees.
C. Extend the child's shoulders.
D. Dorsiflex the child's ankles.

25. A COTA needs to explain to the parents of a child with cerebral palsy the importance of a correct sitting position for use of the hands in activity. Their child uses compensatory movements due to an inability to sit independently. What aspect of therapeutic positioning does the COTA need to emphasize as crucial for this child?
A. Stabilizing the trunk.
B. Weight on the arms.
C. Stabilizing the pelvis/hips/legs.
D. Stabilizing the head/neck.

26. When preparing a home program for independent toileting for a 4-year-old boy with postural instability, the MOST important adaptation the COTA can recommend is:
A. replacing zippers and buttons with Velcro closures.
B. mounting a safety rail next to the toilet.
C. introducing toilet paper tongs.
D. placing a colorful "target" in the toilet bowl.

27. The use of a power-driven wheelchair is contraindicated for a child with:
A. low muscle tone.
B. limited active movement.
C. impairment in response time.
D. low frustration tolerance.

28. Which one of the following children with neuromotor impairment would benefit from using a prone scooter for exploratory play:
A. the child with cerebral palsy with predominant extensor tone.
B. the child with low tone who is easily fatigued.
C. the child with cognitive limitations and poor sensory awareness.
D. the child with spina bifida with LE paralysis.

29. An 18-month-old girl demonstrates poor head control, mild to moderate hypertonicity in the trunk, shoulders, and legs (extensor patterns) and mild to moderate hypertonicity in arms and hands (flexor pattern). The piece of adaptive equipment that would BEST meet her positioning needs during eating and feeding is a:
A. prone stander with lateral trunk supports.
B. corner chair with head support and padded abductor post.
C. supine on a wedge with hips flexed 15 degrees.
D. bolster chair without back support.

30. Julio is 8 years old and has a diagnosis of spastic quadriplegia. When teaching his parents how to position him in sitting so that he can participate in family games, the MOST important point to make is to make sure his:
A. head is upright.
B. arms are on the armrests.
C. back is straight.
D. hips are secured against the back of the seat.

31. David has increased tone and demonstrates tongue thrust (suckling tongue movement) when food is placed in his mouth. Which type of cup should his parents be told to AVOID when beginning cup drinking with him:
A. cup with a lip.
B. cup with a weighted base.
C. cup with a lid with small holes.
D. cup with a spout.

32. Jennifer is in second grade and shows signs of tactile defensiveness and social withdrawal. When involving her in group games, which games should the COTA AVOID:

A. Bingo.
B. 20 Questions.
C. Pin the Tail on the Donkey.
D. Charades.

33. Mina is in sixth grade and has a diagnosis of juvenile rheumatoid arthritis. In order to maintain her ROM, which leisure activity would be recommended:

A. swimming.
B. basketball.
C. soccer.
D. aerobics.

34. Jeremy is seven years old and has a diagnosis of mental retardation. He is currently learning to tie his shoes independently. To facilitate generalization of this skill, his COTA:

A. fits his shoes with Velcro closures.
B. has him practice tying shoes at home as well as in school.
C. uses a backwards chaining technique.
D. provides brightly colored shoelaces.

35. Amy is 4 years old and wears a below-elbow prosthesis on her left upper extremity. When consulting with her preschool teacher, the COTA recommends:

A. offering toys that Amy can manipulate with one hand.
B. stressing bilateral activities incorporating the prosthesis.
C. teaching Amy one-handed manipulation techniques.
D. involving Amy in non-manipulatory activities such as sing-along.

Evaluating the Treatment Plan

36. The COTA has placed a child in prone position on a wedge in order to develop vertical head righting. However, the child fatigues rapidly. What adjustment can the COTA make to the wedge that will make working in this position more successful for the child?

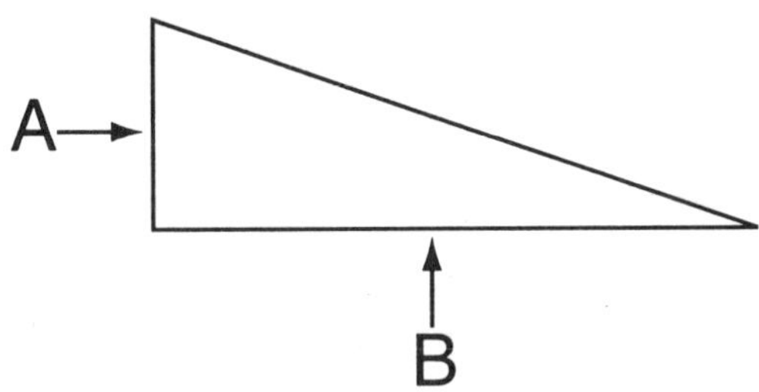

A. Increase the height of the wedge (side A on diagram).
B. Decrease the height of the wedge (side A on diagram).
C. Shorten the length of the wedge (side B on diagram).
D. Lengthen the wedge (side B on the diagram).

37. The COTA observes that a child with a learning disability demonstrates an unusually tight grip and frequently breaks his pencil from applying too much pressure on the paper. This type of problem would MOST likely be caused by inadequate sensory information from the:

A. vestibular system.
B. auditory system.
C. somatosensory system.
D. visual system.

38. Martin is a 1-year-old child working on increasing neck flexor strength. At this time, he can maintain head alignment when tilted backward from an upright, supported sitting position to a 45 degree incline but loses control when tilted further back. The next step in intervention is to work on head/neck alignment:

A. in sidelying while batting a toy.
B. prone while watching a peek-a-boo game.
C. tilted backward up to 60 degrees while rocking.
D. in supine while watching an overhead mobile.

39. Marie-Louise has been working on learning to activate the switch for her communications device needed in her fourth grade classroom. The switch is mounted on her wheelchair tray, but she has difficulty operating it due to her increased muscle tone. Despite practicing for an extended period of time, she is not making any progress. The COTA decides to:

A. work on coordinated reach in side-lying first, then transfer the skill to sitting.
B. passively stretch her upper extremity to increase her ROM.
C. use a brightly colored switch to increase visibility.
D. use systematic behavioral reinforcement through shaping.

40. Cesar is 6 years old and has a diagnosis of attention deficit disorder - hyperactivity type. In order to work on increasing his attention span, his COTA introduced a construction activity. When the blocks were placed in front of Cesar, he swept most of them onto the floor and started throwing the remaining ones around the room. How can the COTA restructure the activity for more success?

A. Use soft foam blocks.
B. Provide blocks of one color only.
C. Use interlocking blocks.
D. Present only a few blocks at a time.

41. Julian is 3 years old and has feeding difficulties due to reduced oral-motor control and oral defensiveness. His parents would like him to be able to eat family meals with them, including such foods as meats (cut up), sandwiches, and vegetables. The COTA explains that the parents can start to introduce these foods when Julian is able to handle the following foods:
A. apple sauce and mashed bananas.
B. dry cereals with milk.
C. strained fruits and vegetables.
D. scrambled eggs.

42. Max is 6 years old and has a diagnosis of muscular dystrophy. He has been learning to operate his manual wheelchair, but progress has been slow due to muscle weakness. The COTA should consider discussing a powered wheelchair with the OTR when:
A. Max starts Junior High school and needs to switch classrooms often.
B. his speed for long distances becomes less than that of a walking person.
C. his home can be made accessible for a power chair.
D. Max becomes unable to propel himself in his manual chair.

43. Javan is 11 years old and socially withdrawn. He has been attending a puppetry group structured on a project group level to increase his social interaction skills. At the last session, Javan verbally attacked a fellow group member, blaming her for not doing her work right. The COTA documents this incident as a sign of:
A. onset of behavioral problems.
B. beginning of spontaneous social interaction.
C. an outbreak of aggressive acting out.
D. the development of group leadership skills.

Discharge Planning

44. An 18-year-old student with mental retardation is being discharged from an occupational therapy program in a large metropolitan school to a community sheltered workshop. The MOST important information for the COTA to communicate to the workshop manager is the student's:
A. leisure interests.
B. ability to follow rules/instructions.
C. preferred grasp patterns.
D. level of reflex integration.

45. A COTA is discussing discharge plans for 6-year-old child with developmental dyspraxia with her parents. The COTA wants to recommend activities that provide proprioceptive input for the parents to carry out with their daughter after discharge. The MOST appropriate activity would be:
A. walking barefoot on textured surfaces.
B. rocking over a large therapy ball.
C. playing in a large box full of styrofoam pellets.
D. pushing or pulling weighted objects while in a quadruped position.

46. Lucy is in third grade and is being discharged from direct OT services provided through the public schools. What activities should the COTA recommend to the gym teacher to help consolidate Lucy's skills in spatial organization and motor planning?
A. Relay races.
B. Obstacle courses.
C. Balance beam.
D. Freeze tag.

47. A COTA has been working in a medical setting with a 6-year-old boy who is s/p traumatic brain injury. At what point should the COTA recommend discharge to the OTR?
A. When age level skills have been achieved.
B. When he is ready to make the transition to first grade.
C. When a maintenance level has been achieved.
D. When he is considered cured.

48. The COTA is preparing for the discharge of a 12-year-old with limited strength and endurance. Which adaptations are MOST important to recommend?
A. Mounting lever handles on doors and faucets.
B. Removing all throw rugs.
C. Placing non-skid pads on steps.
D. Mounting a table top easel for written home work.

49. Which after school activity would be LEAST helpful for a 6-year-old child after discharge for treatment for spatial organization and motor planning difficulties:
A. ballet lessons.
B. karate classes.
C. gymnastics.
D. computer games.

50. As part of discharge planning, the COTA consults with the parents of a 9-year-old child with attention deficit disorder regarding modifications to make to his bedroom. In order to help him with self organization, the COTA would recommend:
A. providing open storage space for clothing and school supplies for easy access.
B. painting walls and furniture in bright colors to facilitate visual focus.
C. adding cabinets with labeled compartments to store items out of sight.
D. placing his bed on the floor for ease of transfer out of bed.

PHYSICAL DISABILITY QUESTIONS

Data Collection

Questions 51–54 pertain to this case study:

Mrs. S. has just been admitted to the rehabilitation unit following a RCVA which resulted in hemiplegia. The COTA has been assigned to administer parts of the initial evaluation.

51. The correct technique to use in assessing light touch sensation with Mrs. S. is:
A. test her affected extremity before the unaffected extremity.
B. demonstrate the procedure on her unaffected extremity, then occlude her vision.
C. demonstrate the procedure on her affected extremity, then establish rapport with her.
D. interview her and assess only the areas she reports are impaired.

52. The BEST evaluation for the COTA to administer to determine if Mrs. S. has unilateral neglect is:
A. six-block assembly.
B. line bisection.
C. proverb interpretation.
D. identification of the square in four overlapping figures.

53. During ADL evaluation, Mrs. S. demonstrates constructional apraxia, body scheme disturbances and unilateral neglect. Combined, these deficits may result in a self-care problem called:
A. spatial relations.
B. dressing apraxia.
C. anosagnosia.
D. figure-ground discrimination.

54. Observing Mrs. S. during the evaluation, the COTA notes that her right arm lays limply by her side. In documenting this observation, the COTA would use the term:
A. paralysis.
B. flaccidity.
C. subluxation.
D. spasticity.

55. The COTA is preparing to administer part of an evaluation to an individual whose diagnosis is cerebrovascular accident. The sensory portion of the test would be invalid for an individual with which one of the following impairments:
A. expressive aphasia.
B. receptive aphasia.
C. agnosia.
D. ataxia.

56. The instrument used to measure range of motion of the hand is a(n):
A. goniometer.
B. dynamometer.
C. pinch meter.
D. aesthesiometer.

57. The COTA is working on dressing skills during a home visit to a patient who has had a CVA. She observes that the patient has difficulty finding white socks on a bed with white sheets. She reports this as a deficit in:
A. figure-ground discrimination.
B. depth perception.
C. position in space.
D. topographical orientation.

58. During manual muscle testing of shoulder flexion, the individual is able to move the arm through the full range of motion but can tolerate only minimal resistance against gravity. The strength according to the manual muscle test (MMT) is:
A. fair minus.
B. fair.
C. fair plus.
D. good minus.

59. The correct position for measuring tip pinch is placing the thumb against the:
A. tip of the index finger.
B. side of the index finger.
C. tips of the index and middle fingers.
D. tips of all the fingers.

60. When conducting a structured interview with an individual, it is important for the COTA to:
A. add additional questions as indicated.
B. rephrase questions when the individual is unable to answer.
C. change the order in which the questions are asked.
D. ask the questions just as they are written.

Treatment Planning

Questions 61–63 pertain to this case study:

James is a 21-year-old man with complete T8 paraplegia resulting from a gunshot wound.

61. The COTA can predict that James will PROBABLY achieve the following level of independence in bathing, dressing and transfers:
A. Complete independence with self-care and transfers.
B. Independence with self-care and minimal assistance with transfers.
C. Minimal assistance with self-care and moderate assistance with transfers.
D. Dependence with both self-care and transfers.

62. The adaptive equipment the COTA will most likely need to provide James with upon discharge is:
A. reacher, sock aid, and dressing stick.
B. sock aid, dressing stick.
C. dressing stick.
D. no equipment.

63. To practice sliding board transfers with a James, the COTA must use a wheelchair with:
A. detachable footrests.
B. detachable arms.
C. antitip bars.
D. brake handle extensions.

64. The COTA is performing a home visit for an elderly man who lives alone. He exhibits severe hand weakness. When addressing safety in the home, the COTA will be most concerned with his ability to:
A. work locks and latches on doors and windows.
B. use built-up utensils while eating.
C. demonstrate energy conservation techniques.
D. manipulate fasteners on clothing for easy donning and doffing.

65. The COTA is beginning training in meal preparation with a 35-year-old homemaker following a TBI. The activity that should be introduced FIRST is:
A. making a peanut butter and jelly sandwich.
B. preparing a hot cup of tea with sugar.
C. pouring a glass of orange juice.
D. cooking a grilled ham and cheese sandwich.

66. The BEST candidate for a wrist driven flexor hinge splint is a(n):
A. artist with a C5 spinal cord injury
B. teacher with a C7 spinal cord injury
C. student with a T2 spinal cord injury
D. computer programmer with a T10 spinal cord injury

67. A COTA is working with a man in a work hardening setting. His program is most likely to include:
A. recreational activities.
B. pain management techniques.
C. driver reeducation.
D. joint protection techniques.

68. Which of the following would be MOST difficult for an individual with limited shoulder abduction and external rotation when doing macramé?
A. Working with short cords.
B. Working with long cords.
C. Working with fine cords.
D. Working with thick cords.

69. A COTA is working on keyboarding activities with a man with asymmetrical muscle tone who keeps falling to the side while sitting in his wheelchair. The wheelchair adaptation that would BEST stabilize his upper body in a midline position would be a(n):
A. reclining wheelchair.
B. arm trough.
C. lateral trunk support.
D. lateral pelvic support.

70. A flight attendant with a back injury is participating in a work hardening program. She demonstrates that she can successfully simulate distributing magazines to all passengers in a plane using proper body mechanics. To gradually upgrade her program, the NEXT activity the COTA would ask her to perform is to simulate:
A. putting blankets in the overhead compartments.
B. distributing meals to the passengers.
C. distributing magazines to half of the passengers in the plane.
D. putting luggage in the overhead compartments.

71. A woman who is s/p hip arthroplasty needs to be independent in kitchen activities. Initially, she is only able to prepare a peanut butter and jelly sandwich. The appropriate grading sequence would be:
A. prepare a tossed salad, make garlic bread, make spaghetti sauce and meatballs.
B. prepare a can of soup, make a grilled cheese sandwich, make instant pudding.
C. broil a steak, bake a potato, steam asparagus.
D. scramble eggs, toast bread, prepare a bowl of cereal and milk.

72. Agatha is an older adult with diabetes, poor vision, and peripheral neuropathy. She has difficulty identifying each of her medications. The BEST adaptation for the COTA to provide to Agatha is:
A. Braille labels.
B. white print on black background labels.
C. a pill organizer box.
D. brightly colored pills, each type of medication a different color.

Treatment Implementation

73. Inga is a 19-year-old woman with quadriplegia. She works with the COTA each morning for ADL training. The first day the COTA works with her on arranging the shirt on her lap. When this is mastered, they work on sliding her arms into the sleeves and pushing the shirt up past her elbows. When this is mastered, they will work on gathering the shirt up at the collar and pulling it on over her head. This technique is known as:
A. repetition.
B. cueing.
C. rehearsal.
D. chaining.

74. The best method of compensation for both unilateral neglect and absence of sensation in an upper extremity is to:
A. avoid using sharp tools or scissors and to avoid extreme water temperature.
B. wear noisy bracelets on the wrist or ankle as a reminder to visually scan toward the affected side.
C. use an electric shaver.
D. cue the individual to look to the involved side,

75. The COTA is working with an individual on writing skills. He instructs the individual to stabilize her forearm on the table when writing because she demonstrates:
A. decreased vision.
B. poor endurance.
C. limited fine movement.
D. incoordination.

76. The COTA is working on transfer training activities with a woman with hemiplegia and her family. The COTA will teach them to perform transfers:
A. only to her unaffected side of the body.
B. only to her affected side of the body.
C. to both sides of her body.
D. only to the side from which the commode will be approached.

77. When a patient returns for a follow-up visit one week after receiving a resting hand splint, he complains that perspiration is causing his thermoplastic splint to be uncomfortable. The BEST action for the COTA to take is to:
A. recommend putting talcum powder in the splint.
B. line the splint with moleskin.
C. fabricate a new resting hand splint using perforated material.
D. provide a stockinette for him to wear inside the splint.

78. A COTA is providing caregiver training to the husband of an elderly woman with Alzheimer's disease who has difficulty following multiple step instructions. The BEST method for the COTA to advise the husband to use when giving his wife instructions is:
A. give one or two step instructions and repeat frequently.
B. give three step instructions and use gestures to demonstrate.
C. write down any instructions that are over three steps for her to read as needed.
D. have her repeat all instructions after the therapist gives them.

79. While in occupational therapy, an individual with C6 quadriplegia complains of a headache, chills, and sweating. The COTA should immediately:
A. tip the individual's chair backwards to increase his/her blood pressure.
B. take the individual's heart rate and blood pressure.
C. give the individual fruit juice to increase his blood sugar levels.
D. unclamp the individual's catheter and tap over the bladder.

80. The occupational therapist is training an individual in the principles of joint protection prior to discharge. These principles would include:
A. using the strongest joint, avoiding positions of deformity, and ensuring correct patterns of movement.
B. massaging a joint before exercise.
C. practicing vivid imagery/relaxation exercises during difficult functional activities.
D. application of heat before and application of cold after range of motion.

81. A COTA is instructing an individual with left hemiplegia how to remove a tee-shirt. The correct sequence would be:
A. (1) remove shirt from unaffected arm; (2) remove shirt from affected arm; (3) gather shirt up at the back of the neck; (4) pull gathered back fabric off over head.
B. (1) remove shirt from affected arm; (2) remove shirt from unaffected arm; (3) gather shirt up at the back of the neck; (4) pull gathered back fabric off over head.
C. (1) gather shirt up at the back of the neck; (2) pull gathered back fabric off over head; (3) remove shirt from affected arm; (4) remove shirt from unaffected arm.
D. (1) gather shirt up at the back of the neck; (2) pull gathered back fabric off over head; (3) remove shirt from unaffected arm; (4) remove shirt from affected arm.

82. Mr. G. has Parkinson's disease and is at risk for aspiration. When instructing his caregivers in proper positioning during feeding, the COTA should recommend:
A. feeding Mr. G. in bed in a supine position.
B. seating Mr. G. upright on a firm surface with his chin slightly tucked.
C. positioning Mr. G. in a semi-reclined position in a reclining chair.
D. feeding Mr. G. in bed in a side-lying position.

83. The BEST cup to use with an individual who tends to drink too quickly is a:
A. vacuum feeding cup.
B. Nosey Cup (cut out for nose).
C. mug with two handles.
D. cup with a large drinking spout.

84. A COTA has provided a Nosey Cup to an individual with dysphagia. She explains to family members that the purpose of the cut-out in the Nosey Cup is to:
A. slow the drinking process.

B. allow the chin to remain tucked when drinking.
C. allow the caregiver to control the flow of liquid.
D. minimize biting reflexes when the cup is placed in the mouth.

85. Sharon, a young woman with MS, is about to be discharged to home. She is independent in tub transfers using a grab bar. The MOST important recommendation for the COTA to give Sharon regarding bathing is to:
A. use cool water temperature.
B. use moderate water temperature.
C. take baths; avoid showers.
D. shower; avoid baths.

Evaluating the Treatment Plan

Questions 86–88 pertain to this case study:

Mr. G. is an elderly man hospitalized following a CVA. He exhibits decreased sensation and flaccidity in the LUE and unilateral neglect. He lives alone and plans on returning home after discharge.

86. The COTA enters Mr. G's room to perform a bedside treatment for upper extremity PROM and notes marked pitting edema of the left hand. The FIRST thing the COTA should do is:
A. perform PROM, then position and elevate the affected extremity.
B. fabricate a resting splint for the affected extremity.
C. no action required at this time; wait for edema to subside.
D. have the individual attempt to squeeze a ball.

87. Mr. G. is beginning to experience sensory return in his left upper extremity. The COTA should recommend modifying the treatment plan to include:
A. remedial treatment, such as rubbing or stroking the involved extremity.
B. remedial treatment, such as the use of hot mitts to avoid burns.
C. compensatory treatment, such as testing bath water with the uninvolved extremity.
D. compensatory treatment, such as using a one-handed cutting board to avoid cutting the insensate hand.

88. The COTA is writing a progress note on Mr. G. using the SOAP note format. The statement that is an example of subjective information is:
A. The COTA will establish a daily self-feeding routine using verbal and physical cues to encourage Mr. G. to open containers on the lunch tray.
B. Mr. G. has been able to identify closed liquid beverage containers on the meal tray for four of six presentations.
C. Mr. G. is able to identify and drink liquids presented in cups without lids but leaves beverages in closed containers untouched.
D. Mr. G. asks for more beverages during meals, and appears surprised when the COTA indicates beverages in closed containers are on the meal tray.

89. The outcome that should be expected after an individual has implemented an energy conservation program is the ability to:
A. get dressed without becoming fatigued.
B. lift heavy cookware without pain.
C. do handicrafts without damaging joints.
D. dust and vacuum more quickly.

90. Ivan is a 60-year-old man who has experienced an MI. He is generally deconditioned and fatigues easily. A long-term goal is to be able to dress independently applying energy conservation techniques. He has achieved the short-term goal of completing upper extremity dressing independently. Which statement is the BEST example of a revised short-term goal?
A. "Pt. will demonstrate energy conservation techniques during performance of all ADLs."
B. "Pt. will perform lower extremity dressing with assistance for shoes and socks."
C. "Pt. will perform lower extremity dressing with verbal cueing 50% of the time for energy conservation techniques."
D. "Instruct patient in the use of energy conservation techniques that apply to dressing."

91. Jaime is s/p TBI and demonstrates deficits in sequencing and problem solving, among other things. She has successfully prepared a cold meal. The NEXT meal preparation activity the COTA should plan for Jaime is preparing:
A. a fruit salad.
B. instant soup.
C. a casserole.
D. a spaghetti dinner with salad and garlic bread.

92. Claudia's weight has changed and her wheelchair seat is now 2.5 inches wider than her hips on each side. What should the COTA recommend regarding wheelchair fit?
A. Obtain a wider wheelchair because this one is too narrow.
B. The patient should lose weight.
C. The sides of the chair should be padded to improve the fit.
D. Obtain a narrower wheelchair, because this one is too wide.

93. An individual has demonstrated competence in heating canned soup. The COTA recommends to the supervising OTR modifying the treatment plan and upgrading the cooking activity to:
A. baking brownies.
B. making an apple pie.

C. making toast.
D. making a fresh fruit salad.

Discharge Planning

94. During a home visit for an individual about to be discharged, the family asks the COTA about building a ramp to the front door. The proper grade for the ramp is:
A. one inch of ramp for every foot of rise in height.
B. one foot of ramp for every inch of rise in height.
C. ten inches of ramp length for every two inches in height.
D. one foot of ramp for every foot of rise in height.

95. An individual who is being discharged home after participating in an inpatient pulmonary rehabilitation program for chronic obstructive pulmonary disease (COPD) is given a list of "tips" to use in the home to promote function. Which one of the following items is most likely to be on the list?
A. Perform pursed lip breathing when performing activities.
B. Use a long-handled sponge while in the shower.
C. Take hot showers to reduce congestion.
D. Perform UE exercises to prevent deconditioning, avoiding overhead movements with the UEs.

96. An individual with a high level spinal cord injury is returning home. What type of adaptive technology would the individual need to ensure safety?
A. An environmental control unit.
B. A call system for emergency/nonemergency use.
C. A remote control power door opener.
D. An electric page turner.

97. A man who has a fractured radial head has his arm immobilized by a cast from above the elbow to below the wrist. He wants to maintain his strength in the elbow and forearm muscles of the affected arm after discharge, and has asked the COTA for some exercises. The COTA instructs him in performing:
A. isometric exercises.
B. isotonic exercises.
C. progressive resistive exercises.
D. passive exercises.

98. Kathleen is about to be discharged from occupational therapy following rehabilitation for a hand injury. She has not been able to work for 3 months, and remains unable to perform her job as a sales manager in a clothing store. What should the OTR/COTA team recommend concerning occupational therapy services?
A. Kathleen should continue to perform her home program.
B. Home health OT.
C. A work hardening program.
D. Discontinuation of OT services.

99. Bunny uses a wheelchair and requires minimal assistance with transfers and basic ADLs. She is expected to remain at this functional level. The most appropriate community living option for her would be a(n):
A. cradle-to-grave home.
B. transitional living center.
C. adult day program.
D. clustered independent living arrangement.

100. Which of the following is the BEST example of the "Plan" section of a discharge summary using a SOAP note format?
A. "Pt. reports he will continue to practice proper body mechanics at work."
B. "Pt. demonstrates independence in his home exercise program."
C. "Pt. has expressed his desire to return to work but does not yet demonstrate the capacity for sitting tolerance required."
D. "Pt. has been provided with a lumbar support and a written copy of his home program."

PSYCHOSOCIAL QUESTIONS

Data Collection

101. The COTA is participating in an evaluation of an older adult in the early stage of Alzheimer's Disease. The functional deficit most likely to be evident is:
A. aphasia
B. incontinence.
C. memory impairment
D. inability to dress and undress.

102. The most appropriate ADL assessment instrument for an adult in an acute care psychosocial setting is the:
A. Kohlman Evaluation of Living Skills (KELS).
B. Milwaukee Evaluation of Daily Living Skills (MEDLS).
C. Occupational History Interview
D. Routine Task Inventory

103. The COTA asks an individual to repeat a list of random numbers one minute after hearing the list. This would be accurately documented as which performance component?
A. Short term memory.
B. Attention.
C. Hearing.
D. Orientation.

104. The COTA is reviewing the history of a new patient, an elderly man in the early stages of Alzheimer's Disease. The COTA is most likely to encounter a report of:
A. difficulty swallowing food.
B. forgetting to turn the stove burner off.
C. angry outbursts at close family members.
D. restless pacing around the house.

105. The COTA is collecting information from a new patient's chart. The psychiatrist has written "observe for side effects with current course of anti-anxiety medications." The side effect the COTA is most likely see is:
A. akathesia.
B. confusion.
C. extrapyramidal syndrome (EPS).
D. tardive dyskinesia.

106. The COTA has been assigned to conduct a structured interview. When doing this type of interview it is important for the COTA to:
A. rephrase the written questions in her own words.
B. ask questions that she thinks are pertinent to this patient.
C. ask the questions as they are stated on the interview sheet.
D. ask additional questions, other than those listed, to gain further insight into the patient.

107. The COTA has been asked to conduct a structured assessment that will provide information about the patient's body concept. The best evaluation for the COTA to use is the:
A. Kinetic Self-Image.
B. Person-Symbol Assessment.
C. House-Tree-Person.
D. Kinetic Family.

108. The COTA's contribution to an initial note should include:
A. the treatment and changes in the patient's condition.
B. the source of referral, reason for referral, and the date referral was received.
C. a summary and analysis of the patient's assets and deficits.
D. the projected outcome of treatment.

109. Which of the following is the BEST example of a measurable statement of a patient's attendance in OT?
A. The patient frequently attends occupational therapy.
B. The patient attended 4 out of 5 OT sessions during a 1-week period.
C. The patient attended OT once since the initial session.
D. The patient likes to attend OT, as indicated by consistent attendance.

110. The instrument that would be best for recording observations about a client's task and interpersonal behaviors and how these behaviors remained stable or changed for 15 sessions is the:
A. Routine Task Inventory (RTI)
B. Comprehensive Occupational Therapy Evaluation Scale (COTE)
C. NPI Interest Inventory
D. Weekly SOAP progress notes

Treatment Planning

111. The performance components that are particularly important to consider when analyzing activities for use with adults with psychosocial problems are:
A. amount of self-control demands, time management demands, self-expression opportunities, and interest in the activity.
B. age appropriateness, prehension patterns required, presence of small pieces that could be mistakenly swallowed.
C. tactile, kinesthetic, visual, and olfactory properties.
D. space requirements, equipment and supply needs, cost, and safety considerations.

112. The COTA is working with a woman who has difficulty being assertive. The MOST appropriate activity for learning and developing assertiveness skills is:
A. record in a diary or log book interactions during which she was passive.
B. role play assertiveness skills in simulated situations proposed by the COTA.
C. apply the problem solving process to her nonassertive behaviors under the guidance of the COTA.
D. imitate the COTA demonstrating the techniques of "broken-record" and "I statements".

113. The COTA is planning a food preparation activity for a 68-year-old woman with major depression. It is important to select a simple activity that will result in a successful experience. The SIMPLEST activity would be preparing:
A. a can of soup.
B. a casserole.
C. brownies from a box mix.
D. a meal with two side dishes and an entree.

114. In carrying out inpatient treatment groups for individuals with schizophrenia, the COTA should routinely:
A. use projective media such as clay to facilitate expression of feelings.
B. allow individuals to work in isolated areas away from the group.
C. use simple, highly structured activities.
D. discuss the individuals' delusions with them.

115. The primary purpose of therapeutic group is to:
A. decrease the sense of alienation among group members.
B. bring about change among the members.
C. enable members to experience several points of view.
D. decrease costs in the health care setting.

116. The COTA is planning a community-living program for patients who are to be discharged following an average of 25–30 years of hospitalization. One of the goals of this program is to train the patients to manage their money. Which of the following activities should be INITIALLY used to address this goal?
A. Providing each patient with 25 dollars to spend during a group trip to the local shopping center.
B. Providing samples of coins and paper money.
C. Using a board game to introduce the concept of receiving and spending money.
D. Establishing a hospital based community store where the patients could buy clothing.

117. The COTA has been asked to develop a program of self-awareness activities for a group of substance abusers. A graded program to develop an individual's self-awareness must include activities that:
A. encourage self-awareness.
B. are structured by the COTA to encourage self-awareness and feedback.
C. provide opportunities for the patient to be self-aware.
D. allow for increasing social interaction.

118. The COTA is working with a 20-year-old man diagnosed with schizophrenia. He states that his main goal is to "have a girlfriend." The most appropriate short-term goal is:
A. The client will find a job and move into his own apartment within 8 months.
B. The client will identify the ways in which his disability has interfered with his thinking processes following each group session.
C. The client will initiate appropriate, casual greetings when beginning casual conversations with female staff.
D. During a conversation with a female group member, the client will make eye contact for 8 to 10 second periods two times in each ½ hour socialization group.

119. The COTA read a goal written by the OTR which stated, "The client will identify two strengths and one limitation about his performance at the close of each group". This goal addresses the component of occupational performance referred to as:
A. termination of activity.
B. intrinsic values.
C. self concept.
D. self expression.

120. The COTA is planning a group where he will involve group members in a game of chance. The only game listed that is a game of chance is:
A. baseball card collecting.
B. bingo.
C. charades.
D. balloon volleyball.

121. The BEST approach to use for encouraging problem solving in a craft media group is to:
A. begin with activities that have obvious solutions and high probability of success, then gradually increase the complexity.
B. begin with activities that require gross motor responses and progress to activities that require fine motor responses.
C. structure the number and kinds of choices available.
D. gradually increase the time used in the activity by 15 minute increments.

122. The COTA is working with an adult with schizophrenia who has tactile defensiveness. The aspect of ceramics that would be MOST intolerable for this client would be:
A. wedging the clay.
B. imprinting a design using a rolling pin.
C. glazing.
D. firing.

Treatment Implementation

123. The most common feature of occupational therapy task groups is that:
A. group members work independently, developing skills such as attending to a task, using tools safely and without waste, and recognizing errors and problems.
B. they simulate a work environment, and group members actually produce a product or service.
C. they prepare low functioning individuals to function in groups that require a higher level of social interaction.
D. they focus on the effects of stress, stress analysis, and stress management.

124. The COTA is leading a stress management group which includes a woman who is schizophrenic and actively hallucinating. The following stress management technique is CONTRAINDICATED for this individual:
A. aerobic exercise.
B. communication skill training.
C. mental imagery.
D. deep breathing.

125. An individual who is HIV-positive cuts his finger while working on a copper tooling project. According to universal precautions, the COTA should:

A. throw the piece of copper tooling into the trash can and get the individual a new piece of copper to use.
B. get out the clinic's first aid kit and put a band-aid on the individual's cut finger.
C. locate a puncture resistant container that the copper piece could be placed into before disposing of it.
D. wipe up any blood that is on the countertop with a paper towel.

126. A COTA is running an ongoing group for assertiveness training. The element MOST helpful in developing group cohesion would be for the COTA to:
A. provide the group with definitions of assertiveness, passivity, and aggression.
B. allow and encourage all group members to physically and verbally release their aggressive feelings towards inanimate objects.
C. demonstrate common assertiveness techniques to the group members.
D. encourage group members to share similar situations and reactions with one another.

127. The COTA is working on a copper tooling project with an individual on an inpatient psychiatric setting who is HIV positive. While placing the piece of copper over the template, the patient cuts his finger on the edge of the copper. The COTA should immediately follow:
A. suicidal precautions.
B. universal precautions.
C. escape from unit precautions.
D. medical precautions.

Questions 128–131 pertain to the following case study:

Miriam, a married 33-year-old mother of two children, ages 14 and 12, was admitted to the acute care mental health unit after several months of depression, withdrawal and refusal to leave her home. This is her first hospitalization. She was referred to occupational therapy for general evaluation of task skills and a stress assessment. Evaluations revealed that Miriam frequently experiences severe stress and depression occasioned by frustration at being alone most of the week while her husband travels for his business. Miriam feels she has no real accomplishments, sees herself as unattractive, and is afraid to leave her home. Just prior to admission she was unable to perform basic daily living skills. Goals for treatment include: identifying, expressing and gratifying personal needs, developing self-awareness as pertains to personal need fulfillment, and effective stress management.

128. Which activity would be MOST effective in initiating self-awareness:
A. designing a craft activity for her husband.
B. designing a craft activity for her children.
C. magazine collage focusing on "who am I".
D. parenting group on how to be a better parent.

129. Miriam's collage was filled with pictures and words depicting anger and sadness. When Miriam finished the collage, she began to cry and said to the COTA, "I didn't realize how much anger I had in me, I'm frightened. Tell me what I should do." The appropriate response would be:
A. "We'll give you an activity to do so you can get the anger out."
B. "We have many different discussion groups and activities for dealing with anger. I'll get you a list of the groups and the times they meet. You can choose the one that interests you."
C. "With your permission, I would like to share with my supervisor the concerns you have, and together we can explore which groups and activities would be beneficial for you."
D. "I should tell your doctor about this immediately."

130. The group that would be most beneficial for Miriam to address the goal of identifying and expressing personal needs and developing effective stress management techniques would include:
A. older women who can share experiences on how they handled similar problems in their pasts.
B. woman between the ages of 28 and 40, who are experiencing stress related symptoms.
C. men between the ages of 45 and 55, who are experiencing stress related symptoms.
D. individuals with post traumatic stress syndrome secondary to sexual abuse.

131. Miriam is participating in a focus group to explore methods of identifying and expressing anger. The LEAST appropriate activity for this group would be:
A. role playing exercises.
B. designing papier mache masks.
C. paint-by-number.
D. journal writing.

132. The COTA is working with a 75-year-old woman diagnosed with an organic mental disorder, admitted after accidentally setting fire to her kitchen. The MOST appropriate approach to use with her in addressing homemaking skills would be:
A. teach her how to safely use kitchen appliances.
B. instruct her in organizational time management skills so that she is able to shop for and prepare 2-3 meals a day for herself.
C. discuss with her using a meals-on-wheels service.
D. emphasize the need for her to resume her previous life roles, such as that of independent homemaker.

133. The COTA uses a variety of sensory integration activities, such as rolling in a parachute, swimming, and tossing a ball into a hoop with an

adult client diagnosed with schizophrenia. This type of intervention is best described as:
A. habilitation.
B. rehabilitation.
C. maintenance of function.
D. functional restoration or treatment.

134. A COTA is working on morning ADLs with a man who is s/p TBI. He requires prompting to apply shaving cream to his face and to pick up the razor. He is then able to complete the activity without further prompting. This would be documented as a deficit in which performance component?
A. Impulsivity.
B. Initiation.
C. Memory.
D. Attention.

135. Jose, diagnosed with schizophrenia, is taking a neuroleptic medication to control hallucinations. While in the hospital, he experienced postural hypotension as a side effect to the medication. It is MOST important prior to discharge to advise Jose:
A. to keep time in the sun as brief as possible.
B. to avoid use of power tools and sharp instruments.
C. to get up slowly from a standing, sitting or lying position.
D. about the dehydrating effects of caffeinated drinks and alcohol.

Evaluating the Treatment Plan

136. The COTA is writing a progress note in the chart of an elderly man with dementia. This facility uses the SOAP note format. The statement that is an example of subjective information is:
A. The COTA will establish a daily self-feeding routine using verbal and physical cues to encourage the patient to open containers on the lunch tray.
B. The patient has been able to identify closed liquid beverage containers on the meal tray for 4 of 6 presentations.
C. The patient is able to identify and drink liquids presented in cups without lids, but leaves beverages in closed containers untouched.
D. The patient asks for more beverages during meals, and appears surprised when the COTA indicates beverages in closed containers are on the meal tray."

137. Magdelena has difficulty attending to tasks. The COTA should recommend to the supervising OTR that OT services be discontinued when:
A. her goals have been met, and she can no longer benefit from OT services.
B. her goals have not been met, but she could benefit from continued services.
C. her goals have been met, but she could benefit from continued services.
D. Magdelena feels that she has not made gains despite objective measures to the contrary.

138. A client's initial short-term goal for improving social conversation with peers was: "Client will initiate two requests to other group members for sharing or using group materials within a one week period." When the client was unable to meet this goal, the COTA recommended a change in the treatment plan to the OTR. The best recommendation would be:
A. "Client will initiate two requests to other group members for sharing or using group materials within a two week period."
B. "Client will initiate one request to one other group member for sharing or using group materials within a one week period."
C. "Client will initiate two requests to each of the five group members for sharing or using one group tool within two weeks."
D. Client will say hello to group leader at start of each group session."

139. Rosa is a factory worker participating in a stress management group. The expected outcome is that Rosa will improve her ability to:
A. get through a job performance appraisal.
B. get to work on time.
C. set limits with her employer.
D. resolve conflicts with coworkers.

140. Ralph is a sales executive and the emphasis of his program is on time management skills. An expected outcome would be for Ralph to improve his ability to:
A. control anxiety when he arrives late for a meeting.
B. take responsibility for his actions when he is late with reports.
C. cope with feelings of inadequacy when he misses a deadline.
D. arrive at work on time on a consistent basis.

141. "The patient has taken a more active role in the task group, as evidenced by her willingness to contribute ideas and offer to assist in designing the unit mural." This is an example of which portion of the SOAP note?
A. Subjective.
B. Objective.
C. Assessment.
D. Plan.

142. The COTA is working with a man with impaired memory. When he is unable to follow verbal instructions, the COTA contemplates the individual's strengths and weaknesses, goals, and alternative methods for reaching those goals. This is an example of:
A. activity analysis.

B. activity adaptation.
C. grading the activity.
D. clinical reasoning.

143. Zack's goals are related to increasing his attention span. The COTA frequently observes him watching the person next to him at the work table. The COTA discusses this difficulty with the treatment team and accurately describes Zack's problem as:
A. inattention.
B. alertness.
C. memory impairment.
D. distractibility.

Discharge Planning

144. The MOST important action for the COTA to take when preparing for the discharge of a patient with an eating disorder is:
A. suggesting the patient return to the facility to attend Overeater's Anonymous meetings.
B. referring the patient for family therapy.
C. adapting the kitchen area of the individual's residence to decrease binge eating.
D. referring the patient to a program that helps individuals get and maintain appropriate jobs.

145. The following treatment program format emphasizes discharge planning for individuals with mental health problems:
A. Club house.
B. Community mental health center.
C. Acute care hospitalization.
D. Quarterway house.

146. The COTA is considering possible topics for a discharge planning group for individuals treated in an inpatient psychiatric unit. The MOST important topic to address, because of its significance in reducing rehospitalization, is:
A. managing family conflicts.
B. living skills needed for keeping after-care appointments.
C. coping strategies for continuing medication compliance.
D. education about problems with alcohol and substance use.

147. The COTA is working in an acute care inpatient psychiatric facility. The FIRST step in planning for the discharge of a socially isolated individual is to:
A. provide for a community reentry activities to introduce the individual to community resources to use after discharge.
B. evaluate the individual's occupational performance.
C. educate the family about the individual's ability to return home.
D. make a referral to an outpatient socialization program.

148. The COTA is a member of a treatment team reviewing treatment options for an individual who is experiencing acute psychiatric symptoms but is not suicidal. This individual has been living with family members. The BEST treatment environment for this individual to receive occupational therapy services would be:
A. partial hospitalization.
B. day care.
C. day treatment.
D. community mental health center.

149. A discharge summary note would include the following statement:
A. "The patient was referred for an assessment of leisure time skills."
B. "The patient continues to isolate himself from the group."
C. "The patient completed 10 out of 14 occupational therapy sessions during this 28-day hospitalization."
D. "The patient will voluntarily attend a social skills group two times within the next 5 days."

150. Which of the following would be included in a discharge summary:
A. "The patient has identified music as a major leisure interest. It is recommended that he explore the possibility of enrolling in a music study course at the community college."
B. "The patient will attend two leisure skills groups within the next five days."
C. "The patient has attended two leisure skills groups and has expressed an interest in joining a music group."
D. "The patient stated during the initial interview that he had no hobbies or interests other than work."

PROFESSIONAL PRACTICE QUESTIONS

Promote Professional Practice

151. After working for 1 year in a community mental health program, the COTA accepts a student for Level II fieldwork. As a fieldwork educator, the COTA is responsible for all of the following EXCEPT:
A. administrative and day-to-day supervision of the student program.
B. direct day-to-day supervision of students.
C. acting as a liaison between the academic setting, facility, and students.
D. establishing objectives for the fieldwork site.

152. The BEST description of the COTA's role with the parent of a pediatric client would be:
A. directive.

B. substitute parent.
C. partner.
D. expert.

153. The majority of occupational therapy practitioners working in mental health provide services to individuals with:
A. chronic mental illness.
B. substance abuse disorders.
C. mild mental retardation
D. eating disorders.

154. A COTA with 10 years of experience is working in a rehabilitation unit. This individual has refined her skills and is able to contribute knowledge to others as well as act a resource person. This person will most likely be functioning at a level of:
A. advanced, with general supervision.
B. intermediate, with routine or general supervision.
C. entry level, with close supervision.
D. advanced, with minimal supervision.

155. A COTA is preparing a 30-year-old man with paraplegia for discharge. She presents to him the rights of individuals with physical or mental disabilities concerning employment, housing, public accommodations, and transportation. The law guaranteeing these rights is the:
A. Architectural Barriers Act of 1969.
B. Federal Rehabilitation Act of 1973.
C. Fair Housing Amendment Act of 1988.
D. Americans with Disabilities Act of 1990.

156. National Board for Certification in Occupational Therapy (NBCOT) regulations and state licensure laws regulate the provision of occupational therapy services. The relationship between the two is such that:
A. state licensure laws supersede NBCOT regulations regarding the practice of occupational therapy.
B. NBCOT regulations supersede individual state licensure laws regarding the practice of occupational therapy.
C. NBCOT regulations and state licensure laws are viewed equally and enforced equally.
D. NBCOT regulations are recommended but are not enforceable. However, state licensure laws are enforceable.

157. According to the Occupational Therapy Code of Ethics, a COTA must maintain his/her credentials and participate in professional development and educational activities. The concept addressed by these requirements is:
A. beneficence.
B. duty.
C. justice.
D. veracity.

158. The COTA/OTR team is writing a monthly recertification for an outpatient. After reviewing the progress achieved over the past month, the COTA asks the patient about the goals she would like to achieve in the next month. The inclusion of the patient in the treatment planning and goal setting process is based on the principle of:
A. beneficence.
B. therapeutic privilege.
C. informed consent.
D. competence.

159. The occupational therapist has assessed an individual and developed a treatment plan that addresses functional deficits. Which of the following inpatient services can be billed as occupational therapy services for the client whose hospitalization is covered by Medicare?
A. Treatment from the OTR's plan provided by a COTA.
B. Treatment from the OTR's plan provided by a music therapist.
C. Treatment from the OTR's plan provided by a recreational therapist.
D. Treatment from the OTR's plan provided by an art therapist.

160. An OT supervisor observes a COTA in a local establishment listening to a band after work one day. The supervisor observes the COTA being intimate with a gentleman who is currently being treated on an outpatient basis by the COTA he is with. The response which is MOST consistent with the occupational therapy code of ethics is for the supervisor to:
A. indicate to the COTA that she may maintain the relationship as long as it does not impair the patient's treatment.
B. notify the state licensure board and terminate the employee.
C. notify the NBCOT of the situation and reassign the patient to a different OT practitioner.
D. discipline the employee and refer the patient to another outpatient center.

161. An important milestone in occupational therapy was the year the first assistant program opened. Many aides working in OT departments were grandfathered into the profession as a result of on-the-job training. These activities occurred in:
A. 1917.
B. 1949.
C. 1959.
D. 1981.

162. Occupational therapy assistants must provide information to support their qualifications and authority to practice. The term which MOST accurately describes this process is:
A. credentialing.
B. licensure.

C. certification.
D. registration.

163. A newly graduated COTA and an OTR have been hired as part of a treatment team on an inpatient rehabilitation unit. The entire rehabilitation team includes a physician, a physical therapist, a rehab nurse, a therapeutic recreation specialist and a neuro-psychologist. A patient has just been admitted to the rehabilitation unit with a primary diagnosis of complicated hip fracture and a secondary diagnosis of rheumatoid arthritis. For assessment purposes, the MOST appropriate role delineation would be for the COTA to assess:
A. weight bearing status for ADLs, and the OTR to assess cognition.
B. cognition, and the OTR to assess weight bearing status for ADLs.
C. dynametric grip strength, and the OTR to assess weight bearing status for ADLs.
D. leisure interest, and the OTR to assess weight bearing status for ADLs.

164. The treatment plan for the individual mentioned in the previous question includes splinting, isometric strengthening, paraffin treatments, and home evaluation. The most appropriate intervention for the newly graduated COTA to independently provide is:
A. splinting.
B. paraffin treatment.
C. home evaluation.
D. isometric exercises.

165. A newly graduated occupational therapy assistant is seeking to be licensed and credentialed. The relationship between these two processes is that:
A. the credentialing process is necessary after licensing.
B. licensing is necessary before the candidate may be credentialed.
C. credentialing and licensing are not dependent on each other.
D. the credentialing process is necessary prior to licensing.

166. When there is not a referral for occupational therapy services, it is important for the COTA involved in the provision of services to know that:
A. the OTR is operating outside the scope of practice and regulating agencies should be notified.
B. the OTR must assume responsibility for all occupational therapy services delivered.
C. a written letter of consent must be received from the patient or a significant other.
D. the COTA should seek a referral from the patient's family physician.

167. The hospital photographer wishes to include, in a marketing brochure, a photograph of an individual participating in occupational therapy. Which information would need to be obtained prior to the photography session?
A. The correct spelling of the COTA's and the individual's names for the photograph caption.
B. The individual's written consent to take the photograph.
C. The COTA's written consent to take the photograph.
D. The correct spelling of the individual's diagnosis and name, for the photograph caption.

168. Current trends in American society reveal that use of COTAs will:
A. expand in long-term care facilities and elder care.
B. decrease in provision of home health services.
C. decrease in need for services for the elderly.
D. decline in non-traditional settings.

169. A COTA desires to work on a plan to promote her own clinical growth. The MOST effective way to accomplish this is to:
A. annually develop a plan for professional development.
B. become involved in state and national activities.
C. develop a mentoring relationship with an OT practitioner with a special skill or experience that the COTA wants to become more knowledgeable about.
D. select a workshop regarding a strong area of interest.

170. A staff COTA recognizes a COTA who is applying for a position in the OT department from when they were in school together. The COTA recalls that the applicant failed a Level II fieldwork experience. The applicant is a weak candidate, and the COTA doesn't think she would make a strong contribution to the department. Which of the following actions would be unethical?
A. Call the applicant's previous employer for a reference.
B. Mention the fact that the applicant failed a level II fieldwork when the staff gets together to discuss the applicants.
C. Voice feelings concerning the applicant's weaknesses when the staff gets together to discuss the applicants.
D. Ask the applicant for a resume.

171. A new COTA works in a busy rehabilitation department. Half of the department's OT staff is out with the flu, including her supervisor. The COTA observes an aide carrying out a morning ADL session with the patient who is scheduled for discharge the next day. The most responsible action for the COTA to take is to:
A. allow the aide to finish so the patient will be prepared for discharge.
B. excuse the aide and complete the session herself.

C. bring the issue to the attention of the facility administrator.
D. discuss her concerns with an OTR who is present.

172. At what level should COTAs MINIMALLY participate in the research process?
A. COTAs are not required to participate in research.
B. COTAs should read, interpret and apply OT research.
C. COTAs should participate in the data collection process.
D. COTAs should contribute to the development of a research question.

173. A COTA witnesses an OT practitioner physically abusing a developmentally delayed child during an OT session. Believing that this practitioner should lose her license to practice, the COTA reports the practitioner's actions to the following body:
A. The state regulatory board.
B. AOTA.
C. NBCOT.
D. The local police.

174. The PRIMARY objective of fieldwork education is to:
A. provide students with the opportunity to apply knowledge learned in school to practice.
B. keep facilities abreast of new concepts and techniques.
C. provide additional personnel to facilities.
D. prepare students to work in traditional, not nontraditional, practice environments.

175. The association that guides research activities for the profession of occupational therapy is referred to as:
A. AOTA.
B NBCOT.
C. AOTF.
D. AOTCB.

176. Which statement is MOST descriptive of the status of occupational therapy practice in mental health?
A. There is an increasing shortage of occupational therapy practitioners in the area of mental health.
B. Occupational therapy services are not required services in most mental health settings.
C. Inpatient programs, more than community programs, are an area of future growth for occupational therapy practitioners in mental health.
D. The majority of occupational therapy practitioners practice in the area of mental health.

177. A COTA must demonstrate service competency in performing the manual muscle test before performing manual muscle testing on patients. One way for the COTA to demonstrate service competency is to:
A. consistently obtain the same results as a competent OT practitioner performing the same procedure.
B. pass the NBCOT exam.
C. attain a minimum number of continuing education credits related to manual muscle testing.
D. practice for a minimum of 1 year.

Support Service Management

178. The primary purpose of a quality assurance program is to:
A. examine the effectiveness of patient care.
B. determine the cost of running a department.
C. evaluate performance of therapy personnel.
D. maximize reimbursement.

179. A COTA job description will most likely contain:
A. the title of the job, past experience and job requirements.
B. a summary of primary job functions, references, and job requirements.
C. the organizational relationships, personality characteristics desired in a job candidate, and accomplishments of the candidate.
D. the title of the job, organizational relationships, essential job functions, and the job requirements.

180. After working at his first job for 3 months, the COTA meets with his supervisor for a performance appraisal. The primary purpose of this meeting is to:
A. objectively assess the COTA's performance.
B. document any disciplinary issues.
C. award a merit increase.
D. write yearly goals and objectives.

181. The owner of the out-patient facility where a COTA is employed announces that they are expecting a visit from an accrediting agency which surveys inpatient and comprehensive outpatient rehabilitation programs. The agency referred to is:
A. AOTA.
B. JCAHO.
C. CARF.
B. NBCOT.

182. A COTA is about to begin hand rehabilitation activities with a patient with an open wound on the dorsum of his hand. The most appropriate way for her to protect herself from blood borne pathogens is to:
A. wear a mask.
B. wear gloves.
C. refuse to work with the patient.
D. wash her hands prior to treating the patient.

183. A COTA beginning his first job receives close supervision from his OTR supervisor. This COTA has contact with his supervisor:
A. once a day.
B. every two weeks
C. once a month.
D. on an as needed basis.

184. An occupational therapy department in a pediatric setting is reviewing their sterilization policy which is based on universal precautions. The policy will MOST likely state that:
A. all equipment is to be sterilized annually.
B. any equipment which has come into contact with body fluids will be sterilized prior to using the equipment again.
C. all equipment is to be sterilized at the end of each day.
D. all equipment is to be sterilized after each use.

185. Medicare will reimburse for equipment issued by a COTA if it is essential for:
A. increasing functional independence.
B. medical necessity.
C. maintaining patient function.
D. reducing deformity.

186. A COTA works in a school based setting providing OT services to children with learning disabilities. His supervising OTR suddenly resigns. The most appropriate action for the COTA to take is to:
A. ask the PT, with whom he has worked for the past three years, to supervise him.
B. request supervision from the other COTA on site, who is an advanced level practitioner, until a new OTR is hired.
C. discontinue provision of OT services until appropriate supervision is available.
D. encourage the school to place an advertisement for a new OTR as quickly as possible. He would continue providing OT services to students without medical conditions until the new OTR arrives.

187. A physician's referral for occupational therapy services may be required by:
A. AOTA, federal, and state governmental agencies.
B. federal and state governmental agencies, and third-party payers.
C. third-party payers, individual facilities, and AOTA.
D. AOTA, third-party payers and state governmental agencies.

188. A COTA receives a referral for OT services for a school-aged child from the child's teacher. The FIRST step the COTA should take is:
A. screen the child for performance deficits.
B. request that the teacher ask a physician to make the referral.
C. explain to the child the purpose of occupational therapy.
D. notify the supervising OTR about the referral.

189. A COTA is responsible for supervising the department's two OT aides. The level of supervision required is:
A. routine supervision.
B. maximal supervision.
C. close supervision.
D. intense close supervision.

190. The most important barrier to infectious materials that COTAs should use while completing self-care bathing and dressing activities would be:
A. latex or vinyl gloves.
B. gown.
C. goggles.
D. face mask.

191. Referrals for occupational therapy services should include the patient's:
A. diagnosis.
B. deficits.
C. treatment plan.
D. discharge plan.

192. The supervisory process between a COTA and his/her OTR supervisor may best be described as a(n):
A. mutual process.
B. evaluative process.
C. counseling process.
D. learning process.

193. Emma was homebound following a stroke and has been receiving OT for self-care and home management training and PT for ambulation and stair training. Emma reported to the COTA on the last visit that she walked to the bus stop alone. This statement is significant in that it indicates that Emma:
A. is making progress toward her goals and home therapy should be continued.
B. has achieved her PT goals.
C. has achieved her OT goals.
D. is no longer homebound.

194. The COTA is filling out an incident report regarding a patient on her caseload. Which of the following scenarios would MOST likely be the incident that the therapist is reporting?
A. A patient complained of nausea during a standing activity.
B. A patient with a spinal cord injury indicated that his hand splints were uncomfortable.
C. A patient who had a total hip replacement did not follow precautions while completing dressing activities but did not complain of discomfort.
D. A patient with a diagnosis of CVA and left neglect caught the left arm in the wheel of the wheelchair, resulting in a cut and bruise.

195. A COTA working in a nursing home does not contribute to the initial evaluation, treatment plan, or reevaluation of residents. She feels she is competent to contribute to the evaluation and treatment planning processes, and is concerned that the OTR, who has never worked with a COTA before, is under-using her skills. The most responsible action for her to take is to:
A. resign from the job.
B. perform part of the initial evaluation and show her supervisor the results in order to demonstrate her competence.
C. discuss the problem with the OTR's administrative supervisor.
D. discuss her concerns with the OTR.

196. "Progress reports will be written on the designated progress report form. They will be placed in the 'Rehabilitation services' section of the patient chart. Notes by COTAs will be co-signed within 24 hours." These statements are an example of:
A. documentation.
B. a policy.
C. a procedure.
D. a job description.

197. The FIRST step in a safe wheelchair transfer is:
A. scoot forward to the front of the seat.
B. position foot plates in the "up" position.
C. swing away the leg rests.
D. lock the brakes.

198. The activity for which good ventilation is MOST important is:
A. painting with acrylic paints.
B. leather tooling.
C. painting ceramics.
D. copper tooling.

199. A COTA in a busy rehabilitation department assigns an aide to monitor a Medicare patient who is performing a food preparation activity. The COTA becomes involved in the treatment of another individual and does not return until the end of the session. Can the COTA bill for this session?
A. Yes, if the aide has been trained in the use of food preparation activities as treatment.
B. Yes, because services were initiated by the COTA.
C. No, because Medicare does not consider services provided by an aide skilled occupational therapy.
D. No, according to the OT Code of Ethics.

200. A federal and state program that funds healthcare for poor and indigent individuals is:
A. Medicare.
B. Medicaid.
C. Worker's Compensation.
D. Education for all Handicapped Children Act.

ANSWERS FOR SIMULATION EXAMINATION 3

1. (B) form constancy perception. Answer B is correct because form constancy refers to the ability to match similar shapes regardless of change in their orientation in space. Answer A is not correct because figure-ground perception refers to the ability to distinguish a form or shape against a distracting background. Answer C is not correct because visual sequencing requires the ability to copy the same sequence of shapes or objects presented to the child. Although the latter is required when stringing the geometric beads, the error described refers to a form constancy error. See reference: Kramer and Hinojosa (eds): Todd, VR: Visual perceptual frame of reference: An information processing approach.

2. (B) Moro. The Moro reflex is characterized by abduction, extension and external rotation of the arms. The rooting reflex involves turning the head toward tactile stimulation near the mouth. Flexor withdrawal reflex is characterized by flexion of an extremity in response to a painful stimulus. Neck righting reaction involves body alignment in rotation following turning of the head. Only the Moro reflex causes an extension movement. See reference: Hopkins and Smith (eds): Simon, CJ. and Daub, MM: Human development across the lifespan.

3. (B) follow test manual directions. When administering a standardized test, directions from the test manual should be followed closely to insure reliability of test results Test environments should *not* be stimulating, or the child may have difficulty concentrating. Test items should be presented to young children with the last item on the table so that the child can make the transition more easily. Although the overall success of an evaluation can depend on the therapist's ability to establish rapport with the child and the family, too much conversation with the child may be distracting and prevent optimal performance. See reference: Dunn, W: Cook, DG: The Assessment Process.

4. (C) social worker's notes. The social worker's notes will "include ... details about the patient's family and occupation, her education, cultural background, financial situation, and "habits." The nurse's notes (answer A) provide information about the patient's adjustment to hospitalization and ongoing functioning in the hospital. The doctor's notes (answer B) document changes in diagnosis or medication. The admitting note (answer D) includes data on circumstances of the hospital admission, tentative diagnosis and any known history. See reference: Early: Data gathering and evaluation.

5. (A) the mother's concerns and goals for her child. The caregiver's concerns are essential in planning effective intervention within the context of the family. Medical management (answer B), equipment needs (answer C) and the physical layout of the home (answer D) are important issues as well, but can be addressed later in relation to the primary concerns identified in the interview. See reference: Case-Smith, Allen, and Pratt (eds): Stewart, KB: Occupational therapy assessment in pediatrics.

6. (D) observes the child as he enters the clinic and takes off his coat and shoes. "In a naturalistic observation, the therapist gathers information in the typical or natural setting that the activity occurs." The most reliable information can be gained by observing the child as she normally does the activity; this is especially true of children with developmental delay who may have difficulty generalizing learning from one situation to another. Therefore, answer B may not provide a sample of the child's true skill level. Answers A and C describe situations in which the COTA is providing assistance, therefore not allowing the child to demonstrate her skill in independent dressing. See reference: Case-Smith, Allen, and Pratt (eds): Shepherd, J, Procter, SA, and Coley, IL: Self care and adaptations for independent living.

7. (A) use of time. By comparing interests and actual participation reported, the COTA may identify discrepancies between interests and actual play/leisure behavior. This can help address the client's use of time and facilitate temporal organization. Answers B, C, and D are not directly addressed using this method. See reference: Case-Smith, Allen, and Pratt (eds): Cronin, AS: Psychosocial and emotional domains of behavior.

8. (C) follow administration instructions and note changes in behavior. "The... characteristic of standardized tests is a fixed protocol for administration." While the tester may not deviate from the protocol, changes in behavior represent important test data and should be recorded. The responses described in answers A, B and D may make the test results invalid by altering the sequence of test items, the grouping of items, or the actual test item itself. These may not be changed unless it is specified in the test manual. See reference: Case-Smith, Allen, and Pratt (eds): Richardson, PK: Use of standardized tests in pediatric practice.

9. (B) objective signs and duration of the seizure. To assess the efficacy of antileptic medication, or during periods of gradual withdrawal, staff is often asked to monitor the child for seizure activity. Type and duration of seizures should be documented carefully. Observations about the child's position (answer A), responsiveness (answer B), and facial expression (answer D) are of somewhat less importance as isolated observations. See reference: Case-Smith, Allen, and Pratt (eds): Gordon, CY, Schanzenbacher, KE, Case-Smith, J, and Carrasco, R: Diagnostic problems in pediatrics.

10. (B) radial-digital grasp. A radial-digital grasp is developed at 9 months and is used for precision control. A pincer grasp (answer B), or tip pinch, is characterized "by opposition of the thumb and index finger tip so that a circle is formed. This pinch pattern is used to obtain small objects." The palmar grasp (answer C) is characterized by flexing digits around an object and stabilizing it against the palm. This is used as a power grip. In a lateral pinch (answer D), the pad of the thumb is placed against the radial side of the index finger near the DIP joint. This pattern is used as a power grip on small objects. See reference: Case-Smith, Allen, and Pratt (eds): Exner, CE: Development of hand skills.

11. (C) following directions about objects located in front, back, and to the side. Answer C is correct because difficulty with position in space refers to difficulty perceiving the relationship of an object to the self. Answers A and B are not correct because they refer to problems of form constancy. Answer D, making judgments about moving through space, is incorrect because it refers to a problem in perceiving spatial relationships. See reference: Case-Smith, Allen, and Pratt (eds): Schneck, CM: Visual perception.

12. (C) change to a power wheelchair to eliminate effort. Considering the progressive nature of the child's disease, as well as strength and endurance, the best recommendation would be to change to a power wheelchair. The child would be better able to participate in the cognitive tasks of school if mobility required less effort. Retaining the manual chair (answer A) would be counter-productive to functioning well at school, and strength will not be improved in a child with this condition. Answer B might make mobility a little easier, but would not solve the long-term problem of decreasing strength and endurance. Answer D would still make demands on strength and energy that would appear unwise considering the nature of Duchenne's dystrophy. The teams recommendation should also be integrated with the family's needs. See reference: Case-Smith, Allen, and Pratt (eds): Johnson, J: School-based occupational therapy.

13. (B) provision of foot support. This is probably the first concern of the therapist, in order for the child to feel secure on the toilet and to be positioned for bowel control. Answer A is not correct since management of fasteners can be developed later, after positioning for stability has been achieved. Answer C is not correct because provision of a seat belt may not be necessary if foot support (or back support) is provided. Answer D is not correct because climbing onto the toilet independently may be developed later (as it occurs with normal developmental progression). See reference: Case-Smith, Allen, and Pratt (eds): Shepherd, J, Procter, SA, and Coley, IL: Self care and adaptations for independent living.

14. (B) high contrast and defined borders. Answer B is correct because it provides the only combination of features when adapting visual material which will assist the child with visual discrimination problems. High contrast of the stimuli (shape, letter, numbers, etc.) in relation to the background, and defining important areas of the stimuli with a border will attract the eye and provide clear input. Answer A is incorrect because low contrast of the stimuli, such as blue ditto lettering, is difficult to discriminate. Answer D is incorrect because undefined borders around the important stimuli makes for less clear input. Answer D is incorrect because both features of the visual stimulus would make it difficulty to discriminate. See reference: Kramer and Hinojosa (eds): Todd, VR: Visual perceptual frame of reference: An information processing approach.

15. (C) interdisciplinary. An interdisciplinary team consists of professionals from various disciplines who collaborate with each other in planning and implementing services. While the goals are developed in collaboration, the actual intervention will be carried out individually, reflecting expertise from each discipline. Unidisciplinary (answer A) is incorrect, since more than one discipline is involved. The multidisciplinary approach (answer B) designates a team of professionals from different disciplines, who plan and carry out intervention with minimal integration across disciplines. In the transdisciplinary approach (answer D), team members from various disciplines interact closely with each other, with one member carrying out treatment and the others acting as consultants. This approach is often used in early intervention to cut down on the amount of professionals the family has to interact with. See reference: Case-Smith, Allen, and Pratt (eds): Stephens, LC and Tauber, SK: Early intervention.

16. (A) promote open-ended symbolic play, such as action figures, puppets, dolls. Toys that elicit feelings and expression can be used to promote beginning play skills and beginning interaction and communication skills. Inherent in open-ended play is the fact that there is no right or wrong way; that failure is not possible. Structured craft activities (answer B) do not provide sufficient opportunity for self expression, and carry the possibility of failure, since there is a right and wrong way to do them. A game of tag (answer C) may be perceived as threatening and overwhelming as an initial activity, especially if it involves peers. Activities that promote tension release (answer D) do not directly address play skills, but rather they focus on the powerful motor action only. See reference: Case-Smith, Allen, and Pratt (eds): Morrison, CD, Metzger, P, and Pratt, PN: Play.

17. (C) avoid resistive materials. Joint protection and energy conservation techniques should be used at all times. Activities involving the manipulation of highly resistive materials such as clay, leather, and copper sheets should be avoided; the pressure applied to the joints could exacerbate the condition. Light touch (answer A) should be avoided in the treatment of a child with tactile defensiveness. Rapid vestibular stimulation (answer B) is contraindicated for a child who is seizure prone. Elevated temperatures (answer D) should not be used for a client with multiple sclerosis, since it exacerbates the symptoms. See reference: Case-Smith, Allen, and Pratt (eds): Gordon, CY, Schanzenbacher, KE, Case-Smith, J, and Carrasco, R: Diagnostic problems in pediatrics.

18. (A) forming letters out of clay. Preschoolers learn best using a multisensory approach. The activity of making letters out of various materials such as clay, bread dough, chocolate pudding, or sand paper uses tactile, kinesthetic, and/or gustatory senses, in addition to the visual sense. In this way, new learning is reinforced through a variety of sensory channels. Flash cards (answer B), matching to a sample (answer C), and coloring (answer D) are methods that rely primarily on visual processing and cognitive skills, and can be used for the older child to strengthen existing skills. See reference: Case-Smith, Allen, and Pratt (eds): Schneck, CM: Visual perception.

19. (D) five out of five common objects, by feel only. "Identifying an object by touch is termed "stereognosis", or "identification of solids". Stereognosis is a relevant tactile discrimination skill needed for the development of fine hand manipulation. Answer A addresses localization of tactile stimuli, answer B, graphesthesia, and answer C tactile discrimination of textures. See reference: Case-Smith, Allen, and Pratt (eds): Exner, CE: Development of hand skills.

20. (A) improve posture, then improve shoulder stability, then improve grasp. Since proximal-to-distal refers to development from the center of the body outward to the extremities, answer A would be correct. Postural stability would be developed first, then shoulder stability, and lastly grasping patterns. Answers B, C, and D would not be correct since they do not follow this order. See reference: Case-Smith, Allen, and Pratt (eds): Exner, CE: Development of hand skills.

21. (D) a therapy ball to sit on during desk work. This answer is the only one that facilitates the development of postural background movement. This is done by requiring Haruka to continually adjust to the subtle movements of an usable surface on an ongoing basis. Answers A, B, and C provide additional external support, i.e. provide adaptations using a compensatory approach; they do not facilitate the development of new skills. See reference: Case-Smith, Allen, and Pratt (eds): Nichols, DS: The development of postural control.

22. (B) Use of a noise machine producing white noise at bedtime. For the child who is easily aroused, the use of constant, monotonous auditory input can be calming to the degree of inducing sleep. The other answers may actually increase arousal. Quick repetitive proprioceptive input as experienced when jumping on a trampoline (answer A) and light touch provided by a fuzzy blanket (answer B) are types of sensory input that have a direct arousing effect on the nervous system. Blocking out all light (answer D) may produce arousal as result of fear generated by total darkness. See reference: Case-Smith, Allen, and Pratt (eds): Cronin, AS: Psychosocial and emotional domains of behavior.

23. (B) can usually handle routine daily functions. Answer B is correct, because it describes the skills of an individual with moderate or trainable-level mental retardation. This child can usually complete activities of daily living, live in a group home setting, and do unskilled work in a sheltered workshop. Answer A describes a child with profound mental retardation. Answer C describes a child with severe mental retardation, and answer D describes a child who is educable or mildly mentally retarded. See reference: Case-Smith, Allen, and Pratt (eds): Gordon, CY, Schanzenbacher, KE, Case-Smith, J, and Carrasco, R: Diagnostic problems in pediatrics.

24. (B) Flex the child's hips and knees. Answer B is correct, because flexing the hips and knees prior to donning socks and shoes provides inhibition of ankle plantar flexion (which makes the task very difficult) through the key point of the hip. Answer A is not correct, because hip and knee extension is the position which already is contributing to the plantar flexion of the ankle and inhibition of plantar flexion could not occur. Answer C is not correct because the shoulder patterns may not influence the ankle patterns as significantly as hip and knee flexion and this is an extension pattern which could not be inhibitory to the abnormal ankle pattern interfering with dressing. Answer D is not correct primarily because the abnormal pattern at the ankle is usually influenced by inhibition from the key point of the hip. See reference: Case-Smith, Allen, and Pratt (eds): Hunter, JG: The neonatal intensive care unit.

25. (C) Stabilizing the pelvis/hips/legs. The correct answer is C because compensatory movements can occur because of a poor central base of support provided by the pelvis, hip, or legs. Answer A is not correct because the pelvis is not stabilized and arm movements may still be compromised. Answer B is not correct because use of a lap board or chair arms for weightbearing of the upper extremities will compromise the use of the arms and hands to stabilize the body. Answer D is not correct because the pelvis continues to be unstable, and provides a poor base for arm movements. See reference: Kramer and Hinojosa: Colangelo, CA: Biomechanical frame of reference.

26. (B) mounting a safety rail next to the toilet. To sit independently on the toilet and relax sufficiently to control muscles needed for elimination, the child has to feel posturally secure. Safety rails next to the toilet, low toilets that allow the child to put both feet on the ground, or reducer rings to decrease the size of a toilet seat, all serve to provide maximum stability for the child with an unstable posture. Answers A, C and D describe adaptations used for other deficits. Replacing zippers and buttons with Velcro closures (answer A) is helpful for a child with reduced strength or fine motor coordination. Introducing toilet paper tongs (answer C) helps increase reach in a child with limited range of motion. Placing a colorful target (answer D) helps little boys aim into the bowl, a difficulty associated with perceptual or cognitive limitations. See reference: Case-Smith, Allen, and Pratt (eds): Shepherd, J, Procter, SA, and Coley, IL: Self care and adaptations for independent living.

27. (C) impairment in response time. A child with delayed reactions could represent a danger to himself and others when operating a power driven wheelchair. Immediate reactions to environmental factors such as people crossing, steps, doorways etc. is a necessity for effective wheelchair use and the avoidance of accidents. Low muscle tone (answer A) is not a contraindication; an alert child with low tone can operate the chair using a low-resistance switch. The child with limited active movement (answer B) may operate the chair using a switch placed within his active movement range. The child with low frustration tolerance (answer D) may be trained to use the chair through carefully graded tasks of gradually increasing difficulty. See reference: Case-Smith, Allen, and Pratt (eds): Wright-Ott, C, and Egilson, S: Mobility.

28. (D) the child with spina bifida with LE paralysis. This child generally has sufficient UE coordination and strength to propel herself on a scooter while the LEs are supported. This child will also have the cognitive and sensory awareness to negotiate a scooter in its environment. Prone scooters may be contraindicated for children described in answers A, B and C. The child with cerebral palsy with predominant extensor tone (Answer A) may increase his abnormal tone through the neck hypertension needed to maintain the position on a scooter. The child with low tone, who is easily fatigued (answer B) may be unable to maintain this very exhausting position for any length of time and become even more fatigued. The child with cognitive limitations and poor sensory awareness (answer C) may injure herself on a scooter due to the possibility of running over her hands or bumping her head into obstacles without the sensory feedback needed and cognitive skills to avoid these situations. See reference: Case-Smith, Allen, and Pratt (eds): Wright-Ott, C, and Egilson, S: Mobility.

29. (B) corner chair with head support and padded abductor post. Answer B is correct because a corner chair provides hip/knee/ankle flexion of 90 degrees, and the abductor post will keep the legs separated when or if extensor tone increases. The corner shape of the chair facilitates shoulder protraction while preventing shoulder retraction, which can prevent a child's hands from coming forward to assist with eating. Placing the child in a standing or extended position (answer A) would not be correct. Answer C is not correct, because the supine position could encourage or facilitate extension. Answer D is not correct, because a child with poor head control and moderate extensor tone, would be unable to sit without support. See reference: Finnie, N: Baby carriages, strollers, and chairs.

30. (D) hips are secured against the back of the seat. The hips are one of the key points of control when positioning Julio. Positioning the hips securely against the back of the seat using a seat belt and/or abductor wedge at the correct angle will serve to break up the extensor pattern and facilitate the positioning of the other body parts (answers A, B and C), so that Julio can participate in family games. See reference: Case-Smith, Allen, and Pratt (eds): Wright-Ott, C, and Egilson, S: Mobility.

31. (D) cup with a spout. Cups with spouts are contraindicated for children with tongue thrust, since stimulation of the tip of the tongue may serve to increase abnormal movement. A cup with a lid (answer C) would be the cup of choice for a beginning drinker, since the small holes will allow for only a limited amount of liquid to be dispensed at a time. A cup with a lip (answer A) is helpful to stabilize lip and jaw while drinking. A cup with a weighted base (answer B) helps with a coordinated release of the cup onto the table surface. See reference: Case-Smith, Allen, and Pratt (eds): Case-Smith, J, and Humphry, R: Feeding and oral motor skills.

32. (C) Pin the Tail on the Donkey. For the defensive child, tactile stimuli may be perceived as extremely threatening if the child cannot anticipate them. Any game that requires blindfolds or other means of occluding vision, therefore, serves to heighten defensiveness and will interfere with Jennifer's socialization and participation in the game. Answers A, B and D are played using vision. While there may be touch involved, the stimulus can be anticipated and actively controlled by the child; therefore, Jennifer could participate more successfully. See reference: Case-Smith, Allen, and Pratt (eds): Parham, LD and Mailloux, Z: Sensory integration.

33. (A) swimming. Swimming provides active movement in large ranges with minimal impact on the joints. Sports mentioned in answers B, C, and D involve bouncing, jumping, and kicking, i.e. resistive motions which place the joints under additional stress. These activities would therefore be contraindicated. See reference: Logigian and Ward (eds): Erlandson, DM: Juvenile rheumatoid arthritis.

34. (B) has him practice tying shoes at home as well as at school. Children with mental retardation often have difficulty generalizing learning from one setting to another, e.g. if they learn to tie their shoes in the OT clinic, they will not be able to perform the same skill at home or at school. The ability to generalize is essential in making the new skill functional in Jeremy's daily life. Answers A, C and D are adaptations or teaching techniques, but do not address generalization. See reference: Logigian and Ward (eds): Ward, JD: Mental retardation.

35. (B) stressing bilateral activities incorporating the prosthesis. Bimanual activities for play, school, and self care should be emphasized to incorporate the prosthesis into the child's body image. Avoiding the use of the prosthesis as suggested in answers A, C and D is counterproductive. See reference: Case-Smith, Allen, and Pratt (eds): Gordon, CY, Schanzenbacher, KE, Case-Smith, J, and Carrasco, R: Diagnostic problems in pediatrics.

36. (A) Increase the height of the wedge (side A on diagram). Answer A is correct because by increasing the height of the wedge from the floor, less weight is born on the arms (which is a source of the heavy work involved in this position). Answer B is not correct, because decreasing the height of the wedge from the floor will increase weightbearing and thus increase the postural work involved in the prone position. Answers C and D are not correct, because shortening or lengthening the wedge will increase or decrease the lower back extension (lumbar curve or tilt) rather than weightbearing on the arms. See reference: Kramer and Hinojosa: Colangelo, CA: Biomechanical frame of reference.

37. (C) somatosensory system. Many children who use an excessively tight grip on the writing tool and press too hard with the pencil on their paper have poor proprioceptive awareness (somatosensory). Answer A, vestibular system, is not the most correct answer (although it is difficult to completely separate any sensory system from another) because it primarily affects balance and general motor coordination. Answer B, the auditory system, is not the most correct answer because this system interprets sound for use in language. Answer D is not correct because, although the visual system can monitor motor control such as pencil grip and pressure, use of the pencil requires unconscious awareness of body position and pressure at times when the task is not monitored visually. See reference: Case-Smith, Allen, and Pratt (eds): Amundson, SJ, and Weil, M: Prewriting and handwriting skills.

38. (C) tilted backward up to 60 degrees while rocking. By lowering Martin backwards from the sitting position, he is required to activate increasing degrees of antigravity control in the neck musculature. As his strength increases, the degree of incline can be increased. Answers A, B and D do not address antigravity control using neck flexor musculature. See reference: Case-Smith, Allen, and Pratt (eds): Nichols, DS: The development of postural control.

39. (A) work on coordinated reach in side-lying first, then transfer skill to sitting. The COTA must consider the optimal position for learning the skill and can then teach the child to transfer the skill to a more functional position. Answer B addresses a limitation in ROM, answer C a visual impairment, and answer D behavioral/cognitive issues, none of which were mentioned as concerns for Marie-Louise. See reference: Case-Smith, Allen, and Pratt (eds): Exner, CE: Development of hand skills.

40. (D) Present only a few blocks at a time. Like other children with his diagnosis, Cesar has poor impulse control and has great difficulty completing a task. By presenting a few blocks at a time, the COTA can help Cesar focus on a few relevant stimuli and make it possible for him to complete a short-term task successfully. This experience will then help him increase his attention span. The use of soft foam blocks (answer A) can help prevent injury if thrown, but is not essential in increasing his attention span. Providing blocks of only one color (answer B) may reduce visual stimulation somewhat and using interlocking blocks (answer C) may make manipulation of the pieces easier, but the presentation of the full amount of blocks all at once would still be perceived as overwhelming to Cesar. See reference: Case-Smith, Allen, and Pratt (eds): Cronin, AS: Psychosocial and emotional domains of behavior.

41. (B) dry cereals with milk. Foods selected for Julian's diet should reflect his current skill level. To increase his oral tolerance and control of food, textures are gradually modified from smooth and consistent (answer C) to smooth and slightly varied (answers A and D) to increasingly resistive foods and a combination of contrasts, for example hard and crunchy mixed with soft or liquid as given in answer B. Once he has mastered this level of control and tolerance, he can safely proceed to an even greater variety of textures, tastes, and temperatures offered at family meals. See reference: Case-Smith, Allen, and Pratt (eds): Case-Smith, J, and Humphry, R: Feeding and oral motor skills.

42. (B) his speed for long distances becomes less than that of a walking person. Max should be considered for a power chair when his current means of locomotion proves less efficient and slower than locomotion by walking. Since he will be experiencing progressive muscle weakness, energy conservation is of primary importance. Answers A and C address valid environmental considerations to be made after determining the general need for a power chair. To wait until he becomes unable to propel himself (answer D) is too long; it would make the transition more difficult and would prevent him from getting around independently in the mean time. See reference: Case-Smith, Allen, and Pratt (eds): Wright-Ott, C, and Egilson, S: Mobility.

43. (B) beginning of spontaneous social interaction. In a project level group, beginning social interaction skills are expected to take the form of conflict and competition among group members. As the focus shifts from group leader to group members, awareness of others emerges, signifying significant progress in social interaction. Answers A and C provide a negative interpretation not applicable to the frame of reference used (developmental groups). The development of group leadership skills (answer D) is too advanced a skill at this level of function. See reference: Ryan (ed): Blechert, TF and Kari, N: Interpersonal communication skills and applied group dynamics. *The Certified Occupational Therapy Assistant.*

44. (B) ability to follow rules/instructions. Answer B is correct because it gives information about the student's basic ability to learn and adapt in a work situation. Answer A, leisure interests, is not correct because although important to the student's life, leisure interest knowledge is not essential to work. Answers C and D are not correct because, although they describe the student's motor control function which can affect which type of job they perform, adaptation can be made to either of these areas of need. See reference: Case-Smith, Allen, and

Pratt (eds): Gordon, CY, Schanzenbacher, KE, Case-Smith, J, and Carrasco, R: Diagnostic problems in pediatrics.

45. (D) pushing or pulling weighted objects while in a quadruped position. Answer D is correct because it is the only activity which provides resistance of additional weight which will give added proprioceptive input needed to improve body awareness. Answers A and C are not correct because they emphasize additional tactile input. Answer B is not correct because it emphasizes slow vestibular input. See reference: Hopkins and Smith (eds): Kinnealey, M and Miller, LJ: Sensory integration/learning disabilities.

46. (B) Obstacle courses. Lucy will need to be exposed to situations in which she needs to problem solve the adjustment of her body to objects in her environment. While all answers involve motor planning in response to the environment (classmates/objects) to some degree, the obstacle courses clearly emphasizes the spatial element the most. Obstacles also consist of static items, and therefore facilitate success in adjustment more easily than moving objects. See reference: Case-Smith, Allen, and Pratt (eds): Parham, LD and Mailloux, Z: Sensory integration.

47. (C) When a maintenance level has been achieved. Since he may never be considered "cured" (answer D), or achieve age level skills (answer A), discharge should be discussed with the OTR when he no longer makes significant progress. Transition to the first grade (answer B) is an educational consideration and is not directly relevant to the provision of services under a medical model. See reference: Case-Smith, Allen, and Pratt (eds): Johnson, J: School-based occupational therapy.

48. (A) Mounting lever handles on doors and faucets. For the child with reduced strength and endurance, using less complex movements and less force will result in energy conservation. Lever handles require less energy than knob handles on doors, faucets and appliances. Answers B and C are environmental adaptations recommended to minimize the danger of slipping and falling for the child with incoordination or postural instability. Answer D is contraindicated, since work at a vertical surface against gravity requires more energy than movement in a horizontal plane. See reference: Case-Smith, Allen, and Pratt (eds): Dudgeon, BJ: Pediatric rehabilitation.

49. (D) computer games. While all activities involve spatial organization, computer games require the least amount of active, total body participation, a key element in effective learning. Answers A, B and C describe activities which involve learning of certain motor routines within closely defined spatial parameters i.e. the mastery of projected action sequences, leading to the experience of success and reinforcement of motor activity. See reference: Case-Smith, Allen, and Pratt (eds): Parham, LD and Mailloux, Z: Sensory integration.

50. (C) adding cabinets with labeled compartments to store items out of sight. In order for the child with attention deficit disorder to optimize self organization skills, the environment should provide a minimum of distractions. Placing items not used out of sight will reduce visual distraction; labeling compartments will help the child retrieve items. Answers A and B add visual distraction, and answer D addresses a limitation in motor function, not self organization. See reference: Case-Smith, Allen, and Pratt (eds): Cronin, AS: Psychosocial and emotional domains of behavior.

51. (B) demonstrate the procedure on her unaffected extremity, then occlude her vision. Due to the compensation that may occur with vision, it is necessary to occlude the individual's vision. The presentation of stimuli in sensory evaluation is extremely important. Stimuli should be presented in a random proximal to distal pattern. Picture cards are helpful in assessing individuals with expressive aphasia. Also, the unaffected extremity should be assessed before the affected extremity, the opposite of answer A, to reduce anxiety and increase understanding of directions. A rapport (answer C) should be established *before* beginning any of the evaluation procedures, also to reduce anxiety. An individual may not be aware of any deficit areas (answer D), so the whole extremity should be assessed to ensure accuracy. See reference: Trombly (ed): Bentzel, K: Evaluation of sensation.

52. (B) line bisection. Line bisection is a paper-and-pencil test used as a method of determining unilateral neglect. The block assembly (answer A) is used to assess constructional apraxia and is not a paper-and-pencil task. Proverb interpretation (answer C) is used to assess abstraction and is typically performed verbally. Overlapping figures (answer D) is used to assess figure-ground discrimination and testing is performed by pointing. See reference: Trombly (ed): Quintana, LA: Evaluation of perception and cognition.

53. (B) dressing apraxia. To some extent, dressing apraxia involves an impaired awareness of the affected side and the relation of body parts to the clothing, as well as assembly of the clothing onto the body. Difficulty with spatial relations (answer A) involves awareness of the relationship of one's self to another object. A person with anosagnosia (answer C) is unaware of any deficits. Figure-ground discrimination (answer D) is the ability to distinguish an object from its background. See reference: Trombly (ed): Quintana, LA: Evaluation of perception and cognition.

54. (B) flaccidity. Flaccidity, or hypotonicity, is often present initially following a stroke, and may later change to spasticity (answer D), or increased muscle tone. The flaccid extremity feels heavy and hangs limply at the individual's side. The weight of the arm may eventually pull the humerus out of the glenohumeral joint, resulting in subluxation (answer C). Paralysis (answer A) may be accompanied by either flaccidity or spasticity, and is not an adequate answer. See reference: Pedretti (ed): Undzis, MF, Zoltan, B and Pedretti, LW: Evaluation of motor control.

55. (B) receptive aphasia. Individuals with receptive aphasia have difficulty comprehending spoken or written words and symbols; therefore, they may not accurately understand verbal directions or consistently respond to stimuli. Individuals with receptive aphasia may be able to imitate or follow demonstration. However, these techniques may not be used with a sensory evaluation. Expressive aphasia (answer A) interferes with an individual's verbal or written expression, but not comprehension of verbal or written information. An individual with expressive aphasia would be able to indicate the response by pointing to the stimulus used or a card which has been marked with the correct response. An individual who has agnosia or ataxia (answers C and D) would be able to understand directions, but unable to accurately indicate an area due to impaired recognition of the body part or impaired coordination. The method of response may be adapted by using verbal description of an area or cue cards. See reference: Trombly (ed): Woodson, AM: Stroke.

56. (A) goniometer. A goniometer measures available joint movement. A pinch meter (answer C) is used to measure available thumb-to-finger pinch strength in all available positions. A dynamometer (answer B) measures grip strength in the hand. An aesthesiometer (answer D) measures two point discrimination. See reference: Trombly (ed): Evaluation of biomechanical and physiological aspects of motor performance.

57. (A) figure-ground discrimination. Figure ground discrimination is the ability to distinguish an object from the background. A person with impaired figure-ground discrimination would have difficulty finding the sock despite its position on the bed. Inability to judge the distance to the sock would demonstrate a problem in depth perception (answer B). Inability to find the sock in relation to the bed would demonstrate difficulty with position in space (answer C). Knowing how to get back to the bed to look for the socks demonstrates topographical orientation (answer D). See reference: AOTA: Uniform terminology for occupational therapy - third edition.

58. (C) fair plus. A person with strength of fair (answer B) or fair minus (answer C) would be unable to tolerate resistance. A person with fair plus strength during manual muscle testing can tolerate minimal resistance. A person whose strength is good minus (answer D) can tolerate less than moderate resistance but more than minimal resistance. See reference: Trombly (ed): Evaluation of biomechanical and physiological aspects of motor performance.

59. (A) tip of the index finger. The correct position for tip pinch is the thumb against the tip of the index finger. The thumb against the side of the index finger (answer B) describes the position for lateral pinch. The thumb against the tips of the index and middle fingers (answer C) describes the test position for three jaw chuck or palmar pinch. The thumb against the tips of all the fingers (answer D) is not a standard test position. See reference: Trombly (ed): Evaluation of biomechanical and physiological aspects of motor performance.

60. (D) ask the questions just as they are written. In structured interviews, which are designed to obtain specific information, it is important to stick to the phrasing and sequence of the questions. Semi-structured interviews, which are often designed to obtain more details and information, offer greater flexibility. Answers A, B, and C are all qualities associated with semi- or unstructured interviews. See reference: Early: Data gathering and evaluation.

61. (A) Complete independence with self-care and transfers. An individual with T3 (or lower) paraplegia will have the trunk balance and upper extremity strength and coordination to complete self-care and work activities independently. See reference: Trombly (ed): Hollar, LD: Spinal cord injury.

62. (D) no equipment. An individual with paraplegia at the T6 level or lower will not require any adaptive equipment for dressing. See reference: Trombly (ed): Hollar, LD: Spinal cord injury.

63. (B) detachable arms. Armrests will need to be removed to allow the individual to place the sliding board and move sideways out of the chair. Footrests (answer A) may be swung away, but do not need to be detached to perform a transfer. Anti-tip bars (answer C) prevent a wheelchair from tipping over backwards, such as when performing a wheelie or when going up or down a step, but not when transferring. Brake handle extensions (answer D) allow the brakes to be locked more easily, but would be in the way during a sliding board transfer. See reference: Trombly (ed): Retraining basic and instrumental activities of daily living.

64. (A) work locks and latches on doors and windows. The ability to manipulate the locks and latches is also a safety concern, as the individual may not be able to open them to let family into their home or close them to keep intruders from entering. Built up handles (answer B), energy conservation techniques (answer C) and adaptations to clothing fasteners (answer D) are not safety issues. See reference: Trombly (ed): Feinberg, JR and Trombly, CA: Arthritis.

65. (C) pouring a glass of orange juice. Meal preparation is graded from cold to hot foods or beverages, and from simple to multiple steps. An individual beginning meal preparation training would start with a cold item involving the least number of steps possible, such as pouring a glass of juice or other cold beverage. Cold sandwich preparation (answer A) adds another step as each topping to the bread is added and as the use of utensils is introduced. After preparation of cold items has been mastered, training in hot food or beverage preparation (answers B and D) may be initiated. See reference: Kovich and Bermann (eds): Van Dam-Burke, A and Kovich, K: Self-care and homemaking.

66. (B) teacher with a C7 spinal cord injury. Although a prehensile grasp is important to students and teachers, artists and programmers, only individual with C7 quadriplegia would benefit from and have adequate wrist extensor strength to operate this orthosis. An individual with a C5 injury lacks the wrist extension strength needed to operate the wrist-driven flexor hinge splint. Individuals with T3 or T10 injuries can grasp and manipulate utensils without difficulty or need for assistance from an orthosis. See reference: Trombly (ed): Hollar, LD: Spinal cord injury.

67. (B) pain management techniques. A work hardening program focuses on returning an individual to work in a physically appropriate setting as quickly as is feasible through reconditioning. As part of that program, pain management techniques are included to assist him with managing and coping with pain during work related activities. A work hardening program would not include recreational activities (answer A) since the focus is on work activities. A person who would need driver reeducation (answer C) would have physical impairments beyond the scope of treatment for work hardening and would be more appropriate for a physical rehabilitation program. A work hardening program would teach proper body mechanics to prevent further injury rather than focus on joint protection techniques (answer D) which are usually taught to someone who has joint pain caused by arthritis. See reference: Pedretti (ed): Burt, CM and Smith, P: Work evaluation and work hardening.

68. (B) Working with long cords. The longer the cords, the more shoulder abduction and external rotation is required; therefore, short cords (answer A) would be easiest for this individual. Fine cords (answer C) would be challenging for individuals with limited finger function. Thick cords (answer D) could be used to downgrade the activity for those individuals. The thickness of the cord, however, would have no bearing on shoulder range of motion requirements. See reference: Breines: Folkcraft.

69. (C) lateral trunk support. A lateral trunk support, in the frontal plane, would provide stabilization at his side to maintain correct alignment of the pelvis and trunk in the chair, counteracting asymmetrical muscle tone. A lateral trunk support would also prevent improper loading onto an unstable shoulder joint through upper extremity support. Answer A, a reclining wheelchair, would shift his weight to the posterior but not prevent the lateral shift of the trunk. An arm trough (answer B) may help maintain a more centered position of the trunk, but the weight of the affected extremity would result in instability and improper alignment of the shoulder, which could result in shoulder pain. A lateral pelvic support (answer D) would provide stabilization of the pelvis to prevent it from shifting sideways, but this support would be too low to prevent the trunk from moving laterally. See reference: Church and Glennen (eds): Harryman, S and Warren, L: Positioning and power mobility.

70. (A) putting blankets in the overhead compartments. When distributing magazines, the flight attendant uses small amounts of reaching and bending. Upgrading the activity would increase the degree of reaching and bending, and add weight to the process greater than lightweight magazines. The weight of meal trays (answer B) is significant, especially when combined with reaching over passengers to the window seat, and would be considered more than a slight upgrade. Putting luggage into the overhead compartments (answer D) would be the final step in the process, as it involves the most weight and the riskiest back position. Distributing magazines to half of the passengers (answer C) is an example of how the activity could be down-graded. See reference: Pedretti (ed): Smithline, J: Low back pain.

71. (A) prepare a tossed salad, make garlic bread, make spaghetti sauce and meatballs. Grading should progress from simple to complex. Using the oven is more complex than using the stove, which is more complex than preparing cold food. Making spaghetti sauce is a complex task which involves making meatballs, frying them, cutting and sautéing vegetables, opening cans and jars, and combining ingredients in a large pot. Making garlic bread requires fewer steps and could be done with a toaster oven. Preparing a tossed salad involves no cooking at all, and is the most simple task in the sequence. In answer B, making a grilled cheese sandwich is more complex than making instant pudding and should be last in the sequence. In answer C, broiling a steak is the most complex of the three tasks and should be last in the sequence. In answer D, scrambling eggs is the most complex task, and should be last. See reference: Boserup (ed): A kitchen training program as an occupational therapy activity.

72. (B) white print on black background labels. White print on a black background is easier for individuals with poor vision to see. Braille labels (answer A) would not be appropriate for individuals with peripheral neuropathy because of the decreased tactile sensation they experience in their fingertips. A pill organizer box (answer C) is useful for taking pills on schedule, and is particularly helpful for individuals with memory deficits or who have a complex medication regimen. It could also be helpful to Agatha in that if the pills were all presorted in the pill organizer, she might not have the need to identify them. It would not, however, address the stated issue of medication identification. Brightly colored pills (answer D) would make it easy for an individual to identify different medications; however, the COTA has no control over how pills are manufactured and what colors are used. See reference: Ryan (ed): Hansvick, B and Saxon, MC: The elderly with hearing and visual impairments. *Practice Issues in Occupational Therapy.*

73. (D) chaining. Teaching a task one step at a time, gradually adding more steps as steps are mastered, is called chaining. Chaining is frequently used when teaching a multiple step task, as it is easier to learn one step at a time than a complete activity. Repetition and rehearsal (answers A and C) involve repeating the whole activity over and over until the activity is learned. Cueing (answer B) uses an external source to remind a person of the next step or part of that step. See reference: Zoltan: Explanations for use of this manual.

74. (B) wear noisy bracelets on the wrist or ankle as a reminder to visually scan toward the affected side. Although hazards may be removed from the environment or padded to prevent injury to an individual, this is only feasible in a person's home. It is best to teach the individual visual scanning of the affected area and the environment, a technique which the person may use anywhere. An individual may avoid using sharp tools or extreme water temperature (answer A), but this does not teach him or her how to monitor the affected side visually since it is a precaution which only addresses the problem with sensation. Noisy bracelets are one technique that may be used to accomplish this. Visual impairments which are not accompanied by sensory or perceptual deficits are more readily overcome with retraining. Using an electric shaver (answer C), may be recommended for an individual with insufficient coordination to shave safely. Cueing the individual to look to the involved side (answer D) is a technique the COTA uses when addressing unilateral neglect, but it is not a method of compensation. See reference: Trombly (ed): Quintana, LA: Remediating perceptual impairments.

75. (D) incoordination. A person who has tremors or poor coordination could reduce instability by stabilizing the limb proximally before working distally. Stabilization adds a secure base of support from which to work. Reduced vision, poor endurance, and limited fine movement (answers A, B and C) would not require stabilization when writing, but would require stronger contrast of guiding lines or ink on paper, more frequent rests, or built-up writing tools. See reference: Trombly (ed): Retraining basic and instrumental activities of daily living.

76. (C) to both sides of the body. Answer C is correct because the individual will need to be able to transfer to both sides of her body at home. Layouts of many home fixtures do not lend themselves to transferring the individual only from one side. If the transfers are not practiced to both sides, the individual may find it easy to transfer to the commode, but not from the commode. The family also needs to know the differences in the way the individual is handled, with more or less support. Thus, answers (A) to the unaffected side, (B) to the affected side and (D) to the side the commode will be approached, are all incorrect because they all involve transfer to only one side. See reference: Trombly (ed): Retraining basic and instrumental activities of daily living.

77. (D) provide a stockinette for him to wear inside the splint. A stockinette liner worn inside the splint keeps perspiration from irritating the skin by absorbing the perspiration and shielding the skin from the damp plastic. A stockinette liner is inexpensive enough to dispense several to the patient at a time, so he can always have a clean one available. Putting talcum powder in a splint (answer A) works well with a small splint, but a large splint would require a considerable amount, and the skin would feel muddy when the powder and perspiration mix. Moleskin as a liner (answer B) does not clean well after it's been worn for a short time. Although it may be comfortable, it usually is discarded because of the soiled appearance and smell. An individual using a splint made with perforated material (answer C) will continue to have perspiration and will need to use another method to keep the damp plastic from irritating the skin. See reference: Ryan (ed): Schober-Branigan, P: Thermoplastic splinting of the hand. *The Certified Occupational Therapy Assistant.*

78. (A) give one or two step instructions and repeat frequently. The best method to use with an individual with Alzheimer's disease is short, one or two step instructions, keeping them to the point and repeating them frequently. Multiple step instructions accompanied with demonstration (answer B) provides too much stimulation and can be confusing. Multiple step written instructions (answer C), which can be easily misplaced, are unlikely to be retained in the individual's short term memory after reading. It is also unlikely the sequence would be correctly retained. Verbally repeating directions (answer D), or rehearsal, does not enable a person with Alzheimer's to retain information in her memory, and she may not repeat the instructions properly. See reference: Glickstein: Working with dementia clients.

79. (D) unclamp the individual's catheter and tap over the bladder. The individual is suffering from a condition called autonomic dysreflexia. If not promptly addressed, death may result. This condition may be caused by a bowel impaction, plugged catheter, or suppository insertion. Do not recline the individual in that this may result in a higher cerebral blood pressure. The condition must be treated promptly so taking a heart rate and blood pressure postpone action on the condition. A drop in blood sugar is usually associated with diabetes which is counteracted by having the individual consume fruit juice to raise the blood sugar level. Autonomic dysreflexia causes the blood pressure to increase to dangerous levels, so no actions should be performed to the individual which would cause the blood pressure to rise. See reference: Trombly (ed): Hollar, LD: Spinal cord injury.

80. (A) using the strongest joint, avoiding positions of deformity, and ensuring correct patterns of movement. These principles of joint protection are beneficial for all individuals. The significance of utilizing these principles for individuals with pre-existing joint deformities and/or adverse musculoskeletal changes may help to restore function as well as prevent further impairments. Answers B, C, and D involve muscle relaxation and stress management. See reference: Trombly (ed): Bear-Lehman, J: Orthopedic conditions.

81. (D) (1) gather shirt up at the back of the neck; (2) pull gathered back fabric off over head; (3) remove shirt from normal arm; (4) remove shirt from affected arm. Answers A, B and C are examples of incorrect sequences that would result in failure to remove the shirt successfully. See reference: Pedretti (ed): Foti, D, Pedretti, LW, and Lillie, S: Activities of daily living.

82. (B) seating Mr. G. upright on a firm surface with his chin slightly tucked. The best position for feeding an individual with a swallowing disorder is upright and symmetrical, with the chin slightly tucked. "Correct positioning normalizes tone, thereby facilitating quality motor control and function of the facial musculature, jaw and tongue movement, and the swallow process, all of which minimize the potential for aspiration" (p. 180). Supine, semi-reclined and side-lying positions all place Mr. G at greater risk for choking and aspiration (entry of food material into the airway). See reference: Pedretti (ed): Nelson, KL: Dysphagia: Evaluation and treatment.

83. (A) vacuum feeding cup. Individuals with impulsive behavior or poor judgment often attempt to drink too quickly. Limiting the rate of intake can be accomplished by using a drinking spout with a small opening, pinching a straw, or using a vacuum feeding cup with a control button. A cup with a large drinking spout (answer D) would increase the rate of intake, which could result in choking or spills. A Nosey Cup (answer B) allows individuals with dysphagia to maintain a tucked chin position while drinking, which is necessary for a good swallow. A mug with two handles (answer C) would benefit an individual with limited grasp or coordination. See reference: Trombly (ed): Konosky, KA: Dysphagia.

84. (B) allow the chin to remain tucked when drinking. Tucking the chin toward the chest maximizes airway protection for individuals with dysphagia. Methods the caregiver can use to control or slow the rate of liquid intake for individuals who demonstrate poor judgment or impulsivity (answers A and C) include using a drinking spout with a small opening, pinching a straw, or using a vacuum feeding cup with a control button. Plastic cups and plastic coated utensils are best for individual's with a bite reflex (answer D) to prevent damage to their oral structures. See reference: Trombly (ed): Konosky, KA: Dysphagia.

85. (B) use moderate water temperature. Hot water temperature may contribute to fatigue in individuals with MS, and should therefore be avoided. Moderate water temperature is recommended. Bathing in cool water (answer A) is unnecessary and may cause chilling and increase spasticity. Bathing (answer C) may be recommended for individuals with poor standing tolerance or those with COPD. Showering (answer D) may be recommended for individuals who experience difficulty bending, such as those with hip or knee replacements, or back pain. See reference: Ryan (ed): Jensen, D and Linroth, R: The adult with multiple sclerosis. *Practice Issues in Occupational Therapy.*

86. (A) perform PROM, then position and elevate the affected extremity. Positioning, compression glove, edema massage, and passive range-of-motion exercises are all effective methods for reducing edema and prevention of further edema. The goal is to promote the movement of fluid back into normal circulation rather than allowing it to collect in one area or body part. Gentle passive range of motion is necessary to help maintain joint structure and provide nutrients to the joint. The actual movement of the extremity may serve as a "pump" to assist in moving excess fluid back into the body. These techniques are contraindicated for individuals who have deep vein thrombosis. In addition, edema is partially a result of the loss of movement in an extremity which does not allow the contraction of muscles to pump the fluid back into the body. Splinting (answer B) is effective in preventing deformity, but compression gloves are more effective in reducing edema. In addition, it is beyond the scope of the COTA's practice to independently initiate splint fabrication. Taking no action (answer C) could result in permanent damage to the tissue of the involved extremity. Having the individual attempt to squeeze a ball (answer D), would be futile, since the left arm is flaccid. See reference: Trombly (ed): Woodson, AM: Stroke.

87. (A) remedial treatment, such as rubbing or stroking the involved extremity. When sensation begins to return, it is appropriate to initiate remedial activities for sensory retraining. Stimulating the involved extremity by rubbing or stroking (to provide tactile input), or through weightbearing activities (to provide proprioceptive input), are examples of remedial activities. Compensatory activities are essential for individuals with decreased or absent sensation, and would have been part of the original treatment plan. Answers B, C and D are all examples of compensatory strategies. See reference: Pedretti (ed): Evaluation of sensation and treatment of sensory dysfunction.

88. (D) Mr. G. asks for more beverages during meals, and appears surprised when the COTA indicates beverages in closed containers are on the meal tray. The subjective portion of the SOAP note should contain information which is gained through a chart review or communication with the patient or his family. This information is not measurable and therefore is considered subjective. Answer A would be in the program plan. Answers B and C would be in the objective portion because they are either measurable or based on specific observations. See reference: Trombly (ed): Bentzel, K: Remediating sensory impairment.

89. (A) get dressed without becoming fatigued. Prevention of fatigue is the primary purpose of energy conservation. Energy conservation techniques may often result in slower, not faster (answer D) performance of activities. Using proper body mechanics may enable an individual with back pain to lift heavy cookware without pain (answer B). Using joint protection techniques may prevent further joint damage to arthritic hands when doing handicrafts (answer C). See reference: Pedretti (ed): Hittle, JM, Pedretti, LW, and Kasch, MC: Rheumatoid arthritis.

90. (C) "Pt. will perform lower extremity dressing with verbal cueing 50% of the time for energy conservation techniques." Goals should be functional, measurable, and objective. This answer meets those criteria. Answer B does not provide measurable criteria. "Goals need to be written to show what the patient will accomplish, not what the therapist will do." Answer D describes what the COTA will do. Short-term goals must relate to the long-term goal being addressed. Since the long term goal being addressed is independence in dressing, the short-term goal must relate to dressing, not all ADLs. See reference: AOTA: Writing functional goals. *Effective Documentation for Occupational Therapy.*

91. (B) instant soup. The most basic level of meal preparation is accessing a prepared meal, which involves tasks such as opening a thermos and unwrapping a sandwich. When an individual becomes proficient at this level, she is progressed to a higher level. More advanced meal preparation activities can be structured to increase in complexity in the following sequence: prepare a cold meal (answer B); prepare a hot one-dish meal (answer C); prepare a hot multi-dish meal (answer D). See reference: Hopkins and Smith (eds): Culler, KH: Home and family management.

92. (D) Obtain a narrower wheelchair, because this one is too wide. The recommended wheelchair seat width is two inches wider than the widest point across the hips and thighs when the individual is seated. Two and a half inches is too wide, not too narrow (answer A). In addition, "wheelchairs should be as narrow as possible while allowing for comfort, ease of repositioning, and transfers." The narrower the wheelchair, the easier it is to maneuver. Since a narrower wheelchair would be better, padding the sides (answer C) is a less desirable option. The need to lose or gain weight (answer B) should be discussed first with a patient's physician. Losing weight would only create a worse wheelchair fit in Claudia's situation. See reference: Trombly (ed): Deitz, J, and Dudgeon, B: Wheelchair selection process.

93. (A) baking brownies. Progressive levels of meal preparation include: access a prepared meal; prepare a cold meal; prepare a hot beverage, soup, or prepared dish; prepare a hot one-dish meal; and prepare a hot multi-dish meal. Making a fresh fruit salad (answer D) is a less challenging activity because no cooking is involved. While both involve heating an item, preparing toast (answer C) is more simple than heating soup because opening a plastic bag is a less complex task than opening a can. Baking brownies (answer A) is slightly more complex because of the progression from stove top to oven and the addition of several ingredients that need to be mixed. Therefore, this would be the appropriate upgrade. Making an apple pie (answer B) involves a higher level of task performance and complexity than brownies, and would be an appropriate task after the individual demonstrates competence in the less complex task of baking brownies. See reference: Hopkins and Smith (eds): Culler, KH: Home and family management.

94. (B) one foot of ramp for every inch of rise in height. A foot of ramp for every inch of rise in height provides a gentle slope which may be independently and safely navigated by an individual. Answers A, B and C would all make extremely short and steep ramps which would be either unsuitable or unsafe for an individual independently entering or exiting a home. See reference: Pedretti (ed): Adler, C and Tipton-Burton, M: Wheelchair assessment and transfers.

95. (A) Perform pursed lip breathing when performing activities. Pursed lip breathing is a technique which narrows the passage of air during expiration. This technique helps individuals with COPD to improve breathing efficiency. The overall effect is improved endurance and tolerance for activities. Taking hot showers (answer C) is contraindicated for individuals with COPD. Tepid water temperature is recommended. Utilizing a long handled bath sponge (answer B) may be helpful but is not the MOST likely tip to be on a home program for an individual with COPD. Reaching the arms overhead during UE exercise (answer D) is recommended for individuals with COPD as it helps with inspiration by expanding the chest. See reference: Trombly (ed): Atchison, B: Cardiopulmonary disease.

96. (B) a call system for emergency/nonemergency use. A call system is necessary for a person with a high level spinal cord injury to allow the caretaker to leave the room, but remain available to answer the person's call for assistance for daily needs or an emergency. This is frequently the first oportunity that a person with a spinal cord injury would have to control some part of his or her life, giving some feeling of independence or choice. An environmental control unit does allow independence in operating appliances, lights, etc. through the use of switches or voice control, but would not be a necessity for safety. A remote control power door opener which would allow a caretaker to enter would be useless if the person is unable to call for assistance. An electric page turner is useless without the ability to call for someone to position or replace reading material. See reference: Hill (ed): Jones, R: Home environmental control.

97. (A) isometric exercises. Isometric exercises involve contracting the muscles without joint movement or a change in muscle length. Isotonic exercises (answer B) shorten muscle length, which results in joint movement. Progressive resistive exercises (answer C) are a type of isotonic exercise in which resistance is increased during consecutive exercise repetitions. A person who has a cast obstructing movement would be unable to perform isotonic exercises. Passive exercises (answer D) are performed by an outside force. PROM results in joint motion but does not involve any active muscle contraction. Passive exercises could not be performed to a casted joint. See reference: Pedretti (ed): Pedretti, LW, and Wade, IE: Therapeutic modalities.

98. (C) A work hardening program. Work hardening programs are designed to "move the injured worker from a submaximum level of performance to a level of functioning adequate for entry or reentry into the competitive work force. Practitioners use graded activities and exercises to increase endurance, strength and positional tolerance for ... activity needed by the worker to perform the job." Continuing to perform her home program (answers A and D) or discontinuing OT services would probably not enable Kathleen to return to the work force after a three month absence. Home health OT (answer B) is appropriate for individuals who are unable to leave their homes to attend outpatient therapy. See reference: Ryan (ed): Engh, J and Taylor, S: Work hardening. *Practice Issues in Occupational Therapy.*

99. (D) clustered independent living arrangement. These are usually comprised of "apartment clusters or other types of housing in close proximity to each other, in which groups of residents with disabilities share services such as attendants and transportation." Cradle-to-grave homes (answer A) are houses designed with accessibility in mind at the time of construction. Should an individual begin to use a wheelchair later in life, her home would already be wheelchair accessible. Transitional living centers (answer B) "provide temporary living arrangements for individuals who are in a transitional phase between hospital or institution and independent community living". Adult day programs (answer C) are rehabilitation-oriented day programs for clients who live in the community. They are not residential. See reference: Trombly (ed): Law, M, Stewart, D, and Strong, S: Achieving access to home, community, and workplace.

100. (D) "Pt. has been provided with a lumbar support and a written copy of his home program." The "plan" section of a discharge summary contains the patient's discharge disposition (i.e. to a nursing home, to outpatient therapy), recommendations for additional therapy or actions on the part of the patient (e.g., outpatient therapy, home health, or performing a home program); equipment needs or equipment provided to the patient; and plans for discharge. Answer A is a subjective report. Answer B is an example of a statement that belongs in the "objective" section of a discharge summary. Answer C belongs in the assessment section. See reference: Kettenbach: Writing plans (P).

101. (C) memory impairment. Cognitive abilities such as memory are most often initially affected in individuals with Alzheimer's Disease. Receptive and expressive aphasia, personality changes, and loss of independence in ADLs appear in the middle stage of the disease. Incontinence, inability to recognize family members and inability to walk are evident in the late stage of Alzheimer's disease. See reference Ryan (ed): Brown, I, and Epstein, CF: The Elderly with Alzheimer's disease. *Practice Issues in Occupational Therapy.*

102. (A) Kohlman Evaluation of Living Skills (KELS). The KELS is the only item that was designed for acute care psychiatric settings. The MEDLS (answer B) is most appropriate for long term psychiatric treatment settings. The Occupational History Interview (answer C) is designed to obtain information about the patient's occupational role development. The Routine Task Inventory (answer D) is designed to assess how well an individual is able to function in the community. See reference: Early: Data gathering and evaluation.

103. (A) Short-term memory. Short term memory is the ability to recall information that has just been received and hold it in temporary use from one to five minutes or more. Attention (answer B) refers to the ability to focus on a stimulus for a period of time without being distracted. In assessing attention, the COTA would ask an individual to repeat numbers presented by the COTA immediately, without the one to five minute delay used for assessing memory. A person who is being evaluated for hearing (answer C) would be checked for the accuracy of sound at different pitches, not a specific sound. Orientation (answer D) refers to the accurate awareness of person, place, and time. See reference: Trombly (ed): Quintana, LA: Evaluation of perception and cognition.

104. (B) forgetting to turn the stove burner off. The progression of dementia of the Alzheimer's type is often described by its phases of impairment in functioning. Behaviors linked to memory impairments usually occur in the early stages whereas social and motor impairments occur later. See reference: Early: Human occupation and mental health.

105. (B) confusion. Anti-anxiety medications often cause confusion. Akathesia, EPS, and tardive dyskinesia, (answers A, C and D), are adverse effects commonly linked to anti-psychotic medications. See reference: Early: Psychotropic medications and somatic treatments.

106. (C) ask the questions as they are stated on the interview sheet. A structured interview requires following the procedure, order and wording of the questions to be asked. Answers A, B and D may be used when more details and information are sought while conducting a semi-structured interview. See reference: Early: Data gathering and evaluation.

107. (B) Person-Symbol Assessment. This tool is used to assess the patient's body concept. Answers A, C and D are structured evaluations that are primarily used by psychologists. The Kinetic Self-Image (answer A) requires the individual to draw a picture of himself engaging in an activity. The Kinetic Family (answer D) asks an individual to draw a picture of himself engaging in an activity with his family. The House Tree-Person (answer C) requires an individual to draw pictures of a house, a tree and a person. See reference: Early: Data gathering and evaluation.

108. (B) the source of referral, reason for referral, and the date referral was received. The initial note is used to record basic information, results of initial evaluations, and often the treatment plan. In addition to documenting items in answer B, the COTA may also contribute data collected from assessments he or she has performed. The OTR is responsible for analyzing an individual's assets and deficits and for projecting the outcome of treatment (answers C and D). See reference: Early: Medical records and documentation.

109. (B) The patient attended 4 out of 5 OT sessions during a 1-week period. This statement describes observable and measurable behavior. The word "frequently" (answer A) is not measurable. Answer C gives no indication of how much time has elapsed since the initial session. Answer D is an interpretation and is not measurable. See reference: Ryan (ed): Backhaus, H: Documentation. In Practice Issues in Occupational Therapy.

110. (B) Comprehensive Occupational Therapy Evaluation Scale (COTE). The recording of a series of task and interpersonal behaviors is best done with the COTE scale. The COTE scale can be used to translate observations into numbers that indicate ranges of task behaviors. Approximately 15 sessions can be recorded on one COTE Scale report form. The RTI (answer A) is an evaluation of ADL's, and the NPI (answer C) is an evaluation of leisure interests and are used primarily as evaluation instruments. SOAP notes (answer D) record progress but are not specifically designed to address only task and interpersonal behaviors. See reference: Early: Data gathering and evaluation.

111. (A) amount of self-control demands, time management demands, self-expression opportunities, and interest in the activity. Components that are primarily within the psychosocial areas and skills of occupational performance are most important to consider with psychosocial populations. Answers B and C are performance components one generally analyzes for childhood populations. Answer D does not address performance components. See reference: Hopkins and Smith (eds): Simon, CJ: Use of activity and activity analysis.

112. (D) imitate the COTA demonstrating the techniques of "broken-record" and "I statements". Demonstration and imitation of desired performances is particularly useful when individuals are learning new and difficult behaviors. The COTA should be aware of a need to supplement this strategy with techniques that provide generalization after skills are developed. Answer A is appropriate when the goals are self evaluative versus skills training. Answer B is effective for testing out newly acquired skills. Answer C is effective for helping the patient to generalize their skills to other situations. See reference: Denton: Treatment planning and implementation.

113. (A) a can of soup. Grading activities according to complexity is an important part of the COTA's selection of appropriate activities for an individual's abilities. Complexity increases as the number of steps, number of different ingredients or tools used, and time to complete the task increases. Answers B, C and D all require more steps and materials and time than preparing a can of soup. See reference: Ryan (ed): People, L, Ryan, SE, Witherspoon, DY, Stewart, R: Activity analysis. *The Certified Occupational Therapy Assistant.*

114. (C) use simple, highly structured activities. Projective media, isolation, and discussing delusions are all contraindicated for people with schizophrenia. Projective activities (answer A) are most useful for encouraging expression of feelings. It may be appropriate to separate individuals (answer B) who are violent or unable to tolerate the presence of others nearby. Discussing delusions (answer D) is undesirable as it is likely to reinforce them. See reference: Early: Responding to symptoms and behaviors.

115. (B) bring about change among the members. Change is the overall purpose of therapeutic groups. Answers A and C are both methods by which members may change. Answer D is an advantage of groups but is not a primary purpose. See reference: Early: Group concepts and techniques.

116. (C) Using a board game to introduce the concept of receiving and spending money. This activity provides an opportunity for the individual to experience the value and purpose of money. While it is important to introduce the actual value of coins and paper money, it is essential to combine this with concrete applications. Answers A, B and D are examples of graded activities to be used following the initial introduction of money concepts. See reference: Early: Daily living skills.

117. (B) are structured by the COTA to encourage self-reflection and feedback. When planning a graded program to develop an individual's self-awareness, the most essential ingredient is the opportunity to verbalize one's ideas and feelings and to receive feedback from others in a safe setting. Thus, it is not the activities that are graded but the way the COTA structures the activities to encourage self-reflection and feedback. See reference: Early: Analyzing, adapting, and grading activities.

118. (D) During a conversation with a female group member, the client will make eye contact for 8 to 10 second periods two times in each ½ hour socialization group. The short-term goal that describes appropriate verbal and nonverbal interactions with female peers is the best answer. Attempting to develop skills with staff (answer C) can pose some confusing boundary and ethical questions in a long term goal related to developing future personal relations. The goals of finding employment and housing (answer A) are long-term goals and are not directly linked to the area of personal relationships. Identifying disability related interferences (answer B) is not related to the client's long term goal. See reference: Early: Understanding psychiatric diagnoses.

119. (C) self concept. Self concept refers to the development of value of one's physical and emotional self. Stating one's strengths and limitations about one's own performance is a reflection of an individual's self concept. Values (answer B) are more globally stated ideas or beliefs such as being a "perfectionist." Termination of the activity (answer A) involves knowing when to stop working on the activity. Self-expression (answer D) refers to the expression of one's thoughts, feelings or needs. See reference: AOTA: Uniform terminology for occupational therapy.

120. (B) bingo. Luck is the key element in games of chance. Bingo is a game that uses chance in calling out numbers randomly. Baseball card collecting (answer A) is considered to be a hobby versus a game. Charades and balloon volleyball (answers C and D) are strategy and skill-based games. See reference: Early: Leisure skills.

121. (A) begin with activities that have obvious solutions and high probability of success, then gradually increase the complexity. Beginning with activities that have obvious solutions and are likely to be successful, then gradually increasing the complexity is effective in developing problem solving skills. Gross and fine motor activities (answer B) can heighten awareness of self and develop coordination. Increasing amounts of time spent on the activity (answer D) facilitates development of attention span. Structuring the number and kinds of choices is used for developing decision making. See reference: Early: Analyzing, adapting, and grading activities.

122. (A) wedging the clay. Individuals with tactile defensiveness often have an aversion to materials such as clay, paste and finger paints. They react most strongly to stimulation of the hands, feet, and face. Answers B, C and D involve stimuli that would not be perceived as noxious to the individual with tactile defensiveness. See reference: Reed: Developmental disorders.

123. (A) group members work independently, developing skills such as attending to a task, using tools safely and without waste, and recognizing errors and problems. Answer B describes work groups. Answer C describes directive groups, and answer D describes psychoeducational stress management groups. See reference: Early: Work, home making and child care.

124. (C) mental imagery. Individuals with schizophrenia generally have difficulty with abstract concepts or approaches. Also, they have difficulty accurately perceiving reality. Because imagery involves abstracting and relies on the individual developing alternate perceptions, this strategy is contraindicated. All the other stress management techniques listed would be generally appropriate. See reference: Hopkins and Smith (eds): Neistadt, ME: Stress management.

125. (C) locate a puncture resistant container that the copper piece could be placed into before disposing of it. Answer C is the only action that is consistent with universal precautions guidelines. Answers A and D do not dispose of blood exposed items in a manner that would protect others from contact. Answer B does not include any blood exposure protection for the person applying the bandage. See reference: Occupational Safety and Health Administration.

126. (D) encourage group members to share similar situations and reactions with one another. Answer D is an approach designed to develop cohesiveness and universality among members. Seeing others as similar has been identified by individuals as being very valuable. Answers A and C are approaches designed to impart information. Answer B is an example of catharsis, which may not be helpful to all members and requires the COTA to understand precautions for the use of catharsis. See reference: Early: Group concepts and techniques.

127. (B) universal precautions. Health care personnel are to follow universal precautions when blood or certain body fluids are present. OSHA has identified materials that require universal precautions to be blood, semen, vaginal secretions, cerebrospinal fluid, synovial fluid, pleural fluid, pericaridal fluid, pertoneal fluid, amniotic fluid, any body fluid with visible blood, any unidentifiable body fluid and saliva from dental procedures. Suicidal, escape and medical precautions are guidelines developed for individuals identified with those risks which are not noted in this question. See reference: Occupational Safety and Health Administration.

128. (C) Making a magazine collage focusing on "who am I". The focus of this patient's treatment is on identifying, expressing and exploring methods for self-awareness and personal need fulfillment. The most appropriate choice of the activities listed would be a theme collage that would provide the opportunity for self-expression in a nonthreatening manner. Answers A, B and D all involve doing something for her significant others and do not address the individual's personal needs. See reference: Early: Expressive and coping skills.

129. (C) "With your permission, I would like to share with my supervisor the concerns you have, and together we can explore which groups and activities would be beneficial for you." This is the best choice at this time in the treatment program. It allows the COTA to collaborate with the OTR and with the patient in order to choose discussion groups and activities that would best meet her needs. Answer A is premature at this time in treatment. The patient needs to have more than just an activity release for anger, she needs to explore and identify the sources of her anger and to learn strategies for managing her anger. While it is important to consider the patient's interests and to offer choices for activities (answer B), it is essential to place the patient in groups she will most benefit from. The OTR and COTA design and develop groups with specific protocols to meet a wide range of needs. It would be appropriate at a later point in treatment, i.e. discharge planning, to provide the patient with a list of support groups to pursue following discharge. While it is a good idea to share with the team members the fears and concerns that arise during an OT activity (answer D), it should be done in a less threatening manner that the way stated here. To do so in this manner could increase the anxiety level of the patient. See reference: Early: Expressive and coping skills; also Group concepts and techniques.

130. (B) woman between the ages of 28 and 40, who are experiencing stress related symptoms. The more similar the patients feel toward others in a group when dealing with identifying and expressing personal needs, the greater the likelihood that they will feel understood, relate to each other, gain insight into their own situations, and discuss possibilities for change. While it may be beneficial to have stress management groups with individuals experiencing diverse reasons for stress (answers A, C and D), it would be most beneficial at this time in her treatment program to have the patient relate to individuals with similar roles and situations. See reference: Early: Group concepts and techniques.

131. (C) paint-by-number. The focus of this group is to gain insight into the causes of and methods for expression of anger. Activities, such as role-playing exercises (answer A), designing papier mache masks (answer B) and journal writing (answer D) are creative, expressive activities that offer opportunities for individuals to express their inner thoughts, anxieties, fears, and insecurities. They are used to increase an awareness of self and one's own feelings and needs. Paint-by-number is a highly structured activity which does not allow for freedom of expression as the other choices do. See reference: Early: Expressive and coping skills.

132. (C) discuss with her using a meals on wheels service. Interventions directed toward "improvement" are typically unrealistic in working with individuals diagnosed with organic mental disorders. These disorders are characterized by a deteriorating course. This patient would not benefit from instruction in safety or time management (answers A and B), although individuals who are cognitively impaired could. Role resumption (answer D) is more appropriate for people with mood disorders. See reference: Early: Understanding psychiatric diagnosis.

133. (D) functional restoration or treatment. Treatment or functional restoration address the underlying causes or processes of a disorder such as schizophrenia. Sensory integration treatment is thought to impact the underactive vestibular processing in some individuals with schizophrenia. Habilitation approaches (answer A) focus on building abilities that were never developed due to illness. Rehabilitation approaches (answer B) emphasize the restoration of lost function. Maintenance (answer C) is an approach that guards remaining abilities. See reference: Early: Treatment planning.

134. (B) Initiation. Initiation problems are often seen when an individual is unable to perform the first step of an activity without prompting. A problem with impulsiveness (answer A) during self care would be evidenced by the individual attempting to complete many steps of an activity rapidly, which would probably result in his cutting himself or doing a poor job of shaving. Memory or attention deficits (answers C and D) would be demonstrated by the individual skipping steps of the activity, either because he does not remember the steps or is distracted by internal or external stimuli. Memory deficits could also be evidenced as steps of a task not performed in sequence. The individual with initiation problems may be able to plan or carry out activities, but may be unable to begin until prompted by someone else. An individual who has difficulty with impulsivity, memory or attention would have no difficulty with beginning the activity, but would have difficulty complete the task successfully. See reference: AOTA: Uniform terminology for occupation therapy - third edition.

135. (C) to get up slowly from a standing, sitting or lying position. This strategy can be used to avoid postural hypotension, a sudden drop in blood pressure resulting in feeling faint or loss of consciousness when moving from lying or sitting to standing. Photosensitivity, an increased sensitivity to the sun, is another side effect often associated with neuroleptic medications that can be addressed by limiting sun exposure (answer A). Individuals experiencing extrapyramidal syndrome, which may cause muscular rigidity, tremors, and/or sudden muscle spasms, should avoid using power tools or sharp instruments (answer B). Dry mouth is a common side effect of many drugs and can be intensified by the dehydrating effects of caffeinated drinks and alcohol (answer D). All of the above are possible side-effects of neuroleptic medications, but answer C is most important because it is the only one Jose has experienced. See reference: Early: Psychotropic medications and somatic treatments.

136. (D) The patient asks for more beverages during meals, but appears surprised when the COTA indicates beverages in closed containers are on the meal tray. The subjective portion of the SOAP note should contain information that is gained through a chart review or communication with patient or his or her family. This information is not measurable and therefore is considered subjective. Answer A would be in the program plan. Answers B and C would be the objective portion because they are either measurable or based on specific observations. See reference: Trombly (ed): Bentzel, K: Remediating sensory impairment.

137. (A) her goals have been met and she can no longer benefit from OT services. Discontinuation of occupational therapy should occur when an individual has met her goals, and/or further progress is not anticipated within the therapeutic environment. Frequently, the individual's goals have been met but the individual could benefit from continued services (answer C). In this situation, new goals are established and intervention continues since further progress is anticipated. If the individual's goals have not been met and she could benefit from continued services (answer B), therapy would continue until goals are achieved. Depending on an individuals status at discharge, recommendations may be made for community services, outpatient care, day care, or home health services. A vital role of the occupational therapy practitioner is to provide appropriate linkages to the community for those individuals served. The preparation for discharge planning should include the patient's support system, discharge environment, and possible need for continued health care services. Discharge of an individual should be made based on objective information. If an individual does not "feel" that they are making progress (answer D), the COTA needs to clarify with the individual her status based on objective measurements and observations. See reference: Reed and Sanderson: Direct service functions.

138. (B) "Client will initiate one request to one other group member for sharing or using group materials within a one week period." Reducing the number of requests and the variety or number of individuals the client is expected to interact with is the best simplification of the initial goal. Simply extending the amount of time to accomplish the goal (answer A) does not make the goal easier to achieve. Increasing the number of individuals, and subsequently the number of requests (answer C) makes the goal more difficult to achieve. Directing interactions to the group leader changes the goal away from the original problem area of "peer" social conversation to authority conversations. See reference: Early: Treatment planning.

139. (A) get through a job performance appraisal. Most people find that having their job performance evaluated is a very stressful experience. The fact that Rosa is involved in a stress management group indicates she has difficulty managing stressful situations. Time management training would help Rosa get to work on time (answer B). Assertiveness training would help Rosa set limits with her employer (answer C). Anger management techniques would help Rosa resolve conflicts with coworkers (answer D). See reference: Early: Expressive and coping skills.

140. (D) arrive at work on time on a consistent basis. Time management focuses on analyzing time use patterns and "developing specific skills such as prioritizing, organizing one's day, etc." Answers A, B and C identify ways of coping with being late as opposed to the time management goal of being on time. See reference: Early: Expressive and coping skills.

141. (B) Objective. The "Objective" portion of the SOAP note (answer B) focuses on measurable and/or observable data obtained by the OT practitioner through specific evaluations, observations, or use of therapeutic activities. The "Subjective" portion of a SOAP note (answer A) refers to what the patient reports or comments about the treatment. The "Assessment" part of a SOAP note refers to the effectiveness of treatment and any changes needed, the status of the goals, and justification for continuing occupational therapy treatment. The "Plan" section of a SOAP note includes statements related to continuing treatment; the frequency and duration of the treatment; suggestions for additional activities or treatment techniques; the need for further evaluations; and, when needed, recommendations for new goals. See reference: Ryan (ed): Backhaus, H: Documentation. *Practice Issues in Occupational Therapy.*

142. (D) clinical reasoning. Clinical reasoning is the problem solving process that OT practitioners use in thinking about an individual's treatment. Modifying how directions are provided, such as using demonstration rather than verbal instruction, is an example of activity adaptation (answer B). Activity analysis (answer A) is the process of identifying the aspects, steps and the materials used in performing the activity. Grading activities (answer C) is a gradual progression of steps toward a goal. See reference: Early: Analyzing, adapting, and grading activities.

143. (D) distractibility. Distractibility involves losing one's focus because of other stimuli. Inattention (answer A) refers to difficulty paying attention when there are no distractions present. A problem with alertness (answer B) can appear as if the client is in a fog. Memory impairment (answer C) refers to difficulty recalling things. See reference: AOTA: Uniform terminology for occupational therapy.

144. (D) referring the patient to a program that helps individuals get and maintain appropriate jobs. Most individuals with an eating disorder have not entered the work environment or have had difficulty making appropriate work choices. This is a long-range goal that is usually best continued after the individual's eating disorder has been stabilized. The patient should attend Overeater's Anonymous meetings (answer A) near his or her home. Family therapy referrals (answer B) are typically performed by other disciplines on the team. Adapting the individual's environment (answer C) is an external control strategy that is in conflict with most programs' focus on developing internal controls. See reference: Hopkins and Smith (eds): Beck, NL: Eating disorders: Anorexia nervosa and bulimia nervosa.

145. (C) Acute care hospitalization. The emphasis of acute care hospitalization is on symptom reduction, medications, and discharge planning. The club house format (answer A) emphasizes belonging and security. Community mental health centers (answer B) focus on medication management, crisis intervention and outpatient therapy. Quarterway houses (answer D) emphasize increasing autonomy and decreasing supervision. See reference: Hopkins and Smith (eds): Richert, GZ, and Gibson, D: Practice settings.

146. (C) coping strategies for continuing medication compliance. Studies designed to determine the factors related to frequent re-admission for psychiatric individuals have found medication noncompliance to be the major reason for readmission. The other strategies listed may be important issues for specific individuals however they are not the primary issue. See reference: Early: Daily living skills.

147. (B) evaluate the individual's occupational performance. Discharge planning in short term hospitalizations should begin at admission. Evaluation of occupational performance is the first step in the occupational therapy discharge planning. Answers A, C and D may be enacted later in the treatment or discharge planning process. See reference: Early: Overview of the treatment process.

148. (A) partial hospitalization. Partial hospitalization is appropriate for individuals who are experiencing acute psychiatric symptoms and who have a place or family to stay with at night. Partial hospitalization offers most of the structure, staffing, and services available on an inpatient unit except for overnight provisions. Day treatment (answer C) focuses on assisting individuals to adapt to their illness and develop daily living skills at the program site. Day treatment services are typically verbal activities and group therapy within a 3- to 6-month period. Day care (answer B) is long term care that provides structured daily activities and medications to maintain current levels of functioning. Community mental health centers (answer D) provide a wide range of individual and outpatient services that address a variety of individual goals. See reference: Hopkins and Smith (eds): Richert, GZ, and Gibson, D: Practice settings.

149. (C) "The patient completed 10 out of 14 occupational therapy sessions during this 28-day hospitalization." The discharge summary is a summary of a patient's course of treatment and frequently includes the number of sessions that the patient attended while in treatment. Information concerning the reason for and/or source of a referral (answer A) is found in an initial note. Answer B reflects information about the patient's behavior while involved in a treatment program and would be included in a progress note. Answer D is a treatment goal which reflects the action the patient is to take, as well as a specific time frame, and is included in the treatment plan. See reference: Ryan (ed): Backhaus, H: Documentation. *Practice Issues in Occupational Therapy.*

150. (A) "The patient has identified music as a major leisure interest. It is recommended that he explore the possibility of enrolling in a music study course at the community college." The discharge summary is a summary of a patient's course of treatment and includes recommendations for further services and/or post-hospitalization activities. Answer B is a treatment goal which reflects the action the patient is to take, as well as a specific time frame, and is included in the treatment plan. Answer C reflects information about the frequency and type of activities the patient has been participating in as well as response to the activity and would be included in a progress note. Answer D is a statement that reflects information obtained during the first session and would be included in an initial note. See reference: Ryan (ed): Backhaus, H: Documentation. *Practice Issues in Occupational Therapy.*

151. (C) acting as a liaison between the academic setting, facility, and students. The academic fieldwork coordinator is a representative of the educational institution from which the student is attaining a degree. This individual oversees all of the students from the designated occupational therapy educational program. Responsibilities include identifying fieldwork sites, writing contracts with fieldwork sites, and maintaining a collaborative effort with the fieldwork sites. A fieldwork educator provides administrative and day-to-day supervision of the student program (answers A and B) and establishes fieldwork objectives for the fieldwork site (answer D). See reference: Jacobs and Logigian (eds): Cohn, E: Designing fieldwork programs.

152. (C) partner. The COTA working with children needs to be accepting of parents in order to develop successful working relationships. Answer A is incorrect as a strong authoritarian approach may intimidate parents and decrease effective communication. Answer B is incorrect as COTAs should strengthen the parent-child relationship and not compete with parents. Answer D is incorrect, as one of the major roles in working with parents is to share information about the child so that the child's problems and functional abilities are clearly understood. See reference: Case-Smith, Allen, and Pratt (eds): Humphry, R and Case-Smith, J: Working with families.

153. (A) chronic mental illness. Individuals with mild mental retardation, eating disorders and substance abuse disorders may also receive occupational therapy services, but are not the majority. See reference: Early: Treatment settings.

154. (A) advanced, with general supervision. Advanced is the highest level of skill, requiring only general supervision which is defined in a monthly contact. These individuals have refined skills in their area of expertise and may have participated in research or in providing continuing education. An intermediate therapist (answer B) will have gained skill mastery and have the ability to function as a resource person. However, they have not yet gained the refinement of special skills to be considered advanced. Entry level therapists (answer C) would be developing their skills and accepting responsibilities for relevant professional activities. Minimal supervision (answer D), with supervision on an "as needed" basis, is the level recommended for advanced-level OTRs. See reference: AOTA: Occupational therapy roles.

155. (D) Americans with Disabilities Act of 1990. Also referred to as the ADA, this act provides civil rights protection for disabled individuals in five specific areas. These areas include telecommunications, transportation, public accommodations, employment, and the activities of state and local government. The Architectural Barriers Act of 1969 (answer A) literally opened doors for changes to occur in gaining access for disabled individuals. The Federal Rehabilitation Act of 1973 (answer B) expanded service intervention for those individuals who were more severely disabled. The Fair Housing Amendment Act of 1988 (answer C) expanded the coverage of Title VIII. See reference: Hopkins and Smith (eds): Jacobs, K: Work assessments and programming.

156. (A) state licensure laws supersede NBCOT regulations regarding the practice of occupational therapy. AOTA and NBCOT recommend that therapists contact the state regulatory (licensure) boards since each state has legal jurisdiction over the practice of therapists within the region; therefore, answers B, C and D are incorrect. See reference: Hopkins and Smith (eds): Hopkins, HL: Scope of occupational therapy.

157. (B) duty. Principle 3 of the Occupational Therapy Code of Ethics addresses duty, which includes the issue of competence. This refers specifically to credentialing and functioning within the parameters of the OT practitioner's skill level. OT practitioners are guided to hold the appropriate credentials, participate in continuing education, and refer patients to other service areas when the skills required do not fall within their expertise. Beneficence (answer A) speaks to the OT practitioner's concern for the well-being of those to whom they are providing services. This includes provision of services without discrimination, avoiding harm, and the setting of fair and reasonable fees. The fourth principle in the Code of Ethics addresses the concept of justice, which includes compliance with laws and regulations (answer C). This principle refers to OT practitioners following state, local, and federal laws in addition to facility specific guidelines and requirements for accreditation. Veracity (answer D) addresses the concept of truthfulness, which includes the OT practitioner accurately representing his/her qualifications as well as participating in any fraudulent statements or claims. See reference: Hopkins and Smith (eds): Hansen, RA: Ethics in occupational therapy.

158. (C) informed consent. One of the fundamental components of the Occupational Therapy Code of Ethics is informed consent. The basis of informed consent is that the patient be given relevant medical information so that she may be an active participant in the decision making process. Therapeutic privilege (answer B), the withholding of medical information, is no longer acceptable in reference to the provision of services. Beneficence (answer A) is the concept of demonstrating concern for the well-being of the patient. Competence (answer D) refers to the level of expertise expected from occupational therapy practitioners but does not refer to the involvement of the patient in the treatment plan. See reference: AOTA: Occupational Therapy Code of Ethics.

159. (A) Treatment from the OTR's plan provided by a COTA. Based on the Code of Ethics, Principle 2 (competence), occupational therapy may only be done by "those individuals holding appropriate credentials for providing services." These credentials are certification from NBCOT and, when appropriate, state licensure as an occupational therapist or occupational therapy assistant. Answers B, C and D are incorrect because recreational, music, and/or art therapists do not hold these credentials. See reference: AOTA: Occupational Therapy Code of Ethics.

160. (C) notify the NBCOT of the situation and reassign the patient to a different OT practitioner. According to the Code of Ethics, OT practitioners are responsible for "maintaining a goal directed and objective relationship with all people served" as well as not engaging in behavior which may constitute a "conflict of interest that adversely reflects on the profession". The patient/therapist relationship is compromised when the OT practitioner enters into a social or intimate relationship with a patient. Every OT practitioner is responsible to report behavior that is in conflict with the Code of Ethics to the NBCOT, whether they are a supervisor or not. See reference: Hopkins and Smith (eds): Hansen, RA: Ethics in occupational therapy.

161. (C) 1959. This is the date most recognized by COTAs as a milestone for their role in the provision of occupational therapy. The need for technical professionals in the area of occupational therapy was recognized in 1949 by AOTA (answer B). At that time, the profession worked to develop a one year educational program. These efforts moved slowly and it was not until 1959 that the first educational programs for occupational therapy assistants were established. Answer A, 1917, is when the Constitution for the Promotion of Occupational Therapy was established. Answer D, 1981 is when the COTA task force was developed. See reference: Hopkins and Smith (eds): An introduction to occupational therapy.

162. (A) credentialing. The process of credentialing encompasses answers B, C, and D and therefore is the MOST correct response. Credentialing provides evidence concerning an individual's competence and right to state that they are qualified to practice as an occupational therapy assistant. Certification and registration (answers C and D) require successful completion of the educational requirements. In addition, certification requires the passage of the NBCOT exam. Licensure (answer B) is a process which is completed at the state level, and requirements are unique to each state. See reference: Hopkins and Smith (eds): An introduction to occupational therapy.

163. (C) dynametric grip strength and the OTR to assess weight bearing status for ADLs. A dynamometer, which is a designated standardized assessment tool, is used to measure grip strength and is the only standardized assessment tool included in the choices. Upon establishing service competency, an OTR may delegate to a COTA administration of standardized assessment tools. Weight bearing status (answer A) is usually determined by the physician. Cognition (answer B) would be assessed by the psychologist on the team. Information on leisure interests (answer D) would most likely obtained by a therapeutic recreation specialist on an inpatient rehabilitation unit. See reference: AOTA: Occupational therapy roles.

164. (D) isometric exercises. This question requires the reader to take into account the COTA's level of experience as well as service competency issues. Based on the treatment plan, the COTA may independently direct the patient in purposeful activities designed to enhance the performance component of strength. Because of the ongoing interpretation that is involved in the processes of splinting and providing paraffin treatments (answers A and B), these activities should be done only after service competency has been established. Given that the COTA is a new graduate, service competency has not yet been established. Finally, the COTA may contribute to the process of the home evaluation (answer C), but because of the analytical nature of the task, would not complete the evaluation independently. See reference: AOTA: Occupational therapy roles.

165. (D) the credentialing process is necessary prior to licensing. State licensing requires proof that the candidate has the minimum level of knowledge necessary to be competent in the provision of occupational therapy services. The credentialing process requires a test (the NBCOT examination) which the candidate must pass in order to ensure entry-level knowledge of the field of occupational therapy; therefore, credentialing is required before licensing. See reference: NBCOT: NBCOT Candidate Handbook.

166. (B) the OTR must assume responsibility for all occupational therapy services delivered. An OTR is always responsible for services provided by COTAs he or she is responsible for supervising. AOTA does not require that the patient have a referral for provision of services; however, it is important to note that state licensure laws and accrediting agencies may require a formal referral. Answer A is incorrect in that the OTR is operating within AOTA standards. A written letter of consent (answer C) is not required by either state or accrediting agencies. A COTA would not initiate contacting the physician (answer D) without discussing the case with the supervising

OTR. See reference: Ryan (ed): Ryan, SE: Therapeutic intervention process. *Practice Issues in Occupational Therapy.*

167. (B) The individual's written consent to take the photograph. A photograph of a person who is being treated at a health care facility would release privileged information and would violate her right to confidentiality just as much as releasing her name or diagnosis (answers A and D). No information about a person may be released without a written consent. Hospitals generally have the right to take photographs of their employees (answer C) when engaged in job related duties. See reference: Ryan (ed): Gohl-Giese, A: Video recording. *The Certified Occupational Therapy Assistant.*

168. (A) expand in long term care facilities and elder care. American demographics show that the "baby boomers" are now entering their fourth and fifth decades of life. As this generation grows older, the need for services for the elderly will increase. COTAs will be essential providers of care as the need for occupational therapy services expand. Answers B, C and D are incorrect in that they reflect a decrease in the use of occupational therapy services. See reference: Ryan (ED): Gilfoyle, EM: The future of occupational therapy. *Practice Issues in Occupational Therapy.*

169. (A) annually develop a plan of professional development. A certified occupational therapy assistant may effectively guide his/her career by developing an annual plan. Such plans include goals and objectives which are written much like the goals written for patients. The COTA should think about the goal that s/he wants to attain and how to achieve the goal. In addition, goals should be written to be accomplished within a certain time frame. Answers B, C and D may all be a part of the professional development plan. See reference: Hopkins and Smith (eds): Levine, RE, Corcoran, MA, and Gitlin, L: Home care and private practice.

170. (B) mention the fact that the applicant failed a level II fieldwork when the staff gets together to discuss the applicants. The OT Code of ethics states that "Occupational therapy personnel shall safeguard confidential information about colleagues and staff members." The COTA should recognize the applicant's level II failure as confidential information. Answers A, C, and D are all professional and appropriate responses. See reference: AOTA: Occupational Therapy Code of Ethics.

171. (D) discuss her concerns with an OTR who is present. Although her own supervisor is absent, an OTR present would become the acting supervisor for the COTA for the day. The COTA should always discuss concerns with the supervisor first. Going to the administration (answer C) would not only disregard the chain of command, but could escalate a problem that should be handled internally. ADL training is a skilled service beyond the scope of what an aide can do. The COTA should not allow the aide to finish the treatment session (answer A). It may not be feasible in a busy department for the COTA to complete the session herself (answer B). See reference: Early: Supervision.

172. (B) COTAs should read interpret and apply OT research. While there is no law or regulation requiring any OT practitioner to participate in research (answer A), graduates of OTA programs should be able to read, interpret and apply information from research in occupational therapy. Participating in data collection (answer C) and the development of a research question (answer D) are more advanced levels at which a COTA can participate. See reference: Ryan (ed): Blechert, TF and Christiansen, MF: Intraprofessional relationships and socialization. *Practice Issues in Occupational Therapy.*

173. (A) The state regulatory board. A license to practice is granted by the state regulatory board, therefore the state regulatory board is the only body with the authority to revoke a license to practice occupational therapy. The Commission of Standards and Ethics of the AOTA (answer B) has the authority to revoke membership in AOTA. The NBCOT (answer C) has the authority to revoke certification, and loss of certification most often results in revocation of licensure by a state regulatory board. Some states have laws requiring health care provides to report child abuse, but reporting the practitioner's actions to the police alone (answer D) will not affect his/her license. See reference: Ryan (ed): Gray, M: The credentialing process in occupation therapy. *Practice Issues in Occupational Therapy.*

174. (A) provide students with the opportunity to apply knowledge learned in school to practice. The main purpose of fieldwork education is to compliment the student's academic preparation with practical experience. A benefit to facilities that accept students is that they are frequently exposed to new concepts and techniques students bring with them to the site (answer B). The purpose of fieldwork is NOT to provide additional human resources to the site (answer C); however, this is a benefit that often occurs as part of the student's learning experience. Fieldwork prepares students to work in both traditional and non-traditional practice environment (answer D). See reference: AOTA: Guide to fieldwork education.

175. (C) AOTF. The American Occupational Therapy Foundation raises money and provides research grants in the field of occupational therapy. AOTA (answer A) stands for the American Occupational Therapy Association. AOTA is an organization the promotes the profession. AOTCB (answer D) stands for the American Occupational Therapy Certification Board. This Board changed its name in 1996 to the NBCOT. The National Board for Certification of Occupational Therapists (answer B) is responsible for the testing and certification of all registered occupational therapists and certified occupational therapy assistants. See reference: Ryan (ed): Jones, RA: Service operations. *Practice Issues in Occupational Therapy.*

176. (A) There is an increasing shortage of occupational therapy practitioners in the area of mental health. Current trends in mental health to use recreational, music and/or art therapists has reduced the demand for occupational therapy practitioners in the mental health environment. In addition, an increasing number of occupational therapy practitioners are pursuing positions in pediatrics and physical disabilities. These two issues combined is causing a shortage of occupational therapy practitioners in mental health settings. The inverse is true of answers B, C, and D, therefore making them incorrect. See reference: Hopkins and Smith (eds): Gibson, D and Richert, G:

Mental health: The therapeutic process. Also: Hopkins and Smith (eds): Levy, LL: The health care delivery system today.

177. (A) consistently obtain the same results as a competent practitioner performing the same procedure. The term "service competency" indicates an interrater reliability between two OT practitioners. Service competency is achieved or demonstrated through passing the certification examination (answer B). Continuing education and experience (answers C and D) may contribute to the development of service competency but do not guarantee competence. See reference: Early: Data gathering and evaluation.

178. (A) examine the effectiveness of patient care. Quality assurance is a systematic and objective means of monitoring the effectiveness of services provided. Several accrediting agencies mandate or emphasize program evaluation in their accreditation processes. Cost accounting is the method used to determine the cost of running a department (answer B). Performance appraisals and peer reviews are two methods for evaluating the performance of therapy personnel (answer C). Appropriate documentation and good time management are two ways OT personnel can help to maximize reimbursement (answer D). See reference: Ryan (ed): Jones, RA: Service operations. *Practice Issues in Occupational Therapy.*

179. (D) the title of job, organizational relationships, essential job functions, and job requirements. Job descriptions will most likely contain the title of the job, organizational relationships, essential job functions, work performed, job requirements and environmental risks. Items that are not required but may compliment an individualized job description would be personality characteristics, past experience requirements and accomplishments. Answers A, B, and C include items that are *not* required in a job description but are more appropriately located on a resume. See reference: Jacobs and Logigian (eds): Parisi, R: Managing human resources.

180. (A) objectively assess the COTA's performance. Performance appraisals are for the primary purpose of evaluating an employee's accomplishments. Answer B is incorrect because disciplinary problems are generally handled through the disciplinary process. Disciplinary processes may involve a verbal warning, written warnings, suspension, and termination. Answer C, a merit increase, may accompany a performance appraisal but is not the purpose of the review. Answer D is also incorrect in that many times, writing goals and objectives for the upcoming year is in addition to the performance review and not a primary purpose of the review. See reference: Jacobs and Logigian (eds): Harel, B: Supervision.

181. (C) CARF. The Commission on Accreditation of Rehabilitation Facilities is the regulatory agency for the provision of rehabilitation services. AOTA (answer A) was formed in March of 1917 as the National Society for the Promotion of Occupational Therapy and does not regulate the provision of occupational therapy services. JCAHO (answer B) is the Joint Commission on Accreditation of Healthcare Organizations. The JCAHO reviews the medical care provided by healthcare organizations. The NBCOT (answer D) is the agency which develops and administers the examinations for registration as an occupational therapy practitioner. See reference: Jacobs and Logigian (eds): Cargill, L: Quality assurance.

182. (B) wear gloves. Wearing gloves places a barrier between the COTA and any possible infection on the patient's hand. A mask (answer A) is more effective as a barrier for airborne pathogens or against splashes of bodily fluids. Refusing to work with the patient (answer C) is not an option, as indicated in the OT Code of Ethics. Individuals fearful of infection should educate themselves about appropriate precautions and procedures, and should seek employment in environments where they are capable of providing intervention to all patients/clients served by facility. Hand washing prior to treating all patients is appropriate (answer D), and is effective in protecting the patient from contamination, but would not be effective in protecting the COTA during patient treatment. See reference: Early: Safety techniques.

183. (A) once a day. Supervision is a mutual undertaking by the COTA and OTR, which promotes quality occupational therapy and the professional development of the individuals involved. Close supervision is defined as "daily, direct contact at the site of work." Other levels of supervision are routine, general, and minimal. Routine supervision is provided when direct contact is made every two weeks (answer B) with "interim supervision occurring by other methods such as telephone or written communication. Under general supervision, contact is made monthly (answer C). Minimal supervision is provided on an "as needed" basis (answer D). It is possible that this may be less than once a month. General supervision is the least frequent level of supervision acceptable for COTAs. See reference: AOTA: Supervision Guidelines for Occupational Therapy Personnel.

184. (B) any equipment which has come into contact with body fluids will be sterilized prior to using the equipment again. OSHA has set out strategies to protect individuals from potential exposure to HIV or HBV. This situation would be an example of an engineering control. These controls are designed to modify the work environment to reduce risk of exposure. Other examples would be utilizing sharps containers, eye wash stations, and biohazard waste containers. See reference: Occupational Safety and Health Administration.

185. (B) medical necessity. Medicare defines a medical necessity as "necessary and reasonable to treat an illness or an injury or to improve the functioning of a 'malformed body member.'" Answer B is the MOST correct answer. Answers A, C and D are correct but are a part of the broader statement of medical necessity. See reference: Bair and Gray (eds): Scott, SJ, and Somers, FP: Payment for occupational therapy services.

186. (C) discontinue provision of OT services until appropriate supervision is available. A COTA may not provide OT services unless supervised by an OTR. While advanced level COTAs (answer B) may supervise more inexperienced COTAs, it must be under the supervision of an OTR. Physical therapists (answer A), teachers, psychologists and other staff at the school are valuable resources and team members; however, an OTR must ultimately be responsible for COTA supervision. Encouraging the school to advertise for a new OTR is a good idea (answer D), but the COTA would not be able to continue providing treatment without violating certification, state licensure, the Code of Ethics and the Standards of Practice regardless of diagnosis. See reference: Ryan (ed): Ryan, SE: COTA supervision. *Practice Issues in Occupational Therapy.*

187. (B) federal and state governmental agencies and third-party payers. AOTA (included in answers A, C, and D) does not require physician referral for the provision of OT services. Federal, state, and local governmental agencies, third-party payers, regulatory and state agencies, and individual facilities may require physician referral. See reference: AOTA: Statement of occupational therapy referral.

188. (D) notify the supervising OTR about the referral. The COTA must first notify the OTR of the referral, as the OTR is ultimately responsible for any action taken. Under the supervision of the OTR, that COTA may then initiate screening or explain the purpose of OT to the child (answers A and C). Within school-based practice, it is not necessary for the referral to come from a physician (answer B). See reference: Ryan (ed): Ryan, SE: Therapeutic intervention process. *Practice Issues in Occupational Therapy.*

189. (D) intense close supervision. An OT aide may "perform delegated, selected. skilled tasks in specific situations under the intense close supervision of an OT practitioner." Individual state laws, which would supersede the AOTA position paper, may further restrict the use of aides. The COTA, in collaboration with the OTR, may be responsible for training and supervision of aides. The intensity of supervision is determined by the tasks being performed, the needs of the patient/client, and the skill level of the aide. Intense close supervision is defined as "daily direct on-site contact." Routine and close supervision (answers A and C) are levels pertaining to the supervision of OTRs and COTAs. Maximal supervision (answer B) is not a term used to describe supervisory levels for OT personnel. See reference: AOTA: Position paper: Use of occupational therapy aides in occupational therapy practice.

190. (A) latex or vinyl gloves. Gloves should always be worn in situations where the COTA may come into contact with blood, bloody fluids, or infectious fluids as may occur during an ADL bathing/dressing activity. Answers B, C and D should all be utilized in addition to answer A when there is the possibility of contaminated materials being spilled or splashed. See reference: Occupational Safety and Health Administration.

191. (A) diagnosis. Referrals typically include the individual's diagnosis, frequency of treatment, duration of treatment and treatment interventions requested. Answers B, C, and D, are all items that would be found in the initial assessment. See reference: AOTA: Statement of occupational therapy referral.

192. (A) mutual process. The supervisory process is one which requires the attention of both parties involved. The COTA needs to develop his/her own role and identity within the institution and profession. In addition, the OTR supervisor needs to provide the COTA with opportunities for growth and development. As part of this relationship, ongoing evaluation and counseling may take place to enhance learning and role development. While answers B, C, and D are necessary to the supervisory process, the best answer is A in that it reflects that the process is mutual. See reference: Early: Supervision.

193. (D) is no longer homebound. Most insurance carriers will only cover home care when the individual is unable to leave his/her residence without assistance. Once she is able to leave her residence, she would not be able to continue to receive home care services (answer A) and would be referred to outpatient services. Without knowing Emma's specific goals, it is not possible to say whether she has achieved them (answers B and C). See reference: Hopkins and Smith (eds): Levine, RE, Corcoran, MA, and Gitlin, L: Home care and private practice.

194. (D) A patient with a diagnosis of CVA and left neglect caught the left arm in the wheel of the wheelchair, resulting in a cut and bruise. An incident report should be completed whenever a situation occurs which is harmful to the patient or therapist. This includes but is not limited to falls, burns, cuts, and contact with hazardous materials. See reference: AOTA: Occupational therapy roles.

195. (D) discuss her concerns with the OTR. Bringing concerns to a supervisor for discussion and problem solving is an important way of participating in a collaborative supervisory relationship. Answers A and C all avoid discussion of the issue with the supervisor, which can limit professional growth and damage a supervisory relationship. It is important to respect the administrative chain of command and speak directly with the supervisor before going to a higher authority. A COTA should never perform an evaluation without instruction to do so from the supervising OTR (answer B). See reference: Early: Supervision.

196. (C) a procedure. The steps involved in enacting a policy are the procedure. Procedures state how a policy is carried out, in what sequence and by whom. A policy (answer B) provides information about actions that need to be taken. Documentation (answer A) refers to written reports concerning patient evaluation and treatment. A job description (answer D) includes the job title, organizational relationship, and required skills and functions. See reference: Jacobs and Logigian (eds): Pagonis, J: Documentation in health care.

197. (D) lock the brakes. Brakes should be locked first to stabilize the wheelchair. Answers A, B and C involve movements that could cause loss of balance or wheelchair movement unless the brakes are locked. See reference: Pedretti (ed): Adler, C and Tipton-Burton, M: Wheelchair assessment and transfers.

198. (D) copper tooling. The liver of sulfate used to give a copper tooling project that antiqued look has a noxious odor and can irritate the eyes. There are no odors or fumes associated with acrylic paints (Answer A), ceramic paints (answer C) or leather tooling (answer B). See reference: Drake: Copper tooling and metal craft.

199. (C) No, because Medicare does not consider services provided by an aide as skilled occupational therapy. Without intense close supervision. Medicare does not consider the unskilled services of an aide occupational therapy, and to bill for those services would be fraudulent. Site specific training that is well defined and well documented can provide aides with higher skill levels in some areas (answer A), however, this scenario would still not meet the Medicare requirements. See reference: Hopkins and Smith (eds): Levine, RE, Corcoran, MA, and Gitlin, L: Home care and private practice.

200. (A) Medicaid. Medicaid is a joint federal and state program. Because it is a joint program, benefits vary widely from state to state. These programs must include "Aid to Families with Dependent Children" (AFDC) and "Supplementary Security Income" (SSI). Medicare (answer B) is a federal program that funds health coverage for individuals 65 years or older, disabled individuals, or people in the end stages of renal disease. Workers compensation (answer C) is a state supported program into which employers pay. Beneficiaries will receive coverage for those services which are identified as covered within their respective states. The "Education for All Handicapped Children Act" (answer D) is funded in part through state and federal grants. It does not fund health care, but requires any school receiving federal assistance to provide handicapped children with a free, appropriate education in the least restrictive environment. See reference: Bair and Gray (eds): Scott, S, and Somers, FP: Payment for occupational therapy services.

SIMULATION EXAMINATION 4

Directions: Circle the correct answer to the following questions. When you have completed this examination, check your answers against the answer key that follows. As you will see, an explanation is given for each answer along with a reference for further study; the book author is listed as well as the chapter author. See the bibliography for complete references. Study the areas in which your comprehension was low, then test yourself again by taking Simulation Examination 5.

PEDIATRIC QUESTIONS

Data Collection

1. During occupational therapy treatment, a child has a seizure that barely interrupts activity performance. What type of seizure would the COTA report this as ?

A. Grand mal.
B. Psychomotor.
C. Petit mal.
D. Akinetic.

2. A 9-year-old child with a diagnosis of dyslexia exhibits an inability to:

A. print or write.
B. read.
C. calculate mathematics.
D. plan motor actions.

3. A 2-year-old girl with developmental delay does not finger feed when presented with food in the clinic. The BEST way to obtain further information about her feeding skills is to:

A. interview her parents to determine her favorite foods.
B. observe her in her home during feeding time.
C. review her chart for food allergies.
D. repeat the observation in a quiet area (in order to minimize distractions).

4. The COTA is working with a 7-year-old boy who exhibits tactile defensiveness. Which area of the child's occupational performance is MOST likely to be affected?

A. reading skills.
B. dressing habits.
C. friendships.
D. hobbies.

5. Which toys are MOST appropriate for assessing a child's exploratory play skills?

A. rattles, teething toys, and teddy bears.
B. simple construction toys, dress-up clothes, and props.
C. arts-and-crafts materials and complex construction toys.
D. board games and team sport equipment.

6. The COTA observes a 4-year-old boy for skill in using the toilet. At this age, she would expect him to:

A. be completely independent in using the toilet.
B. be independent, except for needing help with clothing.
C. need reminders to go to the toilet.
D. have daytime control with occasional accidents.

7. While assessing the motor skills of an 8-month-old girl, the COTA observes the child assume a quadruped position and then begin rocking back and forth. The COTA notes this behavior as indicative of:

A. perseverative tendencies.
B. normal development.
C. low muscle tone.
D. limitation in movement repertoire.

8. After watching a 7-year-old, multiply handicapped girl being fed, the COTA reports her observations to the supervising therapist. The BEST example of objective terminology is:

A. "The child apparently did not like the food presented."
B. "The child demonstrated tongue thrust that interfered with eating."
C. "The child was uncooperative and kept pushing the food out of her mouth."
D. "The child was obviously not hungry at the time."

9. While standing and holding onto furniture, a 3-year-old boy with delayed motor development shifts his weight onto one leg and steps to the side with the other. Which movement pattern does this describe?
A. Creeping.
B. Crawling.
C. Cruising.
D. Clawing

10. The COTA is working with a 7-year-old girl with a diagnosis of spina bifida, who has a shunt. Which of the following signs of shunt malfunction should the COTA watch for?
A. Increased head size.
B. Nausea and vomiting.
C. Back pain.
D. Intermittent headaches.

Treatment Planning

11. The COTA is reviewing a problem list based on a child's performance. The problem list is most commonly developed at which point in the occupational therapy process?
A. Following observation or screening.
B. Following the interview.
C. Following the evaluation.
D. Following the writing of the goals and objectives.

12. An individual educational plan is completed for:
A. occupational therapists, as part of the continuing education plan.
B. adults who have sustained a head injury.
C. all children with disabilities before they receive special education services.
D. families before discharge of a significant other from occupational therapy services.

13. A 3-year-old child with a diagnosis of mental retardation is dependent in all areas of dressing. If the COTA uses a developmental approach with this child, which skill will he or she address FIRST?
A. Donning garments with the front and back correctly placed.
B. Donning a T-shirt.
C. Doffing socks.
D. Buttoning and tying bows.

14. When planning a therapeutic program for a child who has deficits in visual discrimination, the FIRST step is to provide "matching" activities that require:
A. discrimination among the colors of objects.
B. discrimination among the shapes of objects.
C. discrimination among the positions of objects.
D. the ability to recognize objects.

15. While developing a treatment plan for a 6-year-old boy with congenital limb deficiency, the COTA would like to discuss adaptations to the child's artificial limb. Which team member should the COTA consult?
A. The physiatrist.
B. The orthotist.
C. The prosthetist.
D. The physical therapist.

16. When choosing treatment goals for an 8-year-old boy with Duchenne's muscular dystrophy, the COTA should keep in mind that an important developmental issue for a child of this age is the:
A. establishment of basic trust.
B. freedom to use his initiative.
C. development of self-identity.
D. reinforcement of competence.

17. The goal for a 12-year-old girl with limited grip strength is to become independent in self-care. To work toward this goal, which is the BEST method to gradually develop hair care skills?
A. Have the client use a weighted brush and gradually decrease the weight.
B. Color-code combs and brushes, beginning with bright colors, and gradually reduce the intensity of the color cues.
C. Have the client use a brush with a thick handle, and gradually decrease the thickness.
D. Give the client physical cues to begin with, then change to gestural cues and finally to verbal cues.

18. Jeremy's manipulation skills are not as developed as is normal for his age, because of lower-than-normal proprioceptive awareness. What is the MOST appropriate therapeutic activity?
A. Making handprints by pushing his palm into clay.
B. Spreading shaving cream over his hands and forearms.
C. Learning to perform a magic coin trick with one hand.
D. Making a necklace by stringing 1-inch beads.

19. Marcy has inadequate playground skills because of poor anticipatory postural control, that is, she loses her balance when trying to anticipate movement, especially with ball skills. The COTA recommends participation in which of the following sport in order to promote the development of skills?
A. Bowling.
B. Soccer.
C. Basket ball.
D. Ping-pong.

20. A 1-year-old girl with cerebral palsy demonstrates poor head control. In order to improve the child's ability to be fed and to eat, what

aspect of postural control should be addressed FIRST?

A. Shoulder.
B. Head.
C. Trunk.
D. Hand.

21. Luisa is a withdrawn 8-year-old girl, whose occupational therapy objectives include increasing her ability to express feelings and conflicts. What is an appropriate projective activity to promote this skill?

A. Drawing a picture titled "This is me."
B. Playing adapted soccer with a large ball.
C. Playing a structured board game, such as Monopoly.
D. Singing folk songs in a group.

Treatment Implementation

22. A child with a diagnosis of spina bifida needs a chair adapted to provide stability while sitting and working at school. Which of the following combinations of hip/knee/ankle position is the correct choice?

A. 45/45/45 degrees at hip/knee/ankle joints.
B. 90/90/90 degrees at hip/knee/ankle joints.
C. 90/45/45 degrees at hip/knee/ankle joints.
D. 125/125/125 degrees at hip/knee/ankle joints.

23. A child normally begins to "cruise" between:

A. 3 and 5 months of age.
B. 6 and 8 months of age.
C. 9 and 12 months of age.
D. 13 and 15 months of age.

24. A child with poor balance is unable to don and doff lower-extremity clothing. Which of the following approaches would BEST deal with the functional problem?

A. Teaching the child to dress in sidelying position.
B. Adding loops to the waistbands of pants and skirts.
C. Using Velcro fasteners in place of zippers.
D. Teaching the child to dress in standing position.

25. A 1-year-old girl demonstrates weak sucking. The COTA uses a shallow spoon when feeding her. This will help develop:

A. jaw opening.
B. jaw closing.
C. lower lip control.
D. upper lip control.

26. A 10-year-old boy demonstrates aggressive and disruptive behavior in school, which is a result of his low sensory threshold. For the upcoming class trip by bus to the zoo, the COTA should advise the teacher to:

A. review the bus rules with the boy and apply consequences consistently.
B. let the boy sit at the front of the bus and use his tape player and earphones.
C. give the boy the responsibility of monitoring his peers as "bus patrol."
D. let the boy set the criteria for a successful trip and reward him if the criteria are met.

27. When instructing the parents of a pre-verbal toddler in the use and care of a hand splint, the COTA should put MOST emphasis on:

A. checking for irritation and pressure problems.
B. avoiding excessive heat exposure.
C. cleansing the splint regularly.
D. adhering strictly to the wearing schedule.

28. A 12-year-old boy with limited fine motor control wants to play checkers with his brother. To allow him to participate using only palmar grasp, the COTA makes the following adaptation:

A. attaching Velcro to the playing board and markers.
B. mounting half-inch-diameter dowels vertically on the markers.
C. placing a magnetic playing board upright.
D. replacing markers with lightweight playing pieces.

29. What is the BEST method for a COTA to use when working with an infant who exhibits tactile defensive reactions?

A. Tickle him during play times.
B. Play loud music when undressing him.
C. Lightly stroke his arms and legs during the bath.
D. Hold him firmly when picking him up.

30. The COTA has fitted a 6-year-old child for an adapted seat for use in the home for mealtime and other tabletop activities. The COTA instructs the parents to:

A. adapt the seat as needed.
B. bring the seat in for each weekly therapy session in order to adjust it according to the child's growth.
C. bring the seat in for reevaluation within 6 months.
D. keep the seat until the end of the IEP.

31. Linda has a diagnosis of ataxic cerebral palsy and exhibits tremors in her upper extremities. When she feeds herself, the tremors cause most of the food to fall off her spoon before it can reach her mouth. Which of the following adaptations should the COTA recommend?

A. Replacing the spoon with a blunt-ended fork.
B. Building up the handle of the spoon.
C. Giving Linda a swivel spoon.
D. Bending the spoon handle 45 degrees.

32. Annie is a preschooler whose poor visual-tracking skills affect her performance on tasks requiring eye-hand coordination. Which of the following activities is MOST appropriate for the COTA to recommend to Annie's parents in order to promote beginning visual tracking skills during summer vacation?

A. Tossing and catching a waterballoon.
B. Catching and bursting soap bubbles.
C. Throwing and catching a beach ball.
D. Playing softball.

33. Ricky is 6 years old and has a diagnosis of autism. He regularly bites his fingers, often so badly that the skin is broken. Which of the following methods would be LEAST effective in reducing his self-injurious behavior?

A. Engaging him in more productive activities.
B. Providing alternative activities involving heavy-pressure touch.
C. Explaining the consequences of his actions to him.
D. Using behavioral techniques to modify his behavior.

34. When adapting a toilet for use by a child with poor postural control, the COTA should pay primary attention to which of the following issues?

A. Can the toilet paper be reached without a major weight shift?
B. Is the flush handle easy to manipulate?
C. Does the seat design provide enough support for the child to relax?
D. Is a nonskid mat placed on the floor to prevent slipping?

35. Ashanti is 3 years old and has a diagnosis of hypertonia with predominant extensor tone. When teaching her mother how to put shoes and socks on her daughter, the COTA recommends first flexing Ashanti's:

A. hips.
B. knees.
C. ankles.
D. toes.

Evaluating the Treatment Plan

36. Shima has athetoid cerebral palsy and is working on self-feeding skills. She is able to grasp a utensil, but the food keeps sliding off her plate when she attempts to pick it up with a fork or spoon. The MOST appropriate piece of equipment for the COTA to recommend is a:

A. swivel spoon.
B. nonslip mat.
C. mobile arm support.
D. scoop dish.

37. A young child with hypertonicity is unable to bring his hands to midline to reach for a toy while in the supine or sitting positions. The best position to try next, in order to reduce the effects of abnormal patterns and facilitate midline grasp, is the:

A. standing position.
B. prone position.
C. sidelying position.
D. quadruped position.

38. A 6-year-old girl with Down's syndrome demonstrates a 3-year delay in the development of fine-motor skills. She has just developed enough stability and strength in her right hand to hold the scissors properly, hold the paper in her nondominant hand, and make snips or single cuts in the paper. The next scissors skill to develop would be cutting:

A. cardboard and cloth.
B. along curved lines to cut out a circle.
C. along straight lines to cut a triangle.
D. the paper in two following a straight line.

39. Leslie is 3 years old and has just learned to sit independently on the floor. The next step in refining her postural reactions in sitting is to have her:

A. sit straddling a bolster with both feet on the floor.
B. maintain sitting balance on a scooter while being pulled.
C. ride a hippity-hop without falling off.
D. maintain floor-sitting position with the therapist providing pelvic support.

40. Larry is a preschooler who has trouble with manipulation because of higher than normal tone. He has just achieved his goal of independently releasing inch cubes into a cup; however, he uses full extension of his arm and a tenodesis pattern to effect the release. The COTA recommends to the OTR that Larry's goal be updated to reflect the next level of achievement. The new goal should read: "Within 3 months Larry will demonstrate increased manipulation skills by releasing:

A. foam balls into a basket placed 3 feet away from his standing position."
B. inch cubes into a cup placed on a tabletop at a distance of 1 foot ."
C. raisins into a bottle placed on a tabletop at a distanced of 1 foot ."
D. beanbags onto a target placed on the floor at his feet."

41. Ellen is 4 years old and has a diagnosis of developmental delay. She is very withdrawn and passive, possibly because of a background of abuse and neglect. While working on toilet skills with her COTA, Ellen reaches out for a toothbrush and

starts to brush her hair with it. The COTA recognizes the importance of this behavior as:

A. demonstrating attention-getting behavior.
B. a sign of cognitive limitation.
C. indicating initiative and beginning task-directed behavior.
D. demonstrating misinterpretation of cues because of a visual deficit.

42. Doug is 7 years old and has a diagnosis of mental retardation. He has just achieved his goal of bathing himself with minimal assistance. He is able to complete 75 percent of the task independently, but needs verbal and some physical cueing when it comes to washing his neck and face. After discussing Doug's progress with the OTR, the COTA updates the treatment plan to the next level of self-care skill independence. The new goal reads:

A. "Doug will bathe himself with supervision."
B. "Doug will bathe himself independently with set-up."
C. "Doug will bathe himself with moderate assistance."
D. "Doug will bathe himself independently."

43. Shira is 8 years old and has multiple handicaps. She is beginning to develop some controlled movement in her upper extremities. The COTA should discuss the introduction of switch-operated assistive technology with the OTR when Shira:

A. develops tolerance of an upright sitting posture.
B. can reach and point with accuracy.
C. demonstrates any reliable, controlled movement.
D. develops isolated finger control.

Discharge Planning

44. A child with a swallowing dysfunction is being discharged with a home program for feeding. The COTA recommends to the parents that they avoid foods that are the MOST difficult to swallow, such as:

A. smooth semisolids (pureed bananas).
B. lumpy semisolids (cottage cheese).
C. liquids and solids combined (minestrone soup).
D. thickened liquids (malted milk).

45. A school-age child with residual visual perceptual deficits is being discharged from occupational therapy. Which compensatory technique for dealing with visual figure-ground problems should the COTA recommend to the child's teacher?

A. Place a red line on the left side of the paper.
B. Use a timer for certain activities.
C. Teach the child to use lists and color-coding of books and folders.
D. Block out all areas of the page except important words.

46. Direct OT services are being discontinued for a student with attention deficit disorder, but consultation will be provided to help her adjust to the new classroom. Which of the following recommendations can the COTA make to help the teacher adapt the environment to promote optimal learning conditions without affecting the girl's classmates?

A. Use dim lighting and reduce glare by turning down lights.
B. Remove all posters and visual aids to reduce visual distractions.
C. Provide a screen to reduce peripheral visual stimuli.
D. Restructure classroom activities into a series of short-term tasks.

47. The COTA is providing information to the OTR concerning the readiness for discharge from outpatient OT services of an 8-year-old with fine-motor difficulties. The MOST important information for the COTA to focus on is the:

A. child's interests and hobbies.
B. child's writing, dressing, and self-feeding skills.
C. child's academic achievement.
D. availability of the child's parent for follow-up services.

48. A COTA is planning for the discharge of a 9-year-old child with incoordination and tremors. What is the MOST appropriate adaptation for hygiene care that the COTA can recommend?

A. A bath mitt.
B A sponge mounted in the tub.
C. A long-handled bath brush.
D. A hand-held shower head.

49. A COTA is discharge planning with a 16-year-old boy with a seizure disorder. Which of the following environments is MOST likely to elicit seizure activity and should therefore be avoided?

A. A sports event.
B. A movie theater.
C. A shopping mall.
D. A disco.

50. Which of the following is the BEST example of the assessment section of a discharge summary written using a SOAP note format?

A. "Pt. reports he can work at the computer much longer and more comfortably than he could initially."
B. "Pt. can work for up to 3 hours at the computer using periodic stretch breaks."
C. "Pt. has improved significantly in his ability to work at the computer by using periodic stretch breaks."
D. "Pt. will take stretch breaks every 30 minutes when working at the computer."

PHYSICAL DISABILITY QUESTIONS

Data Collection

51. The COTA asks a patient to draw a map of the route she takes to work. Which component of performance does such a task address?
A. position in space.
B. figure-ground discrimination.
C. topographic orientation.
D. visual closure.

52. The COTA gives an individual who has suffered a left-hemisphere cerebrovascular accident a paper with typed letters of the alphabet randomly dispersed across the page. She asks the individual to cross out all the Ms. The COTA observes that the individual has missed letters in a random pattern throughout the page and documents this deficit as:
A. a left visual field cut.
B. a right visual field cut.
C. functional illiteracy.
D. decreased attention.

53. When measuring elbow range-of-motion with a goniometer, the COTA must position the axis of the goniometer:
A. at the lateral epicondyle of the humerus.
B. at the medial epicondyle of the humerus.
C. parallel to the longitudinal axis of the humerus on the lateral aspect.
D. parallel to the longitudinal axis of the radius on the lateral aspect.

54. A COTA is working with an individual who is hemiplegic and demonstrates left-side neglect, poor judgment, decreased balance, and dependence in all activities of daily living (ADLs). When the COTA asks the client to describe the problems he has been having and which he would like to work on first, he replies he is not having difficulty with anything and that he would like to return to his room. This response is most likely indicative of:
A. apraxia.
B. noncompliance.
C. anosagnosia.
D. alexia.

55. An individual demonstrates internal rotation of the shoulder to 70 degrees. This should be documented as:
A. within normal limits.
B. within functional limits.
C. hypermobility that requires further treatment.
D. limited mobility that requires further treatment.

56. During morning self-care activities, an individual is able to place his dentures in his mouth but has difficulty applying denture cream to the appropriate place on the dentures and attempts to place the cap on the tube backwards or on the wrong end of the tube. The COTA would report this deficit to the OTR as:
A. constructional apraxia.
B. ideomotor apraxia.
C. dressing apraxia.
D. unilateral neglect.

57. A COTA working in a hospital setting wants to know which medications a patient is taking before she begins working with him. The FIRST step the COTA should take to obtain this information is:
A. asking the physician.
B. asking the nurse.
C. reading the medical chart.
D. asking her supervising OTR.

58. A COTA has been assigned a patient who is s/p BKA. The BEST source of information on this individual's family history is the:
A. physician's admission note.
B. social worker's admission note.
C. nurse's admission note.
D. physical therapist's initial note.

59. A COTA is evaluating the ability of an adolescent girl with quadriplegia to put on a front-opening shirt. She observes that the girl is able to don the shirt completely but with difficulty and requires assistance for buttoning the shirt. The COTA rates the girl's performance as:
A. independent.
B. requiring minimal assistance.
C. requiring supervision.
D. requiring moderate assistance.

60. After evaluating hand function in an individual with arthritis, the COTA reports the results to the supervising OTR. Which of the following is an UNACCEPTABLE method of reporting this information?
A. With a phone call.
B. In a written report.
C. During discussion at lunch in the cafeteria.
D. During discussion in the OT office.

Treatment Planning

61. The BEST time of day to schedule an individual with arthritis for an evaluation is:
A. early morning (8 to 10 AM).
B. afternoon.
C. late morning (10 to 11 AM).
D. early morning and again in the afternoon.

62. The primary role of the COTA when treating an individual who has recently been diagnosed with rheumatoid arthritis (RA) is to:

A. increase strength with resistive exercises.
B. provide positioning and/or adaptive equipment.
C. provide emotional support.
D. prepare the patient for surgical intervention.

63. An individual with joint changes that limit finger flexion would be MOST comfortable using utensils with:
A. regular handles.
B. weighted handles.
C. a universal cuff attachment.
D. built-up handles.

64. Which of the following devices would help a person who uses a mouth stick to work on a computer by keeping the mouth stick from striking other keys accidentally?
A. A moisture guard.
B. A key guard.
C. An auto-repeat defeat.
D. One-finger-access software.

65. Treatment planning involves all of the following EXCEPT:
A. performing assessments.
B. setting goals.
C. selecting methods by which to achieve the individual's goals.
D. activity analysis.

66. An individual with carpal tunnel syndrome has been fitted with a splint. Her long-term goal is to return to work as a secretary. A related short-term goal is:
A. "Pt. will demonstrate an understanding of work simplification techniques."
B. "Pt. will demonstrate ability to don and doff splint correctly."
C. "Pt. will demonstrate ability to type for 10 minutes with wrists in 10 degrees of flexion."
D. "Pt. will use lightweight cookware for meal preparation."

67. Which of the following items is the COTA MOST likely to recommend to a person with fine-motor incoordination who frequently drops small objects?
A. A shirt with contrasting buttons.
B. Spray deodorant.
C. A toothpaste tube with a flip-open cap.
D. Pants with a drawstring waist.

68. The COTA wants to use an activity that will promote crossing the midline for an individual who is s/p TBI. The MOST appropriate activity is:
A. making a coil pot out of clay.
B. making a macramé planter.
C. stringing a bead necklace.
D. weaving on a frame loom.

69. Which of the following is the BEST example of a prevocational activity for a woman who has worked as a cashier in a clothing store?
A. Having her make a grocery list while sitting.
B. Having her fold laundry and put it in a basket while standing.
C. Having her wash dishes while standing.
D. Having her add a column of numbers by hand while sitting.

70. A COTA is working with an individual with AIDS whose goal is independence in homemaking activities. He is deconditioned and fatigues easily. Intervention for this individual should emphasize:
A. maintaining maximal range of motion.
B. use of adaptive equipment.
C. work-simplification techniques.
D. universal precautions.

71. A man with multiple sclerosis is learning how to use a manual wheelchair. After he demonstrates the ability to propel the chair independently on a smooth floor, the COTA will have him practice on a carpeted surface. This process is known as:
A. modifying the activity.
B. grading the activity.
C. adapting the activity.
D. analyzing the activity.

Treatment Implementation

72. The COTA is performing passive range-of-motion exercises with a patient with quadriplegia. In order to encourage the development of tenodesis, the COTA must be sure to position the patient's wrist in:
A. neutral position during finger flexion and extension.
B. flexion during finger flexion and extension.
C. extension during finger flexion and flexion during finger extension.
D. flexion during finger flexion and extension during finger extension.

73. The COTA is performing a stand-pivot transfer with a patient. The correct way for the COTA to perform this transfer is to:
A. move slowly, twisting her body from the trunk.
B. keep her feet shoulder-width apart while lifting the patient with her arms.
C. keep her knees bent and feet planted when moving.
D. maintain a normal curve of the back, slowly shifting her feet as the turn is completed.

Questions 74 through 76 pertain to the following case study:

Dana, a 31-year-old woman, sustained a complete C7 spinal-cord injury in an automobile accident. She has good– to good strength in her shoulders, elbows, and wrists. Her grip strength is 11 pounds. Her goals include independence in feeding, dressing, and grooming.

74. Dana has difficulty opening her make-up containers so that she can apply eye shadow and blush. The BEST adaptation is to:
A. attach a suction cup to each container so she can stabilize them on the sink for easier access.
B. attach finger loops to both sides of each container, making it easier for Dana to pull them open.
C. use a wrist-driven flexor hinge splint to achieve the necessary grasp.
D. use weighted make-up containers to reduce tremor and minimize incoordination..

75. The COTA provides Dana with a leather-working activity. Which component of this activity would be MOST effective in promoting the development of grip strength?
A. Holding the mallet.
B. Holding the stamping tools.
C. Squeezing the sponge to wet the leather.
D. Lacing with a needle.

76. The BEST position for Dana's hands while she is sleeping or at rest is:
A. with volar-resting pan splints, to prevent flexion contractures.
B. in 45 degrees of wrist extension, to promote development of tenodesis.
C. in 25 degrees of wrist extension, to promote development of tenodesis.
D. flat on the bed with wrist in neutral and fingers flat.

77. A man who works as a cashier needs to improve standing tolerance from 10 minutes to 2 hours. To grade activities that will improve his standing tolerance, the COTA should:
A. have him simulate bagging groceries, beginning with lightweight objects and progressing to heavier objects.
B. have him carry a bag of groceries around the gym, increasing the number of trips around the gym each day.
C. stand at a high table while working on a puzzle for increasing amounts of time each day.
D. perform Theraband exercises that emphasize gluteal, hamstring, and quadriceps strengthening, gradually increasing the resistance of the Theraband.

78. The COTA instructs an individual to pick up a cup with his left hand and place it in the sink to his right. The goals of this activity are weight-shifting from the left leg to the right and trunk rotation. Where should the COTA position the cup in order to elicit the GREATEST amount of movement in the desired movement pattern?
A. On the counter to the left.
B. In a cabinet under the counter to the right.
C. On a shelf over the counter to the left.
D. On the counter to the right.

79. A COTA is instructing a woman with hemiplegia in how to don a front-opening blouse. The MOST appropriate way to position the shirt on her lap is with the inside facing:
A. up and the collar toward her body.
B. down and the collar toward her body.
C. up and the collar toward her knees.
D. down and the collar toward her knees.

80. Which of the methods for donning a front-opening shirt described below is correct?
A. (1) Position shirt on lap; (2) place affected hand into sleeve and pull up past elbow; (3) grasp collar with normal hand and swing shirt around and behind neck and shoulders; (4) place normal hand and arm into remaining sleeve.
B. (1) Position shirt on lap; (2) place normal hand and arm into sleeve and pull up past elbow; (3) grasp collar with normal hand and swing shirt around and behind neck and shoulders; (4) place affected hand into remaining sleeve
C. (1) Place affected hand into sleeve and pull up past elbow; (2) position shirt on lap; (3) grasp collar with normal hand and swing shirt around and behind neck and shoulders; (4) place normal hand and arm into remaining sleeve.
D. (1) Place normal hand and arm into sleeve; (2) position shirt on lap; (3) place affected hand into sleeve and pull up past elbow; (4) grasp collar with normal hand and swing shirt around and behind neck and shoulders.

81. Zack, a 16-year-old boy with juvenile rheumatoid arthritis, is ready to begin shaving but has difficulty as a result of limited range of motion in his shoulders and elbows. Which of the following is the BEST adaptation for him to use?
A. An electric razor attached to universal cuff.
B. A safety razor with a built-up handle.
C. A safety razor with an extended handle.
D. A safety razor attached to a universal cuff.

82. Jack has rheumatoid arthritis and exhibits ulnar drift in both hands. When teaching him how to use a Dycem jar opener, the COTA should tell him to:
A. hold the jar in one hand while opening with the other.
B. squeeze the Dycem with the fingers of the right hand and open counter-clockwise.
C. use the right hand for opening jars and the left hand for closing jars.
D. use the left hand for opening jars and the right hand for closing jars.

83. Matthew is in the late stages of AIDS and bedridden. Flexion contractures have begun to develop in his right hand and he has been

referred to OT for splinting. The MOST appropriate splint for the COTA to fabricate is a:
A. dorsal wrist splint.
B. functional-position resting splint.
C. volar wrist-cock-up splint.
D. dynamic finger-extension splint.

84. Antonio has diabetes and is s/p BKA. His primary goal is to improve standing balance and tolerance. Which of the following activities is contraindicated for Antonio?
A. A group ball-toss activity.
B. Baking rolls in a standard oven.
C. Making a wooden birdhouse.
D. Making a latch hook rug.

85. The COTA is ordering supplies for a cooking activity for an individual who has had a stroke following a long history of hypotension. Which of the following dietary concerns should the COTA be MOST aware of?
A. Salt.
B. Sugar.
C. Cholesterol.
D. Food texture.

Evaluating the Treatment Plan

86. The objective section of the SOAP format includes:
A. functional performance levels.
B. analysis of evaluations.
C. conclusions and assumptions of performance measures.
D. quotes from the individual and/or his or her family.

87. A COTA is evaluating an individual's ability to transfer from a wheelchair to a tub bench. During the evaluation, the COTA has to cue the individual to lock his wheelchair brakes and help him lift his legs from the wheelchair into and out of the tub. He is able to scoot himself from the wheelchair to the tub bench with occasional loss of balance. How would the COTA rate his performance?
A. Dependent.
B. Requiring minimal assistance.
C. Requiring moderate assistance.
D. Requiring maximal assistance.

88. An individual has made gains in fine motor coordination in the past week. The statement that belongs in the assessment section of the note is:
A. "Pt. performed the Nine Hole Peg Test in 20 seconds."
B. Pt. reports being able to button the buttons on most items of clothing."
C. "Pt. is demonstrating gradual improvement in fine motor coordination."
D. "Family reports patient is performing more fine motor activities independently."

89. Ken is a 57-year-old man experiencing progressive weakness. A long-term goal is for the family to carry out his feeding program. They have achieved the short-term goal of understanding how Ken's disability affects his ability to feed himself. Which statement is the BEST example of a revised short-term goal?
A. "Pt. will participate in feeding program."
B. "Pt. will feed himself with moderate assistance."
C. "Family will feed pt. safely and independently 100 percent of the time."
D. "Family will demonstrate independence in positioning pt. correctly for feeding so that he can swallow safely."

90. When working with a patient with a fast-growing brain tumor, the COTA notes that has begun ignoring food on the left side of his meal tray. The BEST approach for the COTA to recommend is:
A. focusing on remediation.
B. educating the patient to increase left-side awareness.
C. implementating compensatory strategies.
D. selecting appropriate adaptive equipment.

91. Which of the following outcomes is most likely after an individual has implemented a joint-protection program?
A. The ability to prepare a meal without becoming fatigued.
B. The ability to lift heavy grocery bags without pain.
C. Minimization of joint damage.
D. The ability to knit for sustained periods of time.

92. After instruction in hip precautions following a total hip replacement, the COTA documented that the patient was able to:
A. stand for long enough to make a sandwich and pour a beverage.
B. perform lower-extremity dressing without internally rotating or adducting the involved hip.
C. walk to the bathroom independently.
D. perform tub transfers independently.

93. Tony has been noncompliant with his OT program since he began attending OT 4 days ago. The FIRST action the COTA should take is to:
A. speak with the physician.
B. discharge Tony.
C. collaborate with Tony on setting goals.
D. revise Tony's treatment plan.

Discharge Planning

94. A COTA is preparing to discharge to home a patient who uses a standard-width wheelchair.

She has asked the client's wife to measure doorways in the home to determine if they will be wide enough to get the wheelchair through. In order for the doorways to be wide enough for the wheelchair to get through, they must be at LEAST:

A. 32 inches wide.
B. 34 inches wide.
C. 36 inches wide.
D. 38 inches wide.

95. Alma has advanced lung cancer and is about to be discharged from an acute-care setting to home. She is depressed, and although she remains ambulatory and independent in basic activities of daily living, she tires very quickly and no longer participates in most of her life roles. What should the OTR/COTA team do concerning occupational therapy services?

A. Provide her with a home program.
B. Recommend home health OT.
C. Recommend discontinuation of OT services.
D. Recommend hospice OT.

Questions 96–98 pertain to the following case study:

Rhoda has completed a rehabilitation program following a hip replacement and is about to be discharged.

96. The MOST important recommendation for the COTA to make is to:

A. move items from high cabinets to lower locations.
B. obtain a raised toilet seat.
C. place high-contrast tape at the edge of each step.
D. install a hand-held shower head.

97. Rhoda's fiancé is present at one of her final sessions. The purpose of his attendance is to:

A. ensure that Rhoda follows the necessary hip precautions.
B. provide him with a summary of Rhoda's progress to date.
C. prove to him that Rhoda can perform activities of daily living independently, so that he will refrain from providing unnecessary assistance.
D. give him an opportunity to ask questions.

98. Which piece of equipment is Rhoda most likely to need to continue using at home?

A. Velcro shoelace fasteners.
B. A padded foam toilet seat 1 inch higher than a normal seat.
C. A short-handled bath sponge.
D. A long-handled bath sponge.

99. A COTA is recommending community resources to an individual with multiple sclerosis (MS) who is about to be discharged. All of the following are appropriate EXCEPT a(n):

A. aquatic therapy program led by an OTR in a warm-water pool (bathtub temperature).
B. ROM dance program provided by a COTA through the hospital's outpatient center.
C. list of local restaurants that are wheelchair accessible.
D. nonaerobic exercise program provided by a PT at a local community center.

100. Which of the following is the best example of the subjective section of a discharge summary?

A. "Pt. reports overall pain levels are lower and ability to perform ADLs has improved."
B. "Pt. continues to c/o back pain with activity."
C. "Pt. has improved from minimal assistance to independence in ADL performance."
D. "My back hurts when I get in and out of the tub and when I lift bags of groceries."

PSYCHOSOCIAL QUESTIONS

Data Collection

101. The assessment instrument designed for screening self-care, physical, and social behaviors through the observations of caregivers familiar with the individual's daily care is the:

A. Bay Area Functional Performance Evaluation (BAFPE).
B. Comprehensive Occupational Therapy Evaluation (COTE).
C. Role Checklist.
D. Parachek Geriatric Rating Scale.

102. The COTA needs to evaluate how a client uses her time and how she feels about the activities she performs in a typical week. The BEST evaluation for the COTA to use is the:

A. Lower Cognitive Level.
B. Allen Cognitive Level.
C. Leisure Activity Profile.
D. Activity Configuration.

103. Asking a middle-aged individual about the grade school he or she attended is one way of obtaining data about the individual's:

A. comprehension.
B. orientation.
C. long-term memory.
D. short-term memory.

104. An OTR and COTA share and coordinate therapy for a caseload. One of the roles that the COTA can perform is:

A. completing chart reviews.
B. completing the nonstandardized portions of the evaluation.

C. interpreting the results of the nonstandardized portion of the evaluation.
D. independently designing a treatment plan for the individual.

105. A COTA is working on morning ADLs with a man who is s/p TBI. He requires prompting to apply shaving cream to his face and to pick up the razor. He is then able to complete the activity without further prompting. This is likely to be documented as a deficit in which of the following performance components?
A. Impulsivity.
B. Initiation.
C. Memory.
D. Attention.

106. The COTA is working with an 89-year-old man who is diagnosed with major depression. Which of the following descriptions of complaints and behaviors is MOST characteristic of this type of patient?
A. He has problems sleeping, difficulty with "thinking" or concentrating, describes himself as "dumb" or "stupid," and feels little hope that things will improve.
B. He complains of feeling "blue" or sad, has lost interest in activities he previously enjoyed, and reports decreased libido.
C. His complaints focus on physical concerns, he denies feeling depressed but feels less energetic, he has lost weight, and he complains of some concentration and memory problems.
D. He cannot correctly identify the date or present location, does not recall where he was earlier in the day, and has difficulty sleeping during the night.

107. The best reason to interview someone who is familiar with the patient's daily activities is to:
A. determine the patient's ability to benefit from occupational therapy.
B. determine appropriate activities for the patient.
C. gain an accurate perspective of the patient's ability to function in daily activities.
D. determine the patient's need for equipment.

108. The COTA frequently administers the King's Person-Symbol Assessment and then discusses it with the OTR. The OTR's role is to:
A. provide input on the quality of the drawings.
B. interprete the results, focusing on the use of color and the artistic skill of the patient.
C. interpret the results, focusing on the features and placement of the drawing.
D. encourage the COTA to analyze the patient's needs.

109. The OTR has assigned the COTA to gather data about the patient's family situation, occupational and educational background, cultural background, and expected discharge environment. What is the MOST accurate source for this information?
A. The patient's entire medical record.
B. The patient's family.
C. The patient.
D. The history taken by the social worker.

110. Which of the following is an appropriate statement for the subjective portion of an initial note written in the SOAP format?
A. "Pt. should not be placed in a large group."
B. "Pt. states that she does not feel comfortable in large groups."
C. "Pt. does not appear to be comfortable in large groups."
D. "Pt. is obviously uncomfortable in large groups."

Treatment Planning

111. The COTA plans to use a "no-bake" cookie activity with a group of young adults in a psychosocial treatment setting. The activity will take about 20 minutes. The COTA will gently encourage members to rely on others in the group and reinforce positive behaviors. This activity is representative of which of the following group levels?
A. project group.
B. egocentric-cooperative group.
C. cooperative group.
D. mature group.

112. The primary disadvantage to implementing a group format for occupational therapy services provided in an acute-care psychiatric setting is that:
A. the other group members provide feedback.
B. more clients can be treated by fewer occupational therapy practitioners.
C. cohesiveness is difficult to achieve.
D. each person's individual goals can be met.

113. The COTA is working with Clare, a 16-year-old adolescent diagnosed with depression. Her primary problem is her socialization with peers. Her strength is in the area of task skills. The MOST appropriate goal for Clare would be:
A. "Clare will increase socialization with peers during task groups."
B. "Clare will select and teach two peers a craft activity which she enjoys."
C. "Clare will be provided with opportunity to interact with peers while she demonstrates a familiar craft activity."
D. "Clare will select and demonstrate a craft activity to the COTA and state two positive comments about her demonstration."

114. The COTA is beginning training in meal preparation with a 35-year-old homemaker following a TBI. The activity that should be introduced FIRST is:
A. making a peanut butter and jelly sandwich.
B. preparing a hot cup of tea with sugar.
C. pouring a glass of orange juice.
D. cooking a grilled ham and cheese sandwich.

Questions 115–119 refer to the following sample documentation:

THE COLUMBIA - MADISON HOSPITAL

SECTION A Pt. is a 49 year old WMM admitted to the unit with a diagnosis of major depression. Pt's self-care, work, and leisure involvement were seriously impaired prior to admission as reported by the counselor at CMHC. Pt. was referred to occupational therapy for evaluation and treatment.

SECTION B #5. Pt. is unable to identify leisure interests.

SECTION C Pt. will identify two possible community locations offering leisure activities within 3 miles of pt.'s home prior to discharge. Pt. will identify three new leisure interests that he wants to pursue at discharge.

SECTION D 3-13-94; 4:00 PM: #5: "I really don't have any plans for myself once I go home." Pt. identified four solitary and two leisure interests involving others at the casual interest level on the Interest Checklist. Pt.'s pattern and strength of leisure interests are inadequate to support leisure resource exploration in his community. Schedule pt. to attend leisure group three to four times/week with focus on leisure interest exploration.

Sam Spade, OTR/L

115. In section D of the sample document, the assessment statement is:
A. "I really don't have any plans for myself once I go home."
B. "Pt. identified four solitary and two leisure interests involving others at the casual interest level on the Interest Checklist activity.
C. Pt.'s pattern and strength of leisure interests are inadequate to support leisure resource exploration in his community.
D. Schedule pt. to attend leisure group three to four times/week with focus on leisure interest exploration.

116. In section A of the sample document, CMHC stands for:
A. Central Medical Health Care.
B. Columbia-Madison Hospital Corporation.
C. Community Mental Health Counselor.
D. Community Mental Health Center.

117. In the sample document, the section containing the individual's goals is:
A. section A.
B. section B.
C. section C.
D. section D.

118. In the sample document, the section that contains the database is:
A. section A.
B. section B.
C. section C.
D. section D.

119. In the sample documentation, the section that contains a problem according to the problem-oriented-medical records (POMR) format is:
A. section A.
B. section B.
C. section C.
D. section D.

120. The COTA is planning an activity program to help reduce the physical symptoms of muscle tension associated with anxiety disorders. Which activity would be most appropriate to begin with?
A. copper tooling.
B. aerobic exercise.
C. line dancing.
D. construction of a woodworking kit.

121. The COTA has been asked to structure a crafts group for low-functioning patients operating at a parallel skill level. When setting the environment, it is important to:
A. prepare a limited amount of materials.
B. prepare separate materials for each person.
C. show the group where all materials are stored and have them obtain and return tools as they need them.
D. encourage sharing of materials.

Treatment Implementation

122. Limit setting concerning impulsivity would be MOST important with which of the following diagnoses in an inpatient setting:
A. Depression and anxiety.
B. Alcoholism and anorexia nervosa.
C. Mania and borderline personality disorder.
D. Delirium and dementia.

123. A COTA spends 2 days a week in a setting in which her clients with mental retardation perform simple assembly and packaging tasks with supervision. They are paid $.10 per package produced. This setting is BEST described as:
A. a sheltered workshop.
B. an adult activity center.
C. supervised employment.
D. supervised employment with job coaching.

124. The COTA is organizing a group picnic outing to a park. The most important precaution for the

COTA to implement for those group members taking neuroleptic medications is to:
A. encourage the use of PABA-free sunblock and hats.
B. encourage members to move slowly when changing positions from sitting to standing.
C. encourage members to use an antiperspirant and wear light-colored clothing.
D. take along such low-calorie snacks as carrot sticks and celery sticks.

125. A COTA is providing caregiver training to the husband of an elderly woman with Alzheimer's disease who has difficulty following multistep instructions. What is the BEST method for the husband to use when giving his wife instructions?
A. Give one- or two-step instructions and repeat frequently.
B. Give three-step instructions and use gestures to demonstrate.
C. Write down any instructions that contain over three steps for her to read as needed.
D. Have her repeat all instructions after the COTA gives them.

126. A woman with a head injury is impulsive during self-feeding and frequently attempts to place too much food in her mouth at one time. The BEST method to use to control her rate of intake during self-feeding is to:
A. cut her food into smaller pieces.
B. have her count to 10 between bites of food.
C. have her place the utensil down until her mouth is cleared.
D. serve food in separate containers on the meal tray.

127. Which of the following therapy groups is the BEST example of a psychoeducational group?
A. A stress management group.
B. A directive group.
C. Group therapy.
D. A task group.

128. The COTA is using a sensory integration approach with a group of regressed patients with limited attention spans. Most group members can tolerate a group situation for no more than a half hour. The BEST activity to begin the session with is:
A. ask each patient to introduce himself or herself.
B. pass around a scent box and ask each patient to smell the contents.
C. ask each patient to read a favorite poem.
D. discuss the menu for lunch.

129. The goal of a cooking group for young women with eating disorders is to increase their knowledge and understanding of:
A. weight-loss techniques.
B. the caloric content of different foods.
C. preparing and consuming nutritional and normal-sized portions of food.
D. preparing appealing looking meals.

130. A 22-year-old college student was referred to a day treatment program following hospitalization for an acute schizophrenic episode. He is uncomfortable in social settings, has difficulty sustaining conversations, is unable to make eye contact, and responds with bizarre comments when spoken to. Among the following, what would be the LEAST effective treatment approach?
A. vestibular stimulation and gross-motor exercises.
B. discussion groups.
C. role playing.
D. social-skills training.

131. During discharge planning, the patient asks the COTA, "What should I do when colleagues at work ask me where I have been all this time?" How can the COTA BEST address this concern?
A. Arrange for the patient to discuss this with her social worker.
B. Tell the patient to tell the truth.
C. Suggest that the patient say she has been on an extended vacation.
D. Arrange for the patient to attend a discharge group to discuss her concerns.

132. A COTA is working in a sheltered workshop with adult clients with developmental disabilities. He provides project samples for clients to duplicate. This action is most appropriate for clients at Allen's cognitive level:
A. 3 (manual actions).
B. 4 (goal-directed actions).
C. 5 (exploratory actions).
D. 6 (planned actions).

133. COTAs working in psychosocial settings are responsible for establishing and maintaining a safe environment in craft areas. The BEST way for the COTA to account for all tools at the start and close of groups is to:
A. keep track of the keys to storage cabinets and unit doors.
B. have all materials and supplies ready before the group begins.
C. allow only clients who have no behavioral risk precautions to attend groups.
D. use a tool-storage area, painted with tool shadows or outlines, that can be locked.

134. The COTA is preparing to do a parachute activity as part of a sensory integration program. Several patients in the group are taking antipsychotic medications. The COTA must take precautions for which of the following possible side effects?
A. postural hypotension.
B. photosensitivity.
C. excessive thirst.
D. blurred vision.

135. Which of the following is the best way for a COTA to explain the purpose of a prevocational evaluation program to a client being treated in a psychosocial setting?

A. "This program will help you to learn about your interests, talents, and skills for assembly jobs."
B. "This program will help you to learn about the skills you have that are needed on most jobs and about your potential for work.
C. "This program will help you identify the responsibility you have to your employer while you are in treatment and to inform your employer of these responsibilities.
D. "This program will help you to develop skills necessary for getting a job."

Evaluating the Treatment Plan

136. The COTA is working with an elderly woman with a diagnosis of depression who has difficulty making decisions. When they reach the occupational therapy kitchen, the patient says that she doesn't want to bake. The response that would BEST facilitate better decision making is:

A. "I think baking would be a helpful activity to try. Baking something you like offers you several choices and decisions. You wanted to bake cookies today, didn't you?"
B. "I think baking would be a helpful activity to try. Baking something you like offers you several choices and decisions. What do you want to bake today?"
C. "I think baking would be a helpful activity to try. Baking something you like offers you several choices and decisions. These choices and decisions can help you feel more positive about making other decisions. You can choose between a cake or cookie mix. Which would you like?"
D. "I think baking would be a helpful activity to try. Baking something you like offers you several choices and decisions. These choices and decisions can help you feel more positive about making other decisions. Do you want to bake cookies?"

137. The COTA is working on developing self-esteem with a middle-aged man diagnosed with depression. He has refused to participate in the day's woodworking group. How is the client most likely to phrase his refusal?

A. "I don't know how."
B. "I can't even sand wood the right way."
C. "I'm waiting for my visitors to come."
D. "I'm good at woodworking. I'd like to make a table and four chairs."

138. The COTA is working with an elderly woman with a diagnosis of depression and dementia during the clean-up portion of a cooking activity. The patient begins to dry the plates and utensils she has already dried. The COTA should:

A. tell her that she is redrying the utensils and dishes.
B. put the dried dishes away and begin to hand her wet dishes.
C. ask her to stop the activity because it seems too difficult.
D. ask her to describe what she is doing.

139. An OTR and COTA work in a collaborative relationship. The teamwork between the two professionals is BEST exemplified by which of the following examples?

A. The OTR completes the assessment and instructs the COTA to provide a specific intervention.
B. The COTA updates the OTR on the progress a patient has made in the last week, and both provide information to update the goals.
C. The COTA gives his progress note to the OTR and the OTR writes the discharge summary based upon the progress note.
D. The OTR tells the COTA what type of equipment to order for a patient and the COTA orders the equipment from a medical equipment company.

Questions 140 and 141 are based on the following case study:

The COTA has been working with Ruby, a 32-year-old woman with strong dependency needs. The leather project first chosen, a wallet, required the COTA to sit next to Ruby while providing step-by-step lacing instruction.

140. What is the BEST next step in grading this activity toward decreasing Ruby's dependency needs?

A. Provide Ruby with written instructions on lacing techniques and ask her to continue on her own.
B. Ask Ruby to try some some lacing with distant supervision and praise her for what she has been able to do.
C. Ask Ruby to take the lacing to her room and continue without the COTA's assistance.
D. Tell Ruby to complete a small amount of lacing while the COTA assists another patient in the same room.

141. Ruby successfully completed the leather wallet and said that she might be able to do another project on her own. The COTA and the OTR discussed ways to adapt the instructional method so as to encourage Ruby to work independently. They agreed that the COTA would:

A. instruct Ruby in a more difficult lacing technique.
B. give Ruby a new project kit, with written instructions for a more difficult lacing tech-

nique, and ask her to begin the project on her own.
C. give Ruby a new kit to take to her room, where she will work on it without assistance.
D. give Ruby a new but similar project kit with written instructions and ask her to begin the project on her own while the COTA assists another patient in the same room.

142. "Patient states she is frightened by the anger she feels when doing ceramics." This statement would be found in which portion of the SOAP note?
A. Subjective.
B. Objective.
C. Assessment.
D. Plan.

143. "Patient continues to demonstrate increasing ability to work independently. Occupational therapy should be continued with a focus on increasing opportunities for self-responsibility in assigned tasks." This is an example of which portion of the SOAP note?
A. Subjective.
B. Objective.
C. Assessment.
D. Plan.

Discharge Planning

144. An individual tells the COTA, "I don't know about going home tomorrow. I wanted to be discharged yesterday and the doctor suggested I stay in the hospital another day." The COTA responds by saying, "It sounds as if you're not sure whether you are ready to be discharged." This response is an example of:
A. paraphrasing.
B. social chitchat.
C. proposing a solution.
D. confrontation.

145. The COTA has been working with a young woman whose planned discharge from a psychiatric inpatient service has just been delayed. What is the GREATEST possible risk to this individual posed by this delay?
A. Disruption in the client's continuity of care.
B. Countertransference.
C. Post-traumatic stress disorder.
D. Regression.

146. Mrs. B. has Alzheimer's disease and is about to be discharged to home, where she lives with her husband. She does not always recognize her children, shows a tendency to wander, and has frequent episodes of incontinence. The most important item for the COTA to include in the family discharge-planning conference is:
A. discussion with Mrs. B. of strategies for handling incontinence.
B. strategies Mr. B. can use to prevent Mrs. B. from wandering.
C. strategies Mrs. B. can use to prevent wandering.
D. reality orientation techniques to increase recognition of the children.

147. Mrs. Kaplan, 82 years old, was hospitalized for a total hip replacement and is preparing to be discharged to her daughter's home. The COTA has recommended a program to address her decreased mental abilities, specifically poor memory and difficulty with orientation to place and time. The BEST way for Mrs. Kaplan to receive OT services is:
A. partial hospitalization.
B. adult day care.
C. home health care.
D. a psychosocial rehabilitation center.

Questions 148 and 149 pertain to the following case study.

Mr. Chang is a client with the diagnosis of bipolar disorder manic episode. His behavior changed as the week progressed. On Monday he walked into occupational therapy, stated that his name was John F. Kennedy, and then walked out of the clinic. On Wednesday, he was able to sit briefly at the table in the OT clinic but was noticeably hypermanic and unable to work on any one craft. On Friday Mr. Chang was able to sit with the other clients in the clinic and was cheerful, yet jumped from topic to topic while conversing. He worked quickly on a short-term craft project.

148. The BEST description of this client's overall course of change is:
A. regression.
B. progression.
C. decompensation.
D. recovery.

149. Which thematic group would be the most appropriate for Mr. Chang to attend on Saturday?
A. An assertiveness group.
B. No thematic groups are appropriate at this time.
C. A discharge-planning group.
D. An exercise group.

150. The treatment team are discussing their concerns about John, a client with schizophrenia who is scheduled to be discharged from an inpatient setting next week. The statement that BEST reflects occupational therapy concerns is:
A. "John has been coming to community meeting regularly and telling others about his scheduled discharge date. I'm not sure he's ready, however, as he laughs to himself when he's talking."
B. "John's tendency to discontinue his medications may be less of a problem if I can get his referral

to the outpatient day program completed before he leaves the hospital."
C. "John's medication should be changed from oral administration to the long-acting intramuscular injection before he is discharged."
D. "I'm concerned about John's ability to live on his own unless he is better able to structure his leisure time. Before admission he was rarely in contact with others. Then his voices got worse."

PROFESSIONAL PRACTICE QUESTIONS

Promote Professional Practice

151. The document that provides occupational therapy guidelines for screening, referral, evaluation, treatment planning, implementation, discontinuation of services, quality assurance, indirect services, and legal and ethical issues is called:
A. Uniform Terminology for Reporting Occupational Therapy Services.
B. Standards of Practice.
C. licensure regulations.
D. AOTA Policies and Procedures.

152. The Individuals with Disabilities Education Act (IDEA) states that occupational therapy in school systems:
A. is a primary service for the 5- to 21-year-old students.
B. is provided to any child with a need for an occupational therapy evaluation.
C. can be provided to any child receiving physical therapy services.
D. must benefit the child's ability to participate in special education.

153. In psychosocial frames of reference of occupational therapy, the COTA's relationship with an individual is BEST described as:
A. the central focus of occupational therapy treatment.
B. a therapeutic device in helping.
C. a friendship.
D. sympathy for the individual's problems.

154. A COTA may independently administer standardized tests:
A. as a level II student.
B. once service competency has been established.
C. once licensure has been received.
D. when NBCOT certification is received.

155. A newly graduated COTA is investigating career possibilities. She finds that opportunities in the area of occupational therapy with older adults are:
A. remaining stable.
B. expanding.
C. diminishing.
D. fluctuating.

156. The National Board for Certification in Occupational Therapy (NBCOT) investigates allegations of misconduct by OTRs and COTAs. What is the LEAST punitive action that the NBCOT may take if misconduct is proved?
A. a reprimand.
B. a censure.
C. probation.
D. revocation.

157. The OTR has assessed an individual and developed a treatment plan that addresses functional deficits. The inpatient psychiatric services that may be billed as occupational therapy services for this individual are treatments from the OTR's plan provided by a(n):
A. COTA.
B. music therapist.
C. recreational therapist.
D. art therapist.

158. Upon completion of Level II fieldwork, the COTA student should be functioning:
A. slightly below entry level.
B. at or above the minimal entry level of competence.
C. at an intermediate skill level based on the Occupational Therapy Roles.
D. at an advanced skill level based on the Occupational Therapy Roles.

159. The COTA, while passing by the door of a patient's room, witnesses an OTR in an intimate position with a patient. Responding consistently with the Occupational Therapy Code of Ethics, the COTA will:
A. notify AOTA.
B. notify the state occupational therapy association.
C. notify the state licensure board.
D. discuss the situation privately with the therapist involved.

160. A COTA and OTR jointly decide to discharge an individual after his goal of independence in activities of daily living (ADLs) has been achieved. However, they are instructed by the facility administrator to continue treating, or at least billing, the individual for two sessions per day for the next week, because his insurance will allow it. The COTA and OTR should:
A. continue to work with the individual on activities he particularly enjoys, such as playing bridge twice a day whenever possible.
B. discontinue treatment but continue to bill as directed by the administrator.

C. inform the administrator they are unable to provide services to individuals who can no longer benefit from OT.
D. compromise with the administrator and agree to drop in and check on the individual once a day and bill accordingly.

161. COTAs most frequently work with patients diagnosed with:
A. CVA.
B. cerebral palsy.
C. developmental delay.
D. fractures.

162. The COTA has been following an outpatient with right hemiparesis. The patient has had recent onset of shoulder pain and is exhibiting increased swelling. The FIRST action the COTA should take is to:
A. notify the physician of the patient's change in status.
B. consult with the patient's physical therapist about the cause of the increased shoulder pain.
C. modify the treatment plan to include pain-reduction techniques.
D. notify the occupational therapist of the patient's change in status.

163. A COTA wishes to demonstrate service competency in the use of a standardized test. What is the best way to do this?
A. By observing an OTR perform the standardized test.
B. By observing an OTR, then practicing on his own, then teaching another individual how to administer the test.
C. By following procedures exactly as outlined in the test manuals.
D. By consistently obtaining the same results as another OT practitioner who has demonstrated service competency.

164. An entry-level COTA is most qualified to initiate a referral for an individual with deficits in:
A. activities of daily living (ADLs).
B. work activities.
C. sensory integration.
D. cognition.

165. In which of the following community-based settings do COTAs work most often?
A. public school systems.
B. residential care facilities.
C. day care centers.
D. community mental health centers.

166. A COTA may use physical agent modalities (PAMs) only when:
A. she or he possesses the necessary theoretical and technical background.
B. she or he has practiced providing PAMs with an OTR present for an adequate period of time.
C. an OTR is on-site.
D. she or he has demonstrated service competency.

167. While preparing for his first presentation at a professional conference, a COTA realizes he does not have the name of the author of an article containing critical information he planned on photocopying and distributing. The MOST appropriate action for him to take is:
A. to distribute the handout and apologize for not having the author's name.
B. to show the handout with an overhead projector and apologize for not having the author's name.
C. to use the handout only as a resource while developing the presentation.
D. to refrain from using the handout.

168. After a month at a new job, a COTA finds he is unable to complete the required job responsibilities in the time allotted. He stays after work for up to 2 hours each day just to catch up with paperwork and prepare for the next day. The MOST professional action for the COTA to take is to:
A. continue to stay late so that he will not fall behind.
B. analyze how he is using his time and implement time-management strategies.
C. find a less demanding job.
D. leave at the end of the scheduled day in order to avoid burnout.

169. An entry-level physical therapist assistant asks an entry-level COTA if she is going to participate in the research activity that is about to be implemented at their facility. Which of the following responses is NOT acceptable or correct for a COTA?
A. "COTAs are not qualified to participate in research."
B. "I'll participate in disseminating the results."
C. "I'll be involved in the data-collection process."
D. "I'm helping to develop the research question."

170. A COTA witnesses an OT practitioner practicing under the influence of alcohol. Realizing that this behavior has gone on for several months, the COTA believes the individual needs to be prevented from practicing occupational therapy, at least until the issue is resolved. These individuals are working in an area where three states border each other, and the COTA is concerned that the practitioner may simply go to another state to practice if his license is revoked by the state licensure agency where they work. The most appropriate body for the COTA to report the practitioner to is the:
A. AOTA.
B. state regulatory board.
C. NBCOT.
D. administration of the facility.

171. A patient gives the COTA $50.00 as a token of his appreciation after 3 weeks of intensive rehabilitation. Which of the following responses is MOST consistent with the Occupational Therapy Code of Ethics?

A. Accept the gift and use it to buy a new radio.
B. Decline the gift but accept it if the patient is insistent.
C. Decline the gift and explain that a COTA cannot accept gifts from patients.
D. Accept the gift and use it to buy a textbook for the department.

172. The Standards of Practice for Occupational Therapy (SOP) states that a COTA "may contribute to the assessment process under the supervision of a registered occupational therapist." This should be interpreted to mean that a COTA:

A. must contribute to the assessment process.
B. should contribute to the assessment process.
C. may perform up to 50 percent of the assessment process.
D. may perform variable portions of the assessment process.

173. A COTA has been working at his first job for 6 months. His supervisor has asked him to accept a Level I fieldwork student from a local college, who would attend for 8 consecutive Thursdays. While considering this request, he considers AOTA guidelines concerning fieldwork. He knows all of the following to be false EXCEPT:

A. Only OTRs can train fieldwork students.
B. He must have a minimum of 1 year's experience in order to accept fieldwork students.
C. It is his professional responsibility to train fieldwork students.
D. His facility must be accredited by the school in order to accept fieldwork students.

174. Certified occupational therapy assistants were first officially recognized by the occupational therapy profession in:

A. 1917.
B. 1945.
C. 1959.
D. 1983.

175. A state law requires a COTA to post her license in the facility in which she works. Since she works 20 hours a week in each of two different facilities, she is uncertain about where to post her license and does not post it at all. This is a violation of:

A. state law.
B. state law and the Occupational Therapy Code of Ethics.
C. state law and the Standards of Practice for Occupational Therapy.
D. state law, the Occupational Therapy Code of Ethics, and Standards of Practice for Occupational Therapy.

176. A COTA working for a contract agency is reassigned from the nursing home where she has worked for the last 4 months to a school setting. On her first day in the new setting, the COTA is assigned a student whose treatment program is based on sensory integration. The COTA is uncomfortable working with this child because she has no background in sensory integration. Following the prescribed treatment plan with this child would constitute an ethical violation of all of the following principles EXCEPT:

A. Avoid harming the child.
B. Have an appropriate level of competence.
C. Respect the child's right to refuse treatment.
D. Consult with/refer to others when additional expertise is required.

Support Service Management

177. Health care coverage for disabled individuals, people with end stage renal disease, or those over 65 is MOST likely paid for by:

A. Medicare.
B. Medicaid.
C. third-party payers.
D. Private pay.

178. The first and most effective method occupational therapy practitioners should use to prevent the spread of disease is:

A. wearing gloves.
B. wearing a mask.
C. frequent handwashing.
D. wearing a gown over work clothes.

179. A COTA has been working in the area of mental health for 3 years. He has mastered basic role functions, and under the supervision of an OTR supervises volunteers, OTA students, and COTAs and administers standardized tests. Based on the Occupational Therapy Roles document, this COTA is functioning as an:

A. entry-level COTA with close supervision.
B. intermediate-level COTA with minimal supervision.
C. advanced-level COTA with general supervision.
D. intermediate-level COTA with routine supervision.

180. The term that BEST describes the relationship between an OTR and a COTA is:

A. dependent.
B. independent.
C. collaborative.
D. intuitive.

181. Which of the following is the most appropriate function for a COTA working individually on a quality-improvement plan?
A. identifying the indicators of quality care.
B. reviewing charts to elicit relevant information.
C. identifying problems related to patient care.
D. developing a report in the form of a quality-improvement plan.

182. In order for a school-aged child to receive occupational therapy services in a school system, which one of the following forms must be completed?
A. UB-82
B. FIM
C. IEP
D. HCFA-1500

183. A COTA has been running a "beauty group" with a group of chronically mentally ill older women. The most appropriate action to take with the make-up at the end of the session is to:
A. put all supplies in a basket to be used next time.
B. label any supplies used by individuals with communicable diseases with the individual's name and put the rest in a basket.
C. label lipstick with the individuals' names. Eye make-up and blush can be shared.
D. label each item with the individuals' names. Cosmetics should never be shared.

184. A COTA performs a kitchen check-out with an elderly woman before discharge and documents that it will be safe for her to cook small meals in the kitchen. The supervising OTR cosigns the COTA's note. The COTA is named in a lawsuit months later by the family of the woman, who was severely burned while cooking her own dinner. Which professional(s) could be held accountable?
A. Only the OTR could be held accountable.
B. Only the COTA could be held accountable.
C. Both the COTA and OTR could be held accountable.
D. Neither the COTA or OTR could be held accountable.

185. What is the FIRST step a COTA should take upon receiving a referral for a mental health client?
A. Read the chart.
B. Accept the referral.
C. Notify the supervising OTR.
D. Identify safety issues.

186. Before initiating treatment with an elderly home health patient, the OTR/COTA team will probably need to receive a(n):
A. referral.
B. report from the patient's physical therapist.
C. report from the patient's nurse.
D. initial evaluation.

187. Of the following, the task for which an aide is LEAST suited is:
A. warping the loom.
B. teaching macramé to a patient.
C. transporting patients.
D. getting a glass of water for a patient.

188. While the COTA is performing a shower transfer, the hose on the patient's catheter bag detaches and dark urine spills into the shower. After the patient is securely seated on the shower chair, the COTA's FIRST response should be to:
A. spray down the area of the spill with water, realizing that urine is not an infectious body fluid.
B. treat the area as if an infectious spill had occurred.
C. find and immediately notify the supervisor.
D. reconnect the bag and continue the shower.

189. It is often necessary to obtain screening information from a patient chart upon referral to occupational therapy. At what level may COTAs participate in this task?
A. At entry level.
B. Not until they have achieved intermediate level.
C. Not until they have achieved advanced level.
D. COTAs cannot perform the task.

Questions 190–194 pertain to the following documentation sample:

A COTA is working with an OTR on an acute-care floor. The following statements are part of the discharge note that the team is writing.

A. The patient plans to return home at discharge.
B. Janie M. is a 42-year-old Caucasian woman with diagnosis of CVA. The patient reports that she lives with her 11-year-old son in a ranch home with a basement. Laundry facilities are located in the patient's basement. There are three steps to enter at the front door and five steps to enter at the rear entrance.
C. Discharge plans are that the patient's mother will move in with her temporarily until she is able to complete all self-care and home management activities independently.
D. The patient's LUE grip strength is in the 50th percentile for her age and sex. The RUE is below the 10th percentile for her age and sex.
E. The patient will require a safety transfer tub seat on discharge.

F. The patient is able to don upper- and lower-body clothing with minimal assistance required for fine-motor dressing.
G. It is recommended that the patient receive outpatient occupational therapy services twice a week with a focus on independence in self-care activities.
H. The patient has been seen by occupational therapy for 1 hour daily with an emphasis on functional use of the right upper extremity, independence in self-care skills, patient and family education, and adaptive equipment recommendations/training.
I. The patient indicates that she is employed as a "finisher" in a local furniture factory. Her job requires that she use heavy machinery to sand wood pieces ranging from 5–10 pounds. She handles approximately 400 parts per 8–10 hour day.

190. A COTA is reviewing a discharge note prior to placing it in the patient's record. The facility follows a standard SOAP format for documentation. Where is statement A most likely to be seen in the discharge note?
A. The section of the note that contains subjective information.
B. The section of the note that includes objective patient data.
C. The section of the note that provides an assessment of the patient's status.
D. The section of the note that reviews plans and recommendations for discharge.

191. A COTA describes Janie M.'s self-care performance in statement F. Where is this statement most likely to be found in the discharge SOAP note?
A. The subjective portion.
B. The objective portion.
C. The assessment portion.
D. The plan portion.

192. Which statements are the COTA/OTR team most likely to include in the Plan section of the SOAP note?
A. Statements E, F, and I.
B. Statements C, E, and G.
C. Statements E, D, and F.
D. Statements C, H, and I.

193. Which statement contains a referral for additional services?
A. Statement A.
B. Statement C.
C. Statement E.
D. Statement G.

194. The statement that is appropriate for the Objective section of a SOAP note is:
A. statement A.
B. statement B.
C. statement C.
D. statement D.

195. An advanced-level COTA has taken on some administrative duties in an occupational therapy department. One of the tasks she would be MOST likely to take on would be:
A. independent development of a quality-assurance program.
B. supervision of other OTRs and COTAs.
C. supervision of noncertified personnel.
D. management for efficient occupational therapy operations.

196. Which statement best exemplifies a policy?
A. The OT department will provide inservices on relevant information on a regular basis.
B. Inservice presentation will rotate among OT practitioners within the department.
C. Individuals presenting inservices must sign up for the conference room at least 2 weeks in advance.
D. Inservice content should be approved by the Director of Occupational Therapy 2 weeks before the presentation.

197. Which of the following is the best instruction to impart to a caregiver on how to propel a wheelchair down a steep ramp?
A. Tip the wheelchair backward and guide it down the ramp backwards.
B. Tip the wheelchair backward and guide it down the ramp forwards.
C. Allow the patient to propel the wheelchair independently.
D. Obtain the assistance of a second individual.

198. During a routine transfer, Mr. M.'s legs buckle, causing him and the COTA to fall to the floor. The most appropriate way for the COTA to document this incident is in a(n):
A. incident report.
B. daily progress note.
C. letter to the department head.
D. verbal report to the department head.

199. Most facilities require the following equipment to be checked by the maintenance department annually or semiannually:
A. rehabilitation department wheelchairs.
B. hot-water pans for splinting, hot-air guns, and power tools.
C. adaptive equipment inventory.
D. paints, solvents, and other flammable liquids.

200. A COTA has just begun working in an early intervention program after working on an adult rehab unit for 5 years. The level of supervision this COTA should receive is:
A. close.
B. routine.
C. general.
D. minimal.

ANSWERS FOR SIMULATION EXAMINATION 4

1. (C) Petit mal. Petit mal is the correct name for a seizure that barely interrupts a child's performance. Answer A, grand mal seizure, usually involves loss of consciousness. Answer B, psychomotor or tonic-clonic seizure, affects automatic movements. Akinetic seizures (answer D) involve loss of muscle tone. See reference: Case-Smith, Allen, and Pratt (eds): Gordon, CY, Schanzenbacher, KE, Case-Smith, J, and Carrasco, R: Diagnostic problems in pediatrics.

2. (B) read. The term "dyslexia" literally means dysfunction in reading. Inability to print or write (answer A) is termed "dysgraphia." Inability to perform mathematics (answer C) is known as dyscalcula. Inability to plan motor actions (answer D) is dyspraxia. See reference: Case-Smith, Allen, and Pratt (eds): Gordon, CY, Schanzenbacher, KE, Case-Smith, J, and Carrasco, R: Diagnostic problems in pediatrics.

3. (B) observe her in her home during feeding time. "Considering the context of the child's environments is a critical process in occupational therapy assessments (p. 167)." The reason she does not feed herself may be environmental, for instance, her parents may have taught her not to touch food with her fingers, or she may not have learned to feed herself because her grandmother always feeds her. Or, the girl may not be able to transfer skills learned at home to the clinic, that is, she may believe that "the place to eat is home, not the clinic." Although answers A and C provide useful information for treatment planning, they do not address feeding skills. Answer D does not put the skill to be assessed into environmental context. See reference: Case-Smith, Allen, and Pratt (eds): Stewart, KB: Occupational therapy assessment in pediatrics.

4. (B) dressing habits. Certain dressing habits may be an indication of tactile defensiveness, for instance, the child may show poor tolerance of certain textures or avoid wearing turtlenecks, socks, or shoes. Conversely, some children may never take their shoes off in order to avoid tactile overstimulation. Reading skills (answer A), friendships (answer C), and the choice of hobbies (answer D) could be affected secondarily, as a result of intolerance of certain textures or human touch or the inability to concentrate. However, because of the close connection between dressing and tactile tolerance, knowledge of the child's dressing habits (answer B) will give the COTA the most reliable information. See reference: Fisher, AG, Murray, EA, and Bundy, AC (eds): Royeen, CB: Touch inventory for elementary school age children.

5. (A) rattles, teething toys, and teddy bears. Infant toys with distinct sensory characteristics and actions are typical of exploratory play (for infants to 2-years-old). Simple construction toys, dress-up clothes, and props (answer B) are characteristic of symbolic play (2- to 4-year-olds). Arts-and-crafts materials and complex construction toys (answer C) are typical toys for creative play (4- to 7-year-olds). Board games and team sport equipment (answer D) are associated with games with rules (7- to 12-year-olds). See reference: Case-Smith, Allen, and Pratt (eds): Morrison, CD, Metzger, P, and Pratt, PN: Play.

6. (B) be independent except for needing help with clothing. At 4 years of age, a child is expected to know when he or she has to use the toilet, to be able to get on and off the toilet, to cleanse himself or herself effectively, and to wash and dry his or her hands without supervision. The child may need help in readjusting clothing. Complete independence in using the toilet (answer A) is usually achieved by the age of 5. By the age of 2, most children have daytime control over elimination, with occasional accidents (answer D), so that they still need to be reminded to go to the toilet (answer C). See reference: Case-Smith, Allen, and Pratt (eds): Shepherd, J, Procter, SA, and Coley, IL: Self-care and adaptations for independent living.

7. (B) normal development. Proximal movement on a fixed distal limb component, that is, on hands and knees, is an example of the development of mobility superimposed on stability. This stage is essential in the development of coordinated antigravity movement. The development of this type of movement in the quadruped position occurs between the ages of 7 and 12 months. This pattern is typical of normal development and does not indicate answers A, C, or D. See reference: Case-Smith, Allen, and Pratt (eds): Nichols, DS: The development of postural control.

8. (B) "The child demonstrated tongue thrust that interfered with eating." "Tongue thrust" is an objective, well-defined term, and it is described as interfering with function. The other answers are less objective. Answer A infers the child's emotional reaction. Answer C implies voluntary control and judges behavior. Answer D interprets data based on insufficient evidence. See reference: Early: Medical records and documentation.

9. (C) Cruising. The described pattern is cruising. Cruising occurs at approximately 12 months of age and directly precedes walking. Creeping (answer A) refers to four-point mobility in prone position with only hands and knees on the floor, a pattern that occurs between 7 and 12 months. "Crawling" (answer B) is the term for the ability to move forward while in prone position; this pattern occurs at about 7 months. Clawing (answer D), also called "fanning," is the ability to spread the toes to maintain balance in standing. See reference: Case-Smith, Allen, and Pratt (eds): Case-Smith, J, and Shortridge: The developmental process: Prenatal to adolescence.

10. (D) Intermittent headaches. The major signs of shunt malfunction in the older child are irritability, short attention span, increased paralysis, decreased upper-extremity strength, decreased school performance, and intermittent headaches (answer D is correct). Answers A and B (increased head size and nausea and vomiting) are major signs of shunt malfunction in very young children but not in older children. Answer D (back pain) is not among the symptoms given for this problem. See reference: Hopkins and Smith (eds): Atkins, J: Neural tube defect.

11. (C) Following the evaluation. The problem list is the information acquired through observation, interview, and evaluation that gives the occupational therapy practitioner a comprehensive picture of a child's performance dysfunctions. See reference: Case-Smith, Allen, and Pratt (eds): Case-Smith, J: Planning and implementing services.

12. (C) all children with disabilities before they receive special education services. The federal government requires that an individual educational plan be developed before special education services begin. This plan, prepared once a year, is completed by all members of the team involved in a child's education. Continuing education plans (answer A) vary according to the requirements of the therapist's professional organization, employer, and state licensure board. Some state licensure boards require CEUs (continuing education units) at the time of licensure renewal. As a component of the rehabilitation program for adults with head injury (answer B), the rehabilitation team produces a document known as the treatment plan or plan of care. Occupational therapy practitioners usually involve the family of the patient in family training before the patient's discharge from the rehabilitation unit. The OTR or COTA documents these training sessions, as well as an assessment of the family's ability to follow discharge plans, but this documentation (answer D) is not referred to as an individual educational plan. See reference: Jacobs and Logigian (eds): Pagonis, J: Documentation.

13. (C) Doffing socks. Answer C is correct because, according to most developmental scales, children first learn to remove garments, especially socks. Answer A is not correct, because the ability to don garments with the front and back correctly placed is a skill that is developed later. Buttoning and tying bows (answer D) is incorrect for the same reason. Answer B is incorrect, because children are able to remove garments before they are able to put them on. See reference: Case-Smith, Allen, and Pratt (eds): Shepherd, J, Procter, SA, and Coley, IL: Self-care and adaptations for independent living.

14. (D) the ability to recognize objects. Answer D is correct, because a child must be able to recognize an object before he or she can discriminate among its specific visual attributes. Answers A, B, and C are not correct, because the ability to discriminate among colors, shapes, and positions is a skill that develops later. See reference: Kramer and Hinojosa (eds): Todd, VR: Visual perceptual frame of reference: An information processing approach.

15. (C) The prosthetist. Prosthetists are professionals trained to make and fit artificial limbs. The physiatrist (answer A) is a physician with specialized training in physical medicine. The orthotist (answer B) specializes in fitting and fabricating permanent splints and braces. The physical therapist (answer D) is a rehabilitation professional trained to administer exercise and physical modalities to restore function and prevent disability. See reference: Case-Smith, Allen, and Pratt (eds): Allen, AS: Relationships with other service providers.

16. (D) reinforcement of competence. According to Erikson, an 8-year-old child is usually in the stage of industry versus inferiority, during which he or she develops a sense of competency. For a client who is expected to lose motor function gradually, a treatment plan that will provide him with an ongoing sense of competence (possibly in other areas) is especially relevant. Answers A, B, and C describe other developmental issues identified by Erikson that are typically achieved at other ages: basic trust (answer A) in infancy, initiative (answer B) during the toddler years, and self-identity (answer C) during adolescence. See reference: Case-Smith, Allen, and Pratt (eds): Hinojosa, J, Kramer, P, and Pratt, PN: Foundations of practice: Developmental principles, theories, and frames of reference.

17. (C) Have the client use a brush with a thick handle and gradually decrease the thickness. A thick handle is easier to grasp with limited grip strength. As the client's strength increases, the COTA can gradually reduce the thickness . Using a weighted brush (answer A) helps stabilize an incoordinated limb. Using color-coding (answer B) and using a sequence of physical, gestural, and verbal cues (answer D) are methods better suited for clients with cognitive limitations. See reference: Case-Smith, Allen, and Pratt (eds): Shepherd, J, Procter, SA, and Coley, IL: Self-care and adaptations for independent living.

18. (A) Making handprints by pushing his palm into clay. This activity provides deep pressure into palm and fingers, which stimulates proprioceptive awareness. Answer A addresses tactile perception. Answers C and D address in-hand manipulation skills. See reference: Case-Smith, Allen, and Pratt (eds): Exner, CE: Development of hand skills.

19. (A) Bowling. To promote the development of anticipatory control, movement should be slow, predictable, and controlled from a stable base. Bowling involves control of a ball from a stable base (standing) or slow movement (stepping). The speed of movement can be controlled by the player. Answers B, C, and D are activities that feature faster-moving objects whose speed and direction of movement cannot be controlled by the player and require quick reactions to unpredictable stimuli. See reference: Case-Smith, Allen, and Pratt (eds): Nichols, DS: The development of postural control.

20. (B) Head. Head control must be developed first in order to provide a stable base for oral-motor control. Answer C (trunk control) is not correct, because head control precedes trunk control in developmental progression. Although shoulder control (answer A) and hand control (answer D) both contribute to eating and feeding skills by increasing the possibility of independence in eating through improved arm and hand function, head control must be acquired first. See reference: Case-Smith, Allen, and Pratt (eds): Case-Smith, J, and Humphry, R: Feeding and oral motor skills.

21. (A) Drawing a picture titled "This is me." Children who have trouble expressing their emotions verbally are sometimes able to express their feeling in open-ended drawing activities. Among the answers given, answer A is the only projective activity. Answers B, C, and D are highly structured activities with minimal potential for open-ended expression. See reference: Case-Smith, Allen, and Pratt (eds): Cronin, AS: Psychosocial and emotional domains of behavior.

22. (B) 90/90/90 degrees at hip/knee/ankle joints. Ninety-degree angles at the hip, knee and ankle joints place the body in a neutral position, avoiding excessive flexion or extension that could cause deformity or interfere with function in sitting. Answers A and C are incorrect, because 45-degree angles at any of these joints creates excessive flexion. Answer D is incorrect because 125-degrees puts each joint in excessive extension. See reference: Hopkins and Smith (eds): Erhardt, RP: Cerebral palsy.

23. (C) 9 and 12 months. Children usually begin to "cruise" (walk sideways holding on to a rail) between 9 and 12 months. See reference: Case-Smith, Allen, and Pratt (eds): Case-Smith, J, and Shortridge, SD: The developmental process: Prenatal to adolescence.

24. (A) Teaching the child to dress in sidelying position. The sidelying position eliminates the need for the child to maintain balance in order to dress the lower extremities. Answer B is not correct, because the primary purpose of putting loops on waistbands is to help a child with limited grasp strength pull garments on. Answer C is not correct, because using Velcro in place of zippers is also an adaptation designed to help children with limited ability to grasp and pull ability. See reference: Case-Smith, Allen, and Pratt (eds): Hunter, JG: The neonatal intensive care unit.

25. (D) upper lip control. The use of a shallow spoon encourages the development of upper-lip control, because it makes it easier for the lip to remove all of the food on the spoon, which can help increase oral-motor control during feeding. Jaw opening and closing are not affected by the depth of the spoon (answers A and B are not correct). The lower lip is not involved in drawing food off the spoon, so lower-lip control (answer C) will not be influenced by the use of a shallow spoon. See reference: Case-Smith, Allen, and Pratt (eds): Case-Smith, J, and Humphry, R: Feeding and oral motor skills.

26. (B) let the boy sit at the front of the bus and use his tape player and earphones. If the boy is seated in the front of the bus, he will experience less jostling by peers, so that he will have less tactile and visual stimulation to deal with. Also, the earphones will serve to reduce auditory overload. The method described in answer A is the only one that addresses the underlying problem of the boy's low tolerance for sensory stimulation. Answers A, C, and D are behavioral management techniques that do not take his hypersensitivity into account. See reference: Case-Smith, Allen, and Pratt (eds): Cronin, AS: Psychosocial and emotional domains of behavior.

27. (A) checking for irritation and pressure problems. Because a pre-verbal child cannot communicate her discomfort effectively, skin irritation may go unnoticed for too long. A young child, therefore, is at higher risk for developing skin and pressure problems than an older, more verbal one. Although answers B, C, and D describe important factors in splint care, for the young child, primary emphasis should be placed on answer A. See reference: Case-Smith, Allen, and Pratt (eds): Exner, CE: Development of hand skills.

28. (B) mounting half-inch-diameter dowels verticaly on the markers. This adaptation will enable the client to grasp the markers with a palmar grasp. Attaching Velcro to the board and markers (answer A) is an adaptation that is more useful for a child whose precision gripping skills are limited because of a lack of stability. Placing a magnetic board upright (answer C) can help a child with visual perceptual difficulties or limitations in his or her upper-extremity range of motion. Replacing the markers with lightweight playing pieces (answer D) is an adaptation for a child with limited strength. See reference: Case-Smith, Allen, and Pratt (eds): Exner, CE: Development of hand skills.

29. (D) Hold him firmly when picking him up. Answer D is correct, because holding the child firmly inhibits responses to light touch (which are usually most uncomfortable for children with tactile defensiveness). For the same reason, tickling (answer A) and light stroking (answer C) are not correct. Answer B is not correct, because a strong stimulus such as loud music would cause further startle and discomfort during a time when he is most vulnerable to the sensation of light touch, that is, when clothing is being removed. See reference: Case-Smith, Allen, and Pratt (eds): Case-Smith, J, and Humphry, R: Feeding and oral motor skills.

30. (C) bring the seat in for reevaluation within 6 months. Fit and function of seating and mobility should be reassessed within 6 months to account for the child's growth as well as any changes in posture. The COTA should not instruct the parents to make unsupervised adaptations (answer A), because improper positioning could harm the child. Weekly adjustment (answer B) is usually not necessary, and transporting the seat every week would be an unnecessary inconvenience to the parents. The end of the IEP (answer D) may be more than 6 months away, too long to wait. See reference: Case-Smith, Allen, and Pratt (eds): Wright-Ott, C, and Egilson, S: Mobility.

31. (A) Replacing the spoon with a blunt-ended fork. For a child with incoordination and tremors, stabbing food with a blunt-ended fork is often more effective feeding than using a spoon. The food will not fall off the fork, and the blunt tines will prevent any injury to the child. Building up the spoon handle (answer B) is more appropriate for a child with a weak grasp. A swivel spoon (answer C) and bending the handle 45 degrees (answer D) are more appropriate for a child with limited forearm and wrist motion. See reference: Case-Smith, Allen, and Pratt (eds): Case-Smith, J, and Humphry, R: Feeding and oral motor skills.

32. (B) Catching and bursting soap bubbles. This activity involves visually tracking a slow-moving target and requires minimal fine-motor precision to accomplish a successful "hit." Answers A, C, and D also require visual tracking and eye-hand coordination but involve more fast-moving targets and require immediate, more precise movements. These activities can therefore be used to promote more advanced skills. See reference: Case-Smith, Allen, and Pratt (eds): Dubois, SA: Preschool services.

33. (C) Explaining the consequences of his actions to him. Because of limited understanding, children with autism are least likely to respond to an insight-based approach. Because self-injurious behaviors often occur during unstructured times, engaging the child in more productive activities (answer A) often helps reduce the incidence of these behaviors. Because of their altered sensory perception, children with autism often seek out intense sensations, such as those provided by biting, scratching, head banging, and so on. Alternate activities involving heavy-pressure touch (answer B), such as massaging, and rolling satisfies the child's "sensory hunger" in a less harmful way. The use of behavioral techniques to modify self-injurious behaviors (answer D) has been effective in breaking through autistic barriers and reinforcing positive behaviors such as attending and focusing. See reference: Logigian and Ward (eds): Ward, JD: Infantile autism.

34. (C) Does the seat provide enough support for the child to relax? A relaxed position during toilet use is essential to success in elimination training. A seat design featuring a wide base, back support, and placement at a height that enables the child to place the feet firmly on the ground or on foot supports will give the child a sense of comfort and security. Answers A, B, and D describe other useful considerations that should be addressed after the issue of support has been addressed. See reference: Logigian and Ward (eds): Logigian, MK: Cerebral palsy.

35. (A) hips. Flexing the hips breaks up the extensor pattern and, combined with knee flexion, reduces tone in the lower extremities, thus facilitating dressing. Flexing more distal joints first (answers B, C, and D) is ineffective in reducing tone and may lead to excessive stress on the joints involved. See reference: Case-Smith, Allen, and Pratt (eds): Shepherd, J, Procter, SA, and Coley, IL: Self-care and adaptations for independent living.

36. (D) scoop dish. This is the best answer, because the sides of the scoop dish will aid the scooping movement. The high back of the plate provides a surface to push the food against, which makes it easier to load the food onto the spoon. Answer A is not correct, because the swivel spoon is more appropriate when supination is limited. Answer B is not correct, because the nonslip mat is designed to stabilize the plate. Answer D is incorrect, because the mobile arm support is best used to position the arm and help weak shoulder and elbow muscles position the hand. See reference: Case-Smith, Allen, and Pratt (eds): Shepherd, J, Procter, SA, and Coley, IL: Self-care and adaptations for independent living.

37. (C) sidelying position. The sidelying position reduces the influence of reflexes, extensor tone, and gravity, all of which make protraction of the shoulders and forward reach difficult. Answer A is incorrect, because standing position will not reduce extensor tone, which encourages shoulder retraction and makes forward reaching of both arms to midline more difficult. Answer B is wrong, because in prone position the upper extremities are involved weightbearing; however, this position may help facilitate forward reach by developing shoulder protraction. Answer D is not correct, because in the quadruped position the upper extremities are involved in weightbearing. If, however, the position is attainable, shoulder protraction and forward reach may be facilitated. See reference: Kramer and Hinojosa: Colangelo, CA: Biomechanical frame of reference.

38. (D) the paper in two following a straight line. Answer D is correct, because scissors skills develop from cutting snips to cutting a single straight line. Answer A is not correct, because the ability to cut heavier materials such as cardboard and cloth develops last in the sequence of scissor skills. Answer B is not correct, because the ability to cut along curved lines develops after the ability to cut a straight line. Answer C is not correct, because the ability to cut along straight lines with enough control to cut a triangle develops after the ability to cut a single straight line and before the ability to cut a curved line. See reference: Case-Smith, Allen, and Pratt (eds): Exner, CE: Development of hand skills.

39. (A) sit straddling a bolster with both feet on the floor. Since Leslie has learned to sit independently on the floor, she no longer needs external stabilizing support (answer D). After having developed independent postural reactions on a stable surface, that is, the floor, she can now further refine her skills by learning to maintain posture when placed on an unstable surface. At first, she should be left in control of the movement of this surface, and she should have both feet on the floor for maximal stability. Later, these skills can be refined by placing her on more challenging surfaces, such as on the hippity-hop (answer C) or on a scooter pulled by another person (answer B). See reference: Case-Smith, Allen, and Pratt (eds): Nichols, DS: The development of postural control.

40. (B) inch cubes into cup placed on a tabletop at a distance of 1 foot. Larry needs to demonstrate control in the midranges by releasing objects in a controlled way without using his full extension pattern. This is achieved by placing target containers closer to his body, requiring gradually increasing elbow flexion with wrist extension. Answers A and D involve larger, softer objects for release and require either throwing or gravity-assisted movement, both of which require less control. Answer C requires the manipulation of smaller objects and more precision, that is, a more advanced skill than given in answer B. See reference: Case-Smith, Allen, and Pratt (eds): Exner, CE: Development of hand skills.

41. (C) indicating initiative and beginning task-directed behavior. Because Ellen is so withdrawn, any spontaneous action should be seen as a very positive sign. It is very important to encourage Ellen in independent exploratory behavior in order for her to develop task competence and become less withdrawn. Her use of a toothbrush instead of a hairbrush may indicate cognitive limitations (answer B), possibly caused by a lack of exposure; it could also be caused by a visual deficit (answer D), but the primary importance of the observation lies in C. Attention-getting behavior (answer A) is unlikely in such a withdrawn child. See reference: Case-Smith, Allen, and Pratt (eds): Cronin, AS: Psychosocial and emotional domains of behavior.

42. (A) "Doug will bathe himself with supervision." The levels of self-care skill independence, from lowest to highest, are: dependent, maximal assistance, moderate assistance (answer C), minimal assistance (Doug's current level), supervision (answer A), independent with set-up (answer B), and independent. See reference: Case-Smith, Allen, and Pratt (eds): Shepherd, J, Procter, SA, and Coley, IL: Self-care and adaptations for independent living.

43. (C) demonstrates any reliable, controlled movement. As long as Shira can produce any such movement, switches can be adapted to meet her positioning and mobility needs. Accurate reach and pointing (answer B) or isolated finger control (answer D) are not necessary to use simple pressure switches. An upright sitting position (answer A) would not be required if Shira needed to be positioned in a reclining or sidelying position. See reference: Case-Smith, Allen, and Pratt (eds): Struck, M: Augmentative communication and computer access.

44. (C) liquid and solids combined (minestrone soup). Answer C is correct, because it combines two food consistencies. Liquids are very difficult for children with poor oral-motor organization to manage in eating. When solids are added into the liquid the child will have difficulty managing two different forms of food. Answers A, B, and C, depending on the child's oral-motor skills, will be easier to move and manage within the mouth. See reference: Case-Smith, Allen, and Pratt (eds): Case-Smith, J, and Humphry, R: Feeding and oral motor skills.

45. (D) Block out all areas of the page except important words. Answer D is correct, because this compensatory technique is a way of dealing with visual figure-ground or visual discrimination problems. The child needs to learn how to rule out extraneous stimuli and focus on the important area of a task, such as reading. Answer A is not correct, because this is a technique used to orient the child with left-right visual tracking problems. Answer B is not correct, because it is a technique used to deal with visual attention problems. Answer C is not correct, because it is a technique used to help children deal with visual memory problems. See reference: Kramer and Hinojosa (eds): Todd, VR: Visual perceptual frame of reference: An information processing approach.

46. (C) Provide a screen to reduce peripheral visual stimuli. Although all the answers describe techniques that could assist the student, the use of a carrel is most appropriate in a mainstreamed classroom, because the other methods or adaptations (answers A, B, and D) could have a negative impact on the other children's ability to learn. See reference: Case-Smith, Allen, and Pratt (eds): Schneck, CM: Visual perception.

47. (B) child's writing, dressing, and self-feeding skills. Because the child was being treated for difficulties with fine-motor skills, discharge criteria should focus on fine-motor function. Answers A, C, and D describe information that is relevant in overall discharge planning but is not relevant in determining readiness for discharge. See reference: Case-Smith, Allen, and Pratt (eds): Johnson, J: School-based occupational therapy.

48. (B) A sponge mounted in the tub. Mounting a device on a stable surface and bringing the body part to it, rather than vice versa, provides stability of movement to the child with incoordination. Answers A, C, and D describe adaptations useful for other conditions. A bath mitt (answer A) can help a child with a weak grasp, and a long-handled bath brush (answer C) and hand-held shower head (answer D) extend the reach for the child with limited range of motion. See reference: Case-Smith, Allen, and Pratt (eds): Dudgeon, BJ: Pediatric rehabilitation.

49. (D) A disco. Flashing lights, such as strobe lights, loud music, high room temperatures, and physical exertion are all stressful stimuli that can elicit seizure activity in the seizure-prone individual. Although the environments in answers A, B, and C include crowds, noise, and lighting effects, the disco provides the most intense stimuli. See reference: Case-Smith, Allen, and Pratt (eds): Gordon, CY, Schanzenbacher, KE, Case-Smith, J, and Carrasco, R: Diagnostic problems in pediatrics.

50. (C) "Pt. has improved significantly in his ability to work at the computer by utilizing periodic stretch breaks." The assessment section of a discharge summary identifies the functional performance deficit(s) and indicates whether they have been resolved or, if they still exist, to what degree. Answer A is a subjective report. Answer B is an example of a statement that belongs in the objective section of a discharge summary. See reference: Kettenbach: Writing assessment (A).

51. (C) Topographic orientation. Topographic orientation is the ability to find or follow a familiar place or route. An example is a person finding the therapy department from his or her room or a person finding the way to the bathroom in the night without turning on the light. Position in space (answer A) is the ability to distinguish front from back, down from up, and so on. Figure-ground discrimination (answer B) is the ability to find an object against a background. Visual closure (answer D) is the ability to recognize an object when only part of it has been seen. See reference: AOTA: Uniform terminology for occupational therapy.

52. (D) decreased attention. An attention deficit is indicated if the individual recognizes the letter and marks it accurately on both the right and left sides of the paper but misses letters in a random pattern. A visual field cut (answers A and B) is evidenced by the missed letters appearing close together in one area, on either the left or right side of the page. The COTA would have determined that the client was functionally illiterate (answer C) before the test—during the interview or from the chart review—in which case the COTA would pick a more appropriate test. Some functionally illiterate persons, however, are able to complete the assigned task accurately, depending on the level of illiteracy. See reference: Trombly (ed): Quintana, LA: Remediating perceptual impairments.

53. (A) at the lateral epicondyle of the humerus. The lateral epicondyle of the humerus is the bony prominence on the lateral side of the elbow. The medial epicondyle (answer B) is the bony prominence on the medial side of the elbow. The stationary arm of the goniometer should be positioned parallel to the longitudinal axis of the humerus on the lateral aspect (answer C). The movable arm of the goniometer should be positioned parallel to the longitudinal axis of the radius on the lateral aspect (answer D). See reference: Trombly (ed): Evaluation of biomechanical and physiological aspects of motor performance.

54. (C) anosagnosia. Individuals with anosagnosia demonstrate denial of their deficits. They are usually unsafe during performance of activities and often have difficulty learning compensatory techniques. Apraxia (answer A) is the inability to perform a purposeful movement on command. A person with alexia (answer D) is unable to understand written language. Noncompliant individuals (answer B) refuse to carry out treatment but are usually aware of their deficits. See reference: Trombly (ed): Quintana, LA: Evaluation of perception and cognition.

55. (A) within normal limits. The normal range of motion for internal rotation is 70 degrees. Rotation can be assessed with the humerus adducted against the trunk or with the shoulder abducted at 90 degrees. If the humeral movements for internal or external rotation are observed during the performance of activities and found to be adequate for the performance of any functional activities, the range of motion may be noted as within functional limits (WFL) (answer B). The COTA may choose not to perform a formal joint measurement if the joint is WFL, even though the end of the range may be lacking a few degrees, because the loss of movement may not be significant to the individual. Hypermobility at a joint is motion past the normal range of motion, which at the shoulder would be past 70 degrees of internal rotation. When hypermobility leads to deformity, caused by an unstable joint as might occur after a surgical repair or a disease process, then splinting or another form of stabilization or immobilization can be used to correct the problem (answer C). If the COTA observes hypermobility during range of motion, he or she should compare the range of movement to that on the individual's opposite side in order to assess normal range. A limitation of internal rotation at the shoulder would be less than 70 degrees of motion (answer D). If a limitation is apparent, the rehabilitation team may choose not to treat it unless it interferes with the function of the upper extremity. See reference: Trombly (ed): Evaluation of biomechanical and physiological aspects of motor performance.

56. (A) constructional apraxia. An individual with constructional apraxia may have full sensory awareness of the affected side of the body but be unable to perform the construction of one or more objects onto each other to carry out a verbal command or don clothing in the proper sequence or position. Unilateral neglect (answer D) occurs when the individual neglects the affected side of the body and performs activities toward or with the unaffected side (for example, an individual might comb only one side of his head or shave one side of his face). Ideomotor apraxia (answer C) is when an individual is able to perform an activity (such as brushing his teeth) automatically but is unable to perform the same activity on command. Dressing apraxia (answer D) is usually the result of constructional apraxia, unilateral neglect, and/or body scheme disturbance. Individuals with dressing apraxia are unable to dress themselves. See reference: Trombly (ed): Quintana, LA: Remediating perceptual impairments.

57. (C) reading the medical chart. A physician, nurse, or supervising OT (answers A, B, and D) should refer to the medical record to determine what medications an individual is taking. COTAs are qualified to read medical charts and elicit information about medications. It is more appropriate for the COTA to obtain this information independently than to ask another professional to do it for her. See reference: Pedretti (ed): Occupational therapy evaluation and assessment of physical dysfunction.

58. (B) social worker's admission note. The social worker is the professional on the rehabilitation team responsible for assessing the patient's social and economic background. This information is included in the social worker's documentation. The physician's documentation (answer A) addresses the patient's medical status. The nurse's initial note (answer C) addresses medical and nursing concerns, such as the patient's wound status, vital signs, and response to hospitalization. The physical therapist's initial note (answer D) focuses on musculoskeletal issues. See reference: Pedretti (ed): Pasquinelli, S: Lower extremity amputations and prosthetics.

59. (B) requiring minimal assistance. Requiring minimal assistance is defined as being able to complete a task while requiring supervision, cueing, and/or physical assistance for less than 20 percent of the task. To be considered independent (answer A), an individual must be able to complete the task without supervision, cueing, or any assistance, at normal or near normal speed. Requiring supervision (answer C) is when the individual can perform the task alone but requires someone there for safety. Requiring moderate assistance (answer D) is defined as having the ability to complete the task with supervision and cueing while needing physical assistance for 20 to 50 percent of the task. See reference: Pedretti (ed): Foti, D, Pedretti, LW, and Lillie, S: Activities of daily living.

60. (C) During discussion at lunch in the cafeteria. Confidential information about an individual must be respected by OT practitioners and should not be discussed in public places. Phone calls (answer A), written reports (answer B), and discussion in the OT office (answer D) are all acceptable ways for a COTA to communicate with a supervising OTR. See reference: Early: Data gathering and evaluation; also AOTA: Occupational therapy code of ethics.

61. (D) early morning and again in the afternoon. Individuals with arthritis should be evaluated at both times to assess the functional abilities of the individual during and after morning stiffness. Evaluating the individual only in the morning (answers A and C) or in the afternoon (answer B) accurately reveals the individual's functional level at only one time of day. Individuals with arthritis have many changes in functional status after morning stiffness has disappeared. See reference: Trombly (ed): Feinberg, JR, and Trombly, CA: Arthritis.

62. (B) provide positioning and/or adaptive equipment. Positioning and adaptive equipment are necessary to maintain the integrity of the musculoskeletal system and prevent deformity. Resistive exercises (answer A) arc used cautiously with individuals with RA, because of the potential for tissue damage. A newly diagnosed individual would need some emotional support (answer C), but the primary means of support is the family or a support group. Surgical intervention (answer D) would not be needed in the early stages of rheumatoid arthritis. It may be offered as a corrective measure for long-standing deformities. See reference: Hopkins and Smith (eds): Functional Restoration-Neurologic, Arthritic, Orthopedic, Cardiac and Pulmonary Conditions.

63. (D) built-up handles. Built-up handles, without adding extra weight, allow a comfortable grasp that regular utensils (answer A) do not provide. A weighted handle (answer B) would cause more rapid fatigue and strain to the joints. An arthritic person will have adequate grasp and release with a built-up handle, making it easier to use than a universal cuff (answer C). See reference: Trombly (ed): Feinberg, JR, and Trombly, CA: Arthritis.

64. (B) A key guard. A key guard is a device that covers the keys and provides a guide for a finger or stick without punching extra keys. A moisture guard (answer A) is a flexible plastic cover that protects the keys from drool, moisture, or dirt. An auto-repeat defeat mechanism (answer C) stops repetition of letters or numbers caused by overlong or involuntary depression of keys. One-finger-access software (answer D) allows the user to lock out keys such as the Shift or the Enter key. This enables an individual who uses only one finger or a stick to type capital letters or perform other keyboard funtions that require simultaneous depression of more than one key. See reference: Church and Glennen (eds): Church, G: Adaptive access for microcomputers.

65. (A) performing assessments. The treatment plan is developed after the individual's problems have been identified through evaluation (answer A). Treatment planning involves the development of long-term and short-term goals (answer B). In order for treatment to be appropriate and effective, the individual's goals, values, and cultural influences must be taken into consideration. Finally, the COTA uses activity analysis and frames of reference to select appropriate treatment methods (answers C and D). See reference: Ryan (ed): Therapeutic intervention process. *Practice Issues in Occupational Therapy.*

66. (B) "Pt. will demonstrate ability to don and doff splint correctly." Correctly donning and doffing a splint is crucial for anyone using a splint. Since the patient will wear the splint to prevent further cumulative trauma to the median nerve at work, this goal is directly related to the long-term goal of returning to work. Work simplification (answer A) is modifying task performance to conserve energy, which is important for individuals with limited endurance, such as those with arthritis or COPD. Typing with wrists in flexion (answer C) is contraindicated and would aggravate the individual's symptoms. Lightweight cookware is appropriate for this individual, but it is related to a homemaking goal, not her goal of returning to work as a secretary. See reference: Reed: Carpal tunnel syndrome.

67. (C) A toothpaste with a flip-open cap. A person who frequently drops small items would be able to manage a toothpaste cap that flips open much more easily than a cap that must be removed completely from the tube. Also, tubes with flip-open caps are larger in diameter, which make them easier to manage. A shirt with contrasting buttons (answer A) would be easier to fasten for someone with visual or perceptual impairments but is not helpful to the person who drops small things. A spray deodorant (answer B) would have a small button to push, which would be difficult for someone with incoordination to operate. Pants with a drawstring waist (answer D) would be difficult to tighten or tie for someone with incoordination. See reference: Pedretti (ed): Foti, D, Pedretti, LW, and Lillie, S: Activities of daily living.

68. (D) weaving on a frame loom. Use of and attention to the entire loom area is essential for weaving on a frame loom. The shuttle must slide across the entire width of the loom, which involves crossing the midline. It is possible to build a coil pot (answer A), to make macramé objects (answer B), and string beads for a necklace (answer C) without crossing the midline. See reference: Breines: Folkcraft.

69. (B) Having her fold laundry and put it in a basket while standing. A prevocational activity is one whose performance facilitates the evaluation or training of work-related skills. A cashier stands during the job, removing clothing from hangers, folding it, putting it in a bag, running the price tags through the scanner, and finally operating the cash register and making change. Activities performed while sitting, such as making a grocery list (answer A) or adding a column of numbers by hand (answer D) are not related to her present employment. Washing dishes while standing (answer C) incorporates the standing aspect of her job but not the other aspects. The activity that incorporates the most components of her job is folding laundry and putting it in a basket while standing. See reference: Pedretti (ed): Foti, D, Pedretti, LW, and Lillie, S: Activities of daily living.

70. (C) work-simplification techniques. Individuals with limited amounts of energy should use work-simplification techniques, which include planning ahead, using correct body mechanics, limiting the amount of work, using efficient methods, using the correct equipment, and pacing oneself. Using adaptive equipment (answer B) may be helpful, but it is only a small part of work simplification. Maintaining maximal range of motion (answer A) and strength are important goals but do not directly address the primary goal of independence in homemaking. The COTA should observe universal precautions in any situation in which she might come in contact with body fluids, but this is not the emphasis of intervention. See reference: Trombly (ed): Stewart, C: Retraining housekeeping and child care skills.

71. (B) grading the activity. OT practitioners gradually change, or grade, an activity to make it slightly easier or slightly more difficult, depending on an individual's needs and abilities, in order to progress toward a goal. Grading is a type of modification (answer A) that implies gradual change; not all modifications are gradual. Adapting the activity (answer C), like modification, involves changing the process, tools, or environment in or with which the activity is performed, so that the individual is able to perform the activity. Using an electric wheelchair would be an example of an adaptation or modification. The OT practitioner uses activity analysis (answer D) to break down a process into its smaller parts in order to determine how the activity can be used therapeutically. See reference: Early: Analyzing, adapting, and grading activity.

72. (C) extension during finger flexion and flexion during finger extension. The method used to maintain tenodesis in the hand of a person with quadriplegia is to keep the wrist extended during finger flexion and flexed during finger extension. This allows the finger flexor tendons to shorten so that tenodesis action can occur. The other methods would stretch the tendons too much, which would not allow a tenodesis grasp. See reference: Ryan (ed): Fike, ML, Weiner, M, and Darlak, S: The young adult with a spinal injury. *Practice Issues in Occupational Therapy.*

73. (D) maintain normal curve of the back, slowly shifting her feet as the turn is completed. The correct way to perform a transfer is slowly, with the knees bent and the feet shoulder-width apart, maintaining the normal curve of the back and lifting from the legs. The practitioner should not twist her body at the trunk (answer A), because this could injure the back. Lifting with the arms (answer B) instead of the legs also could injure the COTA's back. It is incorrect technique to keep the feet planted when moving during a transfer (answer C), because this causes twisting of the back and may damage the knees. See reference: Pedretti (ed): Adler, C, and Tipton-Burton, M: Wheelchair assessment and transfers.

74. (B) attach finger loops to both sides of each container, making it easier for Dana to pull them open. An individual with C7 quadriplegia resulting in weak grasp would be able to open the make-up containers by slipping her fingers through the loops and pulling. Stabilizing items with suction cups (answer A) is a compensatory technique usually used by individuals with hemiplegia. A wrist-driven flexor hinge splint (answer C) would help Dana to achieve a stronger prehension grip, but it would not provide her with the strength or coordination required for this task. Weighting an object is a compensatory technique used to provide more control to people with tremors or incoordination (answer D), neither of which are issues for

Dana. See reference: Hopkins and Smith (eds): Kohlmeyer, KM: Assistive and adaptive equipment.

75. (A) Holding the mallet. Holding the mallet is the only activity listed that requires gripping with the entire hand. Holding the stamping tools and needle (answers B and D) requires pinch patterns. Squeezing the sponge offers less resistance than holding the hammer and would therefore be less effective for strengthening. See reference: Breines: Folkcraft.

76. (C) in 25 degrees of wrist extension, to promote development of tenodesis. A tenodesis grasp is developed by allowing the finger flexors to shorten. The individual is then able to achieve a functional grasp by extending the wrist. This improves the ability of an individual with a C6 or C7 spinal cord injury to grasp and hold objects. The resting position used to facilitate development of tenodesis calls for the wrist to be in 10 to 30 degrees of extension, with the thumb opposed and abducted and the fingers partially flexed. Positions that maintain the fingers in extension, such as placing the hands flat on a bed and using resting pan splints (answers A and D), would prevent the development of tenodesis. Forty-five degrees of wrist extension (answer B) is too much. See reference: Trombly (ed): Hollar, LD: Spinal cord injury.

77. (C) stand at a high table while working on a puzzle for increasing amounts of time each day. To increase standing tolerance, or endurance, the cashier needs to stand for progressively longer periods of time each day. Answer A would be appropriate for an individual with a back injury who needs to improve his ability to lift. Answer B would be appropriate for an individual who needs to increase the distance he is able to walk. Answer D would be appropriate for an individual who needs to increase lower extremity strength. See reference: Pedretti (ed): Pedretti, LW and Wade, IE: Therapeutic modalities.

78. (C) On a shelf over the counter to the left. Reaching for objects placed on the left side would use little trunk rotation and no weight shift to the right side, while decreasing weight-bearing to the right upper extremity. Reaching for an object on the right side increases trunk rotation, weight shift to the right, and weight-bearing on the right arm, but the greatest amount of shift is elicited when reaching for objects below waist level. See reference: Trombly (ed): Proprioceptive neuromuscular facilitation (PNF) approach.

79. (A) up and the collar toward her body. Answers B, C, and D are incorrect placements and would result in failure to perform the activity successfully. See reference: Pedretti (ed): Foti, D, Pedretti, LW, and Lillie, S: Activities of daily living.

80. (A) (1) Position shirt on lap; (2) place affected hand into sleeve and pull up past elbow; (3) grasp collar with normal hand and swing shirt around and behind neck and shoulders; (4) place normal hand and arm into remaining sleeve. Answers B, C, and D are examples of incorrect sequences that would result in failure to don the shirt successfully. See reference: Pedretti (ed): Foti, D, Pedretti, LW, and Lillie, S: Activities of daily living.

81. (C) A safety razor with an extended handle. The extended handle is the necessary component to allow Zack to overcome his limited shoulder and elbow range of motion in order to reach his face. Attaching a safety razor or electric razor to a universal cuff (answers A and D) would benefit an individual who is unable to grasp a razor but would not enable Zack to reach his face to shave. A safety razor with a built-up handle would benefit an individual with limited finger flexion or strength, but it would also be ineffective in enabling Zack to reach his face with the razor. See reference: Trombly (ed): Retraining basic and instrumental activities of daily living.

82. (C) use the right hand for opening jars and the left hand for closing jars. Individuals with arthritis should observe joint-protection principles when opening jars and performing other daily tasks that could cause further damage to joints. These principles include "avoid positions of deformity as well as external pressures and internal stresses in the direction of deformity" and "use the largest, strongest joints available for the job (p. 822)." Jars open in a counter-clockwise direction, therefore the right hand should be used so that the fingers are not pushed in an ulnar direction. Using the left hand to open jars (answer D) would push fingers in a direction of deformity. Rather than holding the jar in one hand while opening it with the other (answer A), the COTA should encourage Jack to stabilize the jar on a wet towel or a nonskid pad and press down on the jar lid with his palm to open it. This methods uses the larger joints of the wrist and arm rather than the fingers (answer B) to open the jar. See reference: Trombly (ed): Feinberg, JR, and Trombly, CA: Arthritis.

83. (B) functional position resting splint. Bedridden individuals are often provided with splints to prevent the development of flexion contractures in the hand that can lead to problems with hygiene. A functional-position resting hand splint is most appropriate for Matthew because it will prevent flexion contractures from developing and allow the caregiver access to his hand for cleaning. Neither the dorsal or volar wrist splints (answer A and C) would keep the fingers in extension, which is necessary to prevent development of finger contractures. Dynamic finger-extension splints (answer D) are appropriate for individuals who have active finger flexion but limited active finger extension. See reference: Hopkins and Smith (eds): Fess, EE, and Kiel, JH: Upper extremity splinting.

84. (C) Making a wooden birdhouse. Individuals with diabetes often experience loss of the sense of touch and pain, as well as impaired circulation, which can affect their ability to heal. An unnoticed splinter could result in infection, even amputation. Therefore, a project such as woodworking that would expose Antonio to the risk of splinters would be contraindicated. Baking (answer B) and making latch hook rugs (answer D) could be structured to address standing balance and tolerance, but may be seen as feminine activities by some men. Gender association in itself is not a contraindication, but these activities could be considered poor choices if not meaningful to the individual. A group ball-toss activity (answer A) can also be structured to address standing balance and tolerance. See reference: Drake: Woodworking.

85. (A) Salt. Foods high in salt are contraindicated for individuals with high blood pressure. Foods high in sugar (answer B) should be avoided for individuals with diabetes. High cholesterol levels (answer C) are considered a risk factor for stroke;

however, the information provided refers to a history of hypertension, which is not cholesterol related. Food texture (answer D) is a concern when working on feeding with individuals with dysphagia. See reference: Hansen and Atchison (eds): Bierman, SN: Cerebrovascular accident.

86. (A) functional performance levels. The objective portion of the SOAP format should include the clinical findings of an evaluation. Analysis of evaluations (answer B) should go in the assessment component of documentation. Conclusions and assumptions of performance measures (answer C) are included in the assessment portion of the SOAP format. Quotes from the patient and/or family (answer D), are a part of the subjective portion. See reference: Hopkins and Smith (eds): Perinchief, JM: Service management.

87. (C) Requiring moderate assistance. Requiring moderate assistance is defined as having the ability to complete the task with supervision and cueing while requiring physical assistance for 20 to 50 percent of the task. The individual who requires minimal assistance (answer A) is able to complete a task with supervision and cueing while requiring physical assistance for less than 20 percent of the task. An individual who needs supervision, cueing, and physical assistance for from 50 to 80 percent of the task is performing at the maximal assistance level (answer D). An individual is rated dependent (answer A) when he or she is able to perform less than 20 percent, or a few steps, of the activity independently. This individual may require elaborate equipment, may perform the activity extremely slowly, and may fatigue easily. See reference: Pedretti (ed): Foti, D, Pedretti, LW, and Lillie, S: Activities of daily living.

88. (C) "Pt. is demonstrating gradual improvement in fine-motor coordination." The assessment portion of the note "contains the analysis of plans and goals for the patient . . . and involves the professional judgment of the therapists." It is also where the OT practitioner draws conclusions and justifies decisions. The objective portion of the SOAP note should contain information that is measurable or based on specific observations (answer A). The subjective portion contains information gained from communication with the patient and his or her family (answers B and D). This information is not measurable and therefore is considered subjective. See reference: Kettenbach: Writing assessment (A).

89. (D) "Family will demonstrate independence in positioning pt. correctly for feeding so that he can swallow safely." Goals should be functional, measurable, and objective. In addition, short-term goals must relate to the long-term goal being addressed. This answer meets those criteria. Answer A does not provide measurable criteria, nor does it directly relate to the long-term goal of family training. Answer B, while measurable, does not relate to the long-term goal. Answer C describes the long-term goal of family independence in the feeding program. See reference: AOTA: Writing functional goals. *Effective Documentation for Occupational Therapy.*

90. (C) implementating compensatory strategies. "The compensation approach focuses on the use of remaining abilities to achieve the highest level of function possible . . .". Compensatory strategies include modifying the environment and are most appropriate for this patient because his prognosis is poor and he is unlikely to improve. An example would be placing the food all on the right side of his meal tray. "The focus of remediation (answer A) is to improve or restore the patient's functional performance . . .. This approach is used when a patient's condition [is likely to improve] adequately to allow for task performance." Whereas patient education (answer B) about a visual-field deficit is likely to have little benefit, educating the family is important so that they can implement compensatory strategies. Adaptive equipment (answer D) is a type of compensation, but it too would be neglected if placed to the patient's left. See reference: Hopkins and Smith (eds): Culler, KH: Home and family management.

91. (C) Minimization of joint damage. Using joint-protection techniques may reduce joint stress and pain, preserve joint structures, and conserve energy. Keeping joints in one position for an undue length of time, such as in knitting (answer D), is "fatiguing and can contribute to joint subluxation and dislocation." The ability to prepare a meal without becoming fatigued (answer A) is a likely outcome of using energy-conservation techniques. Using proper body mechanics can enable an individual with back pain to lift heavy grocery bags without pain (answer B). See reference: Pedretti (ed): Hittle, JM, Pedretti, LW, and Kasch, MC: Rheumatoid arthritis.

92. (B) perform lower-extremity dressing without internally rotating or adducting the involved hip. Following hip arthroplasty, positions such as flexion of the hip past 90 degrees, internal rotation, and adduction can result in dislocation of the hip. Occupational therapy practitioners instruct patients in hip precautions and provide them with adaptive equipment so they can safely perform self-care, work, and leisure activities. The ability to stand for long periods of time (answer A) is a likely outcome from participation in an endurance or conditioning program. Although safe hip positions are essential during ambulation and tub transfers (answers C and D), additional training is required for independence in these activities. See reference: Pedretti (ed): Morawski, D, Pitbladdo, K, Bianchi, EM, Lieberman, SL, Novic, JP, and Bobrove, H: Hip fractures and total hip replacement.

93. (C) collaborate with Tony on setting goals. The patient must be involved in the goal-setting process. "Motivation and cooperation often increase when the patient has a thorough understanding of the treatment process and feels he has had an integral part in the planning. . . . Failure to include the patient in planning may result in ineffective or unnecessary intervention strategies." Speaking with the physician revising the treatment plan, and/or discharge (answers A, B, and D) may ultimately be necessary, but these actions should occur only after other corrective measures have failed. See reference: Ryan (ed): The therapeutic intervention process. *Practice Issues in Occupational Therapy.*

94. (A) 32 inches wide. The minimal width necessary for a standard-width wheelchair to pass through easily is 32 inches. See reference: Rothstein, Serge, and Wolf: Wheelchairs and standards for access.

95. (D) Recommend hospice OT. Occupational therapy in hospice care focuses on role performance, quality of life, locus of control, and adaptation. This type of intervention may bring quality and meaning to Alma's remaining days. It is unlikely that Alma, who is depressed about a terminal illness, will actually carry out a home program (answer A). Not all home health OT practitioners (answer B) have the expertise to work with terminally ill patients using a hospice approach. Discontinuing OT services altogether (answer C) would not facilitate continuation of Alma's role performance. See reference: Hopkins and Smith (eds): Pizzi, M: Environments of care: Hospice.

96. (B) To obtain a raised toilet seat. Rhoda will most likely continue to require a raised toilet seat for several months in order to avoid flexing her hip past 90 degrees. A hand-held shower (answer D) is not usually necessary and would be an expensive temporary measure; however, a shower chair with adjustable legs and grab bars could be helpful. High-contrast tape (answer C) may help to make ascending and descending stairs safer for individuals with limitations in vision. Moving items from low cabinets to higher locations may help Rhoda comply more readily with the necessary hip precautions, but moving objects from high cabinets to lower spots (answer A) would not. See reference: Pedretti (ed): Morawski, D, Pitbladdo, K, Bianchi, EM, Lieberman, SL, Novic, JP, and Bobrove, H: Hip fractures and total hip replacement.

97. (D) give him an opportunity to ask questions. A family member or significant other should attend at least one session "so that any questions can be answered. Appropriate supervision recommendations and instruction regarding activity precautions are given at this time." Rhoda is responsible for adhering to her own hip precautions (answer A), unless a cognitive or psychosocial deficit limits her ability to comply with these precautions. Rhoda's progress should be evident to her fiancé, so answer B is incorrect. Rhoda cannot be forced to perform ADLs independently, and if she and her fiancé prefer that he assist her with ADLs (answer C), it would be inappropriate for the COTA to force his or her opinions on the couple. See reference: Pedretti (ed): Morawski, D, Pitbladdo, K, Bianchi, EM, Lieberman, SL, Novic, JP, and Bobrove, H: Hip fractures and total hip replacement.

98. (D) A long-handled bath sponge. A person with a total hip arthroplasty must avoid hip flexion of 90 degrees or more, hip adduction with internal rotation at the knee or ankle, and lifting the knee higher than the hip during self-care or home-management activities. Velcro shoelace fasteners (answer A) are helpful for individuals with impaired fine-motor coordination; they do not remove the need to bend to reach the shoe, which is contraindicated for individuals with hip replacements. Elastic shoelaces, on the other hand, would eliminate the need for bending. A padded toilet seat 1 inch higher than normal or a short-handled sponge (answers B and C) would cause the person to flex the hip past 90 degrees during the performance of self-care activities. See reference: Trombly (ed): Bear-Lehman, J: Orthopedic conditions.

99. (A) aquatic therapy program led by an OTR in a warm-water pool (bathtub temperature). Heat can contribute to symptoms of fatigue in individuals with MS. Although a water-exercise program is an excellent way for individuals with MS to maintain or promote physical fitness, they should avoid environments in which they may become overheated. All other resources mentioned are appropriate. See reference: Ryan (ed): Jensen, D, and Linroth, R: The adult with multiple sclerosis. *Practice Issues in Occupational Therapy*.

100. (A) "Pt. reports overall pain levels are lower and ability to perform ADLs has improved." The subjective section of the discharge summary should indicate "whether the patient believes the goals set were achieved and whether the patient feels ready to function at home." Answers B and D are subjective reports but do not indicate the patient's perception of any changes in status. Answer C is an example of a statement that belongs in the assessment section of a discharge summary. See reference: Kettenbach: Writing subjective (S).

101. (D) Parachek Geriatric Rating Scale. The Parachek Geriatric Rating Scale is a 10-item screening instrument that can be completed in approximately 5 minutes by those familiar with the individual's daily behaviors. The protocol for this assessment contains suggested interventions appropriate for the score levels derived from this assessment. The BAFPE and COTE (answers A and B) are direct observations of an individual's performance. The Role Checklist (answer C) involves a self-assessment format. See reference: Early: Data gathering and evaluation.

102. (D) Activity Configuration. The Activity Configuration charts how an individual spends his or her time during a typical week. Tested individuals then categorize the activity (e.g. work, recreation, rest) and indicate whether the task was required or voluntary, how adequately they believe they performed it, and whether they did it because they wanted to or because someone else wanted them to. The ACL and LCL (answers A and B) assess levels of cognitive disability. The Leisure Activity Profile (answer C) is used to distinguish between alcoholic and nonalcoholic use of leisure time. See reference: Early: Data gathering and evaluation.

103. (C) long-term memory. The ability to recall events from one's distant past is long-term memory. It is usually assessed through verbal interviews and informal testing, such as a question eliciting the individual's recall of childhood events. Comprehension (answer A) can be determined by giving the individual a command to follow. Orientation (answer B) is determined by asking about the current time and date. Short-term memory (answer D) can be determined by asking about meals eaten that day. See reference: Early: Responding to symptoms and behaviors.

104. (A) completing chart reviews. An identified role of the COTA is to complete data collection such as a record review, general observation checklist, or behavior checklist. Answers B and C suggest that the COTA is independently collecting nonstandardized data and interpreting the data. COTAs are not educationally prepared to interpret the results of nonstandardized evaluation. A COTA can contribute to the development of a treatment plan, but it is not within the COTA's scope of practice to develop treatment plans independently. See reference: AOTA: Occupational therapy roles.

105. (B) Initiation. Inability to perform the first step of an activity without prompting indicates that the individual has initiation problems. A problem with impulsiveness (answer A) during self-care would be evidenced by the individual attempting to complete several steps of an activity rapidly, which would probably result in him cutting himself or doing a poor job of shaving. Memory or attention deficits (answers C and D) are demonstrated by the individual skipping steps of the activity, either because he does not remember the steps or is distracted by internal or external stimuli. Memory deficits could also be evidenced by the performance of task steps out of correct sequence. See reference: AOTA: Uniform terminology for occupational therapy.

106. (C) His complaints focus on physical concerns, he denies feeling depressed but feels less energetic, he has lost weight, and he complains of some concentration and memory problems. The general presentation of depression varies somewhat with an individual's age group. Answer A is more descriptive of adolescent depression, and answer B is descriptive of middle-adult depression. It is important for caregivers to be able to distinguish between depression and dementia when working with geriatric patients. Answer D is a description of complaints consistent with dementia. See reference: Hopkins and Smith (eds): Rogers, JC: Geriatric psychiatry.

107. (C) gain an accurate perspective of the patient's ability to function in daily activities. The patient may be unable to assess his or her own behavior or provide accurate information. Someone else may be a more reliable source. Answers A, B, and D are based on the evaluation process and are determined by the occupational therapy staff. See reference: Early: Data gathering and evaluation.

108. (C) interpret the results, focusing on the features and placement of the drawing. The OTR bases his or her interpretations on such features of the drawing as broken lines, erasures, or reinforced lines, which may indicate a problem in body concept or sensory processing. Neither the COTA nor the OTR is expected to offer a value judgment or analysis of the artistic skill of the patient (answers A and B). The COTA's role is to gather information and record observations (answer D). See reference: Early: Data gathering and evaluation.

109. (D) The history taken by the social worker. This includes details about the patient's family situation, occupational and educational background, cultural background, and expected environment. Referring to this document eliminates the need to duplicate this information. Interviews with the patient and his or her family by OT practitioners (answers B and C) are designed to obtain information concerning role and task performance and performance levels in work, self-care, and leisure. It would be a waste of time to review the entire medical record (answer A) just to obtain information about an individual's social status. See reference: Early: Data gathering and evaluation.

110. (B) "Pt. states that she does not feel comfortable in large groups." A subjective report is based on what the patient says, as well as what family members or significant others say. Answers A, C, and D reflect the thought of the OT practitioner, not the statements of the patient or family member. See reference: Ryan (ed): Backhaus, H: Documentation. *Practice Issues in Occupational Therapy.*

111. (A) project group. Project groups should focus on short-term tasks in which the group participants are expected to demonstrate some interaction and sharing. Groups in answers B, C, and D involve more interaction among the members and longer-term tasks and feature less involvement by the COTA. See reference: Ryan (ed): Blechert, TF, and Kari, N: Interpersonal communication skills and applied group dynamics. *The Certified Occupational Therapy Assistant.*

112. (C) cohesiveness is difficult to achieve. The development of cohesiveness is discouraged by the continual addition and subtraction of members in a group in acute settings. Answers A and B state advantages of a group format. Answer D states an advantage of individual treatment. See reference: Denton: Treatment planning and implementation.

113. (B) Clare will select and teach two peers a craft activity which she enjoys. The correct answer, B, is the only option that is measurable and builds upon Clare's strengths to address problem areas. Answer A is an appropriate goal direction, but it is difficult to measure Clare's progress. Answer C describes the COTA's methods. Answer D does not address the problem area of peer socialization. See reference: Hopkins and Smith (eds): Florey, LL: Psychiatric disorders in childhood and adolescence.

114. (C) pouring a glass of orange juice. Meal preparation is graded from cold to hot foods or beverages, and from simple to multiple steps. An individual beginning meal preparation training should start with a cold item involving the least number of steps possible, such as pouring a glass of juice or other cold beverage. Cold sandwich preparation (answer A) adds another step as each topping to the bread is added and as the use of utensils is introduced. After preparation of cold items has been mastered, training in hot food or beverage preparation (answers B and D) may be initiated. See reference: Kovich and Bermann (eds): Van Dam-Burke, A, and Kovich, K: Self-care and homemaking.

115. (C) Pt.'s pattern and strength of leisure interests are inadequate to support leisure resource exploration in his community. This statement is an assessment of the objective findings about the patient's responses to the interest checklist using the SOAP note format. Answer A is the subjective component of the progress note. Answer B is the objective findings, and answer D is the plan section of the note. See reference: Early: Medical records and documentation.

116. (D) Community Mental Health Center. CMHC is an abbreviation for Community Mental Health Center. Individuals are often recommended for hospitalization from outpatient care such as that provided by community mental health centers. See reference: Hopkins and Smith (eds): Richert, GZ: Program planning, development, and implementation.

117. (C) section C. Statements that identify the direction the patient will take and the criteria the patient must meet are goals. Section A contains demographics. Section B contains the problem. Section D contains a SOAP progress note. See reference: Early: Medical records and documentation.

118. (A) section A. The database of a problem-oriented medical record includes demographics such as age, marital status, and diagnosis. This section should also contain an overall statement of the patient's chief complaint. See reference: Early: Medical records and documentation.

119. (B) section B. In the POMR format, problems are numbered descriptions of the individual's problems. Progress should be linked to the problem list (see section D). See reference: Early: Medical records and documentation.

120. (B) aerobic exercise. Gross-motor activities, involving either aerobic exercise or stretching and relaxation, can help to reduce the physical symptoms associated with anxiety. Although line dancing (answer C) involves all of the elements of gross-motor activities, it requires the individual to follow specific steps and movements, which could cause the patient to become more anxious. Activities requiring fine motor coordination often require prolonged muscle contraction (answers A and D) and would not be appropriate for the stated purpose. See reference: Early: Responding to symptoms and behaviors.

121. (B) prepare separate materials for each person. It is important for the group leader to consider the functional level and needs of the group members. When working with lower-functioning groups, the COTA should prepare in advance the tools, supplies, sample projects, and any other materials required during the course of the group. It is necessary to prepare separate materials for each person and to set them up so that each person has his own work area, while sitting at the same table. See reference: Early: Group concepts and techniques

122. (C) Mania and borderline personality disorder. Stabilizing the crisis that precipitated hospitalization is a common goal of short-term psychiatric treatment. Consistent limit setting helps stabilize individuals with mania and borderline personality, whose impaired judgment and impulsive behaviors are common admitting problems. Limit setting concerning denial is more appropriate for alcoholism and anorexia (answer B). For depression and anxiety (answer A), limit setting concerning reassurance is usually appropriate. Delirium and dementia (answer D) usually involve setting limits for decreased confusion. See reference: Hopkins and Smith (eds): Richert, GZ: Program planning, development, and implementation.

123. (A) a sheltered workshop. Sheltered workshops are designed to help individuals master basic work skills. Answers C and D are similar in that they incorporate actual job sites for developing work skills. Answer A focuses on work-related and leisure activities. See reference: Hopkins and Smith (eds): Humphry, R, and Jewell, K: Developmental disabilities.

124. (A) to encourage the use of PABA-free sunblock and hats. Individuals taking neuroleptic medications are prone to photosensitivity and need protection from the sun. The precautions described in answer B are helpful to the individual experiencing postural hypotension, which can be a side effect of neuroleptic medication but is not an issue for a picnic outing. Answers C and D are not linked to the side effects of neuroleptic medications. See reference: Early: Psychotropic medications and somatic treatments.

125. (A) Give one- or two-step instructions and repeat frequently. The best method to use with an individual with Alzheimer's disease is to give short, one- or two-step instructions, keeping them to the point and repeating them frequently. Multistep instructions accompanied with demonstration (answer B) provides too much stimulation and can be confusing. Multistep written instructions (answer C) can be easily misplaced and are unlikely to be retained in the individual's short-term memory after reading. It is also unlikely that the individual will be able to remember the sequence correctly. Verbally repeating directions (answer D), or rehearsal, does not enable a person with Alzheimer's to retain information in her memory, and she may not repeat the instructions properly. See reference: Glickstein: Working with dementia clients.

126. (C) have her place the utensil down until her mouth is cleared. This individual needs to learn to pace herself during feeding. This skill may then be used after discharge from therapy. An individual with problems relating to the rate of intake will put too much food in her mouth in spite of the size of the pieces (answer A). An impulsive person who eats too fast will also have difficulty counting slowly (answer B) enough to have her mouth cleared by the time the count of ten is reached. Food in separate containers (answer D) would slow the meal down if items were presented one at a time but would not necessarily slow the rate of food intake. See reference: Kovich and Bermann (eds): Van Dam-Burke, A and Kovich, K: Self-care and homemaking.

127. (A) A stress management group. Psychoeducational groups focus on specific content areas such as stress management or assertiveness. The purpose of such groups is to educate individuals about specific content areas; such groups are appropriate for short-term treatment facilities. Directive group treatment (answer B) is a highly structured approach that is used in acute-care psychiatry for minimally functioning individuals. This approach is useful for individuals with psychoses and other neurological disorders who demonstrate disorganized and disturbed functioning. Task groups (answer D) involve working on simple tasks for the purpose of developing basic performance skills. Group therapy (answer C) focuses on verbal psychotherapy and sessions are conducted by other professionals from other disciplines. See reference: Early: Expressive and coping skills.

128. (B) pass around a scent box and ask each patient to smell the contents. Sensory integration theory holds that patients can learn by receiving, processing, and responding to sensory stimulation. Starting a group for regressed patients with sensory stimuli such as touch and smell helps to get the patients' attention and arouse their interest. Asking patients in this type of a group to introduce themselves (answer A) can be confusing and time consuming, especially when dealing with regressed individuals with limited attention spans. Reading favorite poems (answer C), and discussing lunch menus (answer D) are activities more suited to patients functioning on higher levels than the group described here. See reference: Early: Group concepts and techniques.

129. (C) preparing and consuming nutritional and normal-sized portions of food. Individuals with eating disorders are generally well versed in weight loss techniques (answer A), as well as making food look appealing for others to eat (answer D). They have extensive knowledge of the caloric content of foods (answer B) but little knowledge of other aspects of food content, such as vitamin and nutritive value. A cooking group would support the experience of preparing and consuming normal-sized portions of food. See reference: Early: Special populations.

130. (A) vestibular stimulation and gross-motor exercises. The sensory integration treatment approach, which aims to improve the reception and processing of sensory information within the central nervous system, uses vestibular stimulation and gross-motor exercise. This approach is best suited to chronic schizophrenics who have proprioceptive deficits. This college student would benefit most from discussion groups, role playing activities, and social-skills training (answers B, C, and D), all of which can be used to help him in relating appropriately and effectively with others. See reference: Early: Models for occupational therapy in mental health.

131. (D) Arrange for the patient to attend a discharge group to discuss her concerns. The COTA can structure a discharge-planning group to encourage patients to share similar concerns regarding post-hospitalization adjustment. The group can provide the support and encouragement of fellow patients as well as opportunities for brainstorming and problem solving issues related to return to community living. Answers A and B do not provide opportunities for the patient to gain the insight and perspective of other patients who may share similar concerns. Suggesting that the patient lie (answer C) is not ethical. See reference: Early: Expressive and coping skills.

132. (B) 4 (goal-directed actions). Individuals functioning at cognitive level 4 are able to copy demonstrated directions presented one step at a time. They find it easier to copy a sample than to follow directions or diagrams. Individuals functioning at cognitive level 3 are capable of using their hands for simple, repetitive tasks but are unlikely to produce a consistent end product. Those functioning at cognitive level 5 can experiment with or explore a variety of ways to use materials. Individuals functioning at cognitive level 6 can anticipate errors and plan ways to avoid them. See reference: Early: Models for occupational therapy in mental health.

133. (D) use a tool-storage area, painted with tool shadows or outlines, that can be locked. Painting a lockable tool cabinet with shadows or outlines to indicate where tools are to be kept is a very effective method that allows easy and accurate identification of missing items. This method also makes it easy to hold clients responsible for returning tools at the end of group sessions. Keeping track of keys (answer A) is an overall safety strategy that is not specific to tools Advance preparation (answer B) is a strategy to reduce the COTA's distractions during groups. Many clients treated for psychosocial problems would be excluded from OT treatment if they had to wait until all of their behavioral risks are being managed (answer C). Clients with severe suicidal or impulsive behaviors should rarely be involved with activities requiring tools that have potential to harm. See reference: Early: Safety techniques.

134. (A) postural hypotension. A frequent side effect of neuroleptic drugs is a drop in blood pressure in response to sudden movements, specifically up and down movements, resulting in faintness or blacking out. The parachute activity involves significant up-and-down body movements and therefore warrants the COTA's attention with this patient population. Answers B, C, and D are also potential side effects of antipsychotic medications but would usually not be problematic with parachute activities. See reference: Early: Psychotropic medications and somatic treatments.

135. (B) "This program will help you to learn about the skills you have that are needed on most jobs and about your potential for work." Prevocational evaluation programs are designed to assess work skills that the client possesses and to identify the client's potential for work. Vocational evaluation programs identify the actual interests and skills for specific types of work, such as assembly line work (answer A). Work-role maintenance programs are for individuals who are employed but whose involvement in treatment has temporarily interrupted their employment (answer C). Developing job-search skills (answer D) is for clients who have job skills but who have difficulty finding employment. See reference: Early: Treatment settings.

136. (C) "I think baking would be a helpful activity to try." Baking something you like offers you several choices and decisions. These choices and decisions can help you feel more positive about making other decisions. You can choose between a cake or cookie mix. Which would you like?" Answer C limits options to one of two acceptable choices and provides the rational for the choices. Answer A is a leading question that really offers only one "choice." Answer B does not provide a limit to the number of options. Answer D is a closed question, offering no real choice for the individual. See reference: Denton: Effective communication.

137. (B) "I can't even sand wood the right way." Individuals with depression usually feel helpless, hopeless, worthless, and/or guilty. Answer B is indicative of feelings of worthlessness and low self-esteem. Answer A reflects the individual's perception of his ability or competence. Answer C expresses interests or values that conflict with the proposed activity. Answer D is a response that could be given by a manic individual, reflecting grandiose ideation. See reference: Early: Responding to symptoms and behaviors.

138. (B) put the dried dishes away and begin to hand her wet dishes. Compensating for mistakes helps to increase the sense of self-worth and integrity of individual's with dementia. This approach is preferable to drawing attention to errors, especially in situations where safety is not an issue. Answers A, C, and D all draw attention to the individual's errors. See reference: Early: Responding to symptoms and behaviors.

139. (B) The COTA updates the OTR on the progress a patient has made in the last week and both provide information to update the goals. A collaborative relationship between an OTR and COTA supports sharing of information and the use of each professional's skills. In this type of relationship, communication is two-way, and both individuals work as a team to the benefit of the patient. Answers A and D demonstrate one-way communication, in which the OTR tells the COTA what to do. In answer C, the OTR takes information from the progress note but does not get input or recommendations from the COTA for the patient's discharge summary. See reference: AOTA: Occupational therapy roles.

140. (B) Ask Ruby to try some lacing on her own and praise her for what she has been able to do. All of the responses are increments of approaches used for decreasing dependency needs, but answer B is the best next step in this case because it allows the patient to attempt some lacing in the presence of the COTA, who in turn offers reassurance that the patient is actually able to do the activity. The step in answer B would be followed by the step in answer D. Here the patient is required to attempt some lacing without benefit of the COTA at her side; the COTA is nearby, but working with another patient. As the patient is able to do more of the activity independently, written instructions (answer A) replace the COTA as instructor. Finally, when the patient is feeling comfortable with self-instruction, asking her to work on the project out of the presence of the COTA (answer C) heightens the level of self-responsibility. See reference: Early: Analyzing, adapting, and grading activities.

141. (D) give her a new but similar project kit with written instructions and ask her to begin the project on her own, while the COTA assists another patient in the same room. Answer D combines the goal of decreasing dependency and the use of an adapted technique (i.e., following written instructions). The patient has the opportunity to attempt a new but similar project on her own, with the aid of written instructions and the security of the COTA nearby. Answer B also includes the use of written instructions, but it requires learning a new lacing technique, which may be too intimidating at this stage of treatment. Answer A does not offer the opportunity for self-instruction as a means of increasing independence and self-responsibility. The approach offered in answer C is best used when the patient has demonstrated a stronger sense of her ability to work without assistance. See reference: Early: Analyzing, adapting, and grading activities.

142. (A) Subjective. The Subjective portion of a SOAP note (answer A) includes what the patient reports or comments about the treatment. The Objective portion of the SOAP note (answer B) focuses on measurable and/or observable data obtained by the OT practitioner through specific evaluations, observations, or the use of therapeutic activities. The Assessment part of a SOAP note addresses the effectiveness of treatment and any changes needed, the status of the goals, and justification for continuing occupational therapy treatment. The Plan section of a SOAP note includes statements related to continuing treatment, the frequency and duration of the treatment, suggestions for additional activities or treatment techniques, the need for further evaluations, and recommendations for new goals as needed. See reference: Ryan (ed): Backhaus, H: Documentation. *Practice Issues in Occupational Therapy*.

143. (C) Assessment. The Assessment part of a SOAP note addresses the effectiveness of treatment and any changes needed, the status of the goals, and justification for continuing occupational therapy treatment. The Subjective portion of a SOAP note (answer A) includes what the patient reports or comments about the treatment. The Objective portion of the SOAP note (answer B) focuses on measurable and/or observable data obtained by the OT practitioner through specific evaluations, observations, or the use of therapeutic activities. The Plan section of a SOAP note includes statements related to continuing treatment, the frequency and duration of the treatment, suggestions for additional activities or treatment techniques, the need for further evaluations, and recommendations for new goals as needed. See reference: Ryan (ed): Backhaus, H: Documentation. *Practice Issues in Occupational Therapy*.

144. (A) paraphrasing. Paraphrasing is repeating what someone has said in your own words. Chitchat (answer B) is a conversational response unrelated to what was said. Confrontation (answer D) is a response that requires the individual to acknowledge difficult or painful issues. Proposing a solution (answer C) does not help the individual improve his or her decision-making skills or sense of competence. See reference: Denton: Effective communication.

145. (D) Regression. In regression the client shows a decreased sense of responsibility, increased dependency, and increased disregard for others. Regression is a risk for clients who remain in treatment settings longer than necessary. Countertransference (answer B) is the development of feelings that practitioner and client experience for and about each other that are interfere with the therapy. Continuity of care (answer A) is a term that describes a range of services differing along treatment structure and intensity. Post-traumatic stress disorder (answer C) is a psychiatric diagnosis, not a risk factor. See reference: Hopkins and Smith (eds): Richert, GZ, and Gibson, D: Practice settings.

146. (B) strategies Mr. B. can use to prevent Mrs. B. from wandering. Although wandering, incontinence, and failure to recognize family members are all issues, wandering is the only potentially dangerous one. Because Mrs. B.'s dementia is advanced, most of the discharge planning is directed toward Mr. B. Discussion with Mrs. B. will have no effect on her ability to manage her incontinence. At this point, environmental adaptation will be more effective than attempting to change Mrs. B.'s behavior. See reference: Early: Understanding psychiatric conditions.

147. (C) home health care. Home health care provides treatment services to individuals in their homes who have chronic or debilitating illnesses, in order to increase their functional independence. Although most individuals who receive home health services have primarily physical disabilities, secondary psychiatric disorders are quite common. Partial hospitalization (answer A) is a type of outpatient program that serves as a transition to community living. It offers most of the structure and services available on an inpatient unit while allowing individuals to live in the community and to receive services by visiting the program. Adult day care (answer B) provides psychosocial programs for the elderly that focuses on avocational skills and social activities. Psychosocial rehabilitation centers (answer D) focus on the social rather than the medical aspects of mental illness. The psychosocial club or rehabilitation center provides socialization programs, daily living skills counseling, prevocational rehabilitation, and transitional employment. See reference: Early: Treatment settings.

148. (D) recovery. Tangential (topic jumping) speech, elated mood, and some hyperactivity are seen in the first stages of manic depressive illness. People in recovery are moving back through the stages of a disease progression to the first stages of the disease. Regression and decompensation (answers A and C) both are processes of decline. Progression (answer B) is a general term of improvement but is not specific enough to describe Mr. Chang's changes. See reference: Bonder: Mood disorders.

149. (C) A discharge-planning group. Discharge-planning group is recommended, because the client's progress toward recovery has been fairly steady and quick. Addressing recurrence prevention is particularly important for individuals with a bipolar disorder. Although assertiveness group (answer A) could be generally helpful, there is no information that indicates Mr. Chang is having difficulty with passive or aggressive communication styles. Exercise group (answer D) is not considered to be a thematic group. See reference: Bonder: Mood disorders.

150. (D) "I'm concerned about John's ability to live on his own unless he is better able to structure his leisure time. Before admission he was rarely in contact with others. Then his voices got worse." Occupational therapy emphasizes functional information. Answer D is an example of functional information about self-management within the area of leisure performance. Answer A reflect concerns of various team members. Answer B is consistent with aftercare referral concerns of social work. Answer C reflects medication concerns of the physician or nurse. See reference: Hopkins and Smith (eds): Gibson, D and Richert GZ: The therapeutic process.

151. (B) Standards of Practice. These standards are a guide to the provision and management of occupational therapy services. The Uniform Terminology for Reporting Occupational Therapy Services (answer A) defines areas of practice and descriptors of services. This document assists in providing consistent documentation in occupational therapy throughout all areas of practice. Licensure regulations (answer C) vary from state to state and are not always consistent with the guidelines for practice. AOTA Policies and Procedures (answer D) guide the activities of the association but do not refer to the provision of services. See reference: AOTA: Uniform Terminology.

152. (D) must benefit the child's ability to participate in special education. Answer D is correct, because the present law (IDEA) requires that any service that can improve a child's educational performance must be provided to children who are receiving special education or "specialized instruction." Answer A is incorrect, because occupational therapy is not a primary service but a "related service," related to special education services. Answer C is incorrect, because physical therapy is also a related service and follows the same guidelines as occupational therapy in that the child must have been receiving special education, and educational performance will probably be improved if physical therapy services are provided. See reference: Case-Smith, Allen, and Pratt (eds): Johnson, J: School-based occupational therapy.

153. (B) a therapeutic device in helping. The occupational therapy practitioner's use of "self" is a tool in the therapy process but not the central focus (answer A) of the therapy. The therapeutic use of self shares a few characteristics of friendship (answer C), but it also requires the therapist to understand and manage some of his or her reactions. Empathy, not sympathy (answer D), is recommended in therapeutic relationships. See reference: Hopkins and Smith (eds): Schwartzberg, SL: Tools of practice: Therapeutic use of self.

154. (B) once service competency has been established. Service competency assures interrater reliability between the OTR and COTA. This concept ensures that professionals working together in a collaborative relationship for patient treatment will obtain the same or equivalent results. Techniques for assuring service competency vary between facilities. Answers A, C, and D are inappropriate, because they do not address the skill level required to administer a standardized test. See reference: Early: Data gathering and evaluation.

155. (B) expanding. The number of older persons in the United States is expected to increase, because individuals are living longer. In addition, "baby boomers" will be reaching middle and older ages in the next two decades. Therefore, opportunities in gerontic OT are expanding and answers A, C, and D are incorrect. See reference: Punwar: Current trends and future outlook.

156. (A) a reprimand. A reprimand is a formal written expression of disapproval of an OT practitioner's conduct; once issued, it is retained in the NBCOT's file. This information is also communicated privately with the individual. A censure (answer B) is a formal, public written expression of disapproval. Probation (answer C) is the period of time a therapist is given to retain the counseling or education required to remain certified. Answer D is permanent loss of NBCOT certification. See reference: Hopkins and Smith (eds): Hansen, RA: Ethics in occupational therapy.

157. (A) COTA. It is fraudulent to bill any other services as occupational therapy services. Billings are limited to charges for services rendered by the OTR and/or COTA for evaluation and treatment of functional deficits. See reference: AOTA: Occupational Therapy Code of Ethics.

158. (B) at or above the minimal entry level of competence. The Guide to Fieldwork Education recommends that entry-level COTAs practice in settings in which they are supervised by an experienced COTA or OTR. Entry-level therapists are more likely to receive coaching and mentoring in development of clinical skills when working in settings that provide the opportunity to be supervised by an experienced OT practitioner. See reference: AOTA: Guide to fieldwork education.

159. (C) notify the state licensure board. Licensure is a regulatory procedure established by legislation and designed to protect the consumer. Any occurrence of unprofessional conduct involving a consumer should be reported to the licensure board. Answers A and B are incorrect, because AOTA and state occupational therapy associations do not have regulatory jurisdiction over therapists. Answer D, discussing the situation with the therapist involved, is appropriate, but does not discharge the responsibility of the COTA to protect the consumer. See reference: Hopkins and Smith (eds): Hopkins, HL: Scope of occupational therapy.

160. (C) inform the administrator they are unable to provide services to individuals who can no longer benefit from OT. Answers A, B, and D involve falsifying documentation, financial exploitation of insurance carriers, and inaccurate recording of professional activities, and are violations of the OT Code of Ethics. It is unethical to bill for services not rendered or to provide services to individuals who can no longer benefit. In this case, the individual reached his full potential for independence in self-care and no longer requires OT services. See reference: AOTA: Occupational therapy code of ethics.

161. (A) CVA. Individuals diagnosed with a CVA represent 44 percent of the populations that COTAs treat. Individuals with fractures account for 11.6 percent, those diagnosed with developmental delay 8.6 percent, and those with cerebral palsy 3.1 percent. See reference: AOTA: 1996 Member data survey.

162. (D) notify the occupational therapist of the patient's change in status. It is the responsibility of the COTA to communicate to the primary therapist any changes in the patient's status. At that time, the COTA and OTR would collaborate on the appropriate intervention, which may include answers A, B, or C. See reference: AOTA: Occupational therapy roles.

163. (D) By consistently obtaining the same results as another OT practitioner who has demonstrated service competency. In order to establish service competency, it is necessary for the COTA to obtain the same results as a competent OT practitioner when performing a treatment technique or evaluative procedure. Demonstrating service competency often requires more than one trial in order to refine techniques to obtain the same results. Answers A, B, and C do not provide the opportunity for the OT practitioners to compare and contrast their techniques and measurements in order to obtain similar results. See reference: Ryan (ed): Ryan, SE: COTA supervision. *Practice Issues in Occupational Therapy.*

164. (A) activities of daily living (ADLs). Activities of daily living include grooming, oral hygiene, bathing, toilet hygiene, dressing, eating and feeding, medication routine, socialization, functional communication, functional mobility; and sexual expression. COTAs receive an emphasis on these areas in their training programs and are therefore able to initiate referrals for individuals with deficits in these areas. COTAs do not receive the necessary in-depth training related to answers B, C, and D. Referrals for work, cognitive retraining, and sensory integration skills are most likely to come from employers, social workers, teachers, OTRs, and psychologists. See reference: Ryan (ed): Ryan, SE: Therapeutic intervention process. *Practice Issues in Occupational Therapy.*

165. (A) public school systems. As of 1996, 14 percent of all practicing COTAs were employed primarily in the school system. Those working in residential care facilities account for 3.8 percent of practicing COTAs. Even smaller percentages account for those employed in day care and community health centers (0.8 percent in each). See reference: AOTA: 1996 Member data survey.

166. (D) she or he has demonstrated service competency. "Physical agent modalities may be used by occupational therapy practitioners when used as an adjunct to or in preparation for purposeful activity by a practitioner who has demonstrated service competency." Service competency in this area includes but is not limited to possessing the theoretical background and technical skills (answer A) for the safe and effective use of the modality. Although study and practice (answer B) are necessary to establish service competency, an OTR must determine that the COTA is competent before he or she can use PAMs. Having an OTR on-site (answer C) is not adequate if service competency has not been established. See reference: AOTA: Policy: Registered occupational therapists and certified occupational therapy assistants and modalities.

167. (C) to use the handout only as a resource while developing the presentation. The OT Code of Ethics states that "Occupational therapy personnel shall accurately represent the qualifications, views, contributions, and findings of colleagues." The options presented in answers A and B do not give the necessary credit to the author for his or her contribution. It is not necessary to discard the article altogether (answer D). See reference: AOTA: Occupational Therapy Code of Ethics.

168. (B) analyze how he is using his time and implement time-management strategies. It is usually possible to use time more efficiently. By analyzing how you spend your time, you may be able to eliminate or modify tasks that are unnecessary or too time consuming. Continuing to stay late (answer A) will probably result in burnout. Finding a less demanding job may ultimately be necessary (answer C), but an individual who does not manage time efficiently will probably have time-management problems in any setting and should attempt to deal with the problem rather than avoid it. Answer D would result in falling behind with documentation and treatment planning and is not an acceptable option. See reference: Early: Organizing yourself.

169. (A) "COTAs are not qualified to participate in research." COTAs may develop entry-level, intermediate-level, or high-proficiency skills in research if they choose to do so, although it is not required. Data collection (answer C) is considered an entry-level skill, and developing the research question and publishing or presenting the results (answers B and D) are considered intermediate-level skills. See reference: AOTA: Occupational therapy roles.

170. (C) NBCOT. The NBCOT grants certification to OT practitioners upon successful completion of the certification exam. Only NBCOT can revoke or suspend certification. An individual may not practice or call himself or herself an OTR or COTA if certification has been suspended or revoked, regardless of location. A state regulatory board (answer B) has jurisdiction only over individuals practicing in that particular state. The AOTA (answer A) has jurisdiction only over its members and can discipline only members. Although it may be important to report the individual to the administration of the facility (answer D), the facility cannot limit the individual's right to practice outside of the specific facility. See reference: Ryan (ed): Gray, M: The credentialing process in occupation therapy. *Practice Issues in Occupational Therapy.*

171. (C) Decline the gift and explain that a COTA cannot accept gifts from patients. Accepting gifts from patients is unprofessional conduct. Fees are established based on a cost analysis of the overhead, supplies, and time required to provide a service. Therefore, answers A, B, and D are incorrect. See reference: Hopkins and Smith (eds): Hansen, RA: Ethics in occupational therapy.

172. (D) may perform variable portions of the assessment process. How much a COTA contributes to the assessment process is determined by the policies of each facility and the level of competence of each COTA. The SOPs are "intended as guidelines" and "serve as a minimum standard for occupational therapy practice." The SOP does not state that a COTA should or must contribute (answers A and B), and it does not limit the degree to which a COTA can contribute to the assessment process (answer C). See reference: AOTA: Standards of practice for occupational therapy.

173. (C) It is his professional responsibility to train fieldwork students. Without the support of practicing OTRs and COTAs, it would be impossible to educate future practitioners. Training fieldwork students is not only a matter of professional responsibility; it is very rewarding and contributes to the professional development of the clinical educator as well. In order to expand the pool of clinical educators and open up valuable opportunities to OT and OTA students, AOTA supports a variety of types of clinical educators (answer A). "Level I fieldwork [students] shall be supervised by qualified personnel including but not limited to [OTRs, COTAs], teachers, social workers, nurses and physical therapists." OTRs and COTAs must have a minimum of 1 year's experience in a practice setting to accept Level II fieldwork students, but there is no such minimum requirement for training Level I students (answer B). Because of the mobility of OTRs and COTAs, OT educational programs do not usually accredit sites (answer D). See reference: AOTA: Essentials and guidelines for an accredited educational program for the occupational therapy assistant.

174. (C) 1959. The first OTA program was approved in 1959, and in the same year 336 occupational therapy aides who had received on-the-job training were grandfathered in as COTAs. The founding of the National Society for the Promotion of Occupational Therapy in 1917 is considered the beginning of occupational therapy. The shortage of occupational therapists at the end of World War II was the impetus for the intensive training of OTAs (answer B). In 1983, COTAs won the right to have a member-at-large in AOTA's Representative Assembly. See reference: Hopkins and Smith (eds): Ryan, SE: Scope of occupational therapy. *The Certified Occupational Therapy Assistant.*

175. (D) state law, the Occupational Therapy Code of Ethics, and Standards of Practice for Occupational Therapy. If required by state law, the COTA must post his license or risk being in violation of the law. If uncertain, he should contact his state regulatory board. The Occupational Therapy Code of Ethics states that "Occupational therapy personnel shall understand and abide by . . . local, state and federal laws" . . . . The Standards of Practice for Occupational Therapy states that occupational therapy practitioners "shall practice . . . in accordance with applicable federal and state laws and regulations." See reference: AOTA: Occupational therapy code of ethics. Also AOTA: Standards of practice.

176. (B) respect the child's right to refuse treatment. It is the COTA, not the child, who does not want to engage in the sensory-integration activities, and therefore the child's right to refuse treatment is not at issue. If an OT practitioner attempted to provide sensory-integration-based treatment without being competent in these specialized techniques, harm to the child (answer A) could result. It would be appropriate for a COTA with demonstrated service competency in sensory integrative techniques to provide treatment to this child, but it would be an ethical violation for this COTA to do so (answer B). Consulting with or referring to another more qualified OT practitioner (answer D) is appropriate and necessary when the OT practitioner does not posses the required skills or expertise. See reference: AOTA: Occupational therapy code of ethics.

177. (A) Medicare. Medicare was established in 1965 by Title XVIII of the Social Security Act. The program consists of two parts. Medicare part A pays for inpatient hospitalization, skilled care, and hospice services. Medicare part B covers outpatient services along with physician and other professional medical services. Medicaid (answer B) provides health care for the poor and medically indigent. Third-party payers (answer C) are the largest source of payment for health care in the United States. These providers, which may be for-profit or nonprofit organizations, adhere to state insurance codes that require set levels of coverage. Private pay (answer D) is the term for situations in which the patient is responsible for the payment for services rendered. See reference: Bair and Gray (eds): Scott, S, and Somers, FP: Payment for occupational therapy services.

178. (C) frequent handwashing. Hands should be washed at specified times during the day, including before and after patient treatment, before and after removing gloves, and before eating or preparing food, to name a few. Specific handwashing procedures have been developed and should be followed. Gloves (answer A), masks, and gowns (answers B and D) are examples of protective barriers to be worn when encountering bodily fluids, but handwashing is the primary and most effective method used. See reference: Early: Safety techniques.

179. (D) intermediate-level COTA with routine supervision. The amount, type, and pattern of supervision depend on the practice setting, practitioner's competence, and type of people being served. An intermediate-level COTA will have mastered basic role functions and have the ability to supervise others. However, the COTA at this level has not yet achieved sufficient refinement of special skills to be considered an advanced-level COTA. See reference: AOTA: Occupational therapy roles.

180. (C) collaborative. The supervision of a COTA is intended to be collaborative. This term takes into account the sharing of information and use of each individual's skills in the process of working with patients. Answer A places the COTA in a role of being unable to provide information or have input into the treatment of the patient. Answer B is not appropriate because the COTA should not work independently without the supervision of an OTR. Answer D is incorrect because open communication between the COTA and OTR is vital for a team approach. See reference: AOTA: Occupational therapy roles.

181. (B) Reviewing charts to elicit relevant information. The five steps involved in a quality-assurance plan are: (1) identifying the indicators of quality care; (2) collecting measurable data, often by chart review; (3) determining the cause of a problem; (4) implementing remedial action; and (5) performing the measurement process again to see if the problem has been solved. The most appropriate steps for the COTA to perform are chart review (answer B) and implementing remedial action as appropriate. OTRs and COTAs in an OT department often work together to determine the design and analysis of the quality improvement plan (answers A and C). The department head is usually responsible for writing a report (answer D). See reference: Hopkins and Smith (eds): Perinchief, JM: Service management.

182. (C) IEP. The individual education plan is a form that must be completed for children receiving services in the school system. This documentation standard was defined in the Education of the Handicapped Act (1975 and 1986). The UB-82 form (answer A), is used to process insurance claims. FIM (answer B), which stands for "functional independence measure" is a method used on rehabilitation units to measure an individual's level of independence. The HCFA-1500 form (answer D) is used to bill Medicare and other insurance carriers for health care services. See reference: Hopkins and Smith (eds): Perinchief, JM: Service management.

183. (D) label each item with the individuals' names. Cosmetics should never be shared. Federal regulations prohibit the sharing of cosmetics if there is any likelihood of them coming in contact with bodily fluids. This likelihood would be high in a geropsychiatric population. See reference: Early: Safety techniques.

184. (C) Both the COTA and OTR could be held accountable. If guilt or incompetence on the part of the COTA is actually established, both could ultimately be held responsible. According to the AOTA document Supervision Guidelines for Certified Occupational Therapy Assistants, the "supervising OTR is legally responsible for the outcomes of all occupational therapy services provided by the COTA." See reference: Supervision guidelines for certified occupational therapy assistants.

185. (C) Notify the supervising OTR. Upon receiving a verbal or written referral, the COTA should notify the supervising OTR. Only then can the referral be accepted (answer B) and evaluation and treatment be initiated. Chart review (answer A) and identification of safety issues (answer D) should both occur very early in the process. Once the case has been accepted, the OTR will determine the role of the COTA in the client's evaluation and treatment. See reference: Early: Overview of the treatment process.

186. (A) referral. Medicare does not view occupational therapy as a primary service; therefore, OT can only enter a case once a primary service, such as nursing, PT, or speech has qualified the patient for home health services and made a referral for occupational therapy services. Reports from the patient's physical therapist and nurse (answers B and C) would provide useful information but are not required before beginning treatment. The initial evaluation (answer D) follows receipt of the referral. See reference: Hopkins and Smith (eds): Levine, RE, Corcoran, MA, and Gitlin, L: Home care and private practice.

187. (B) teaching macramé to a patient. Although the aide may know macramé well enough to teach it to others, she or he does not have the skill or judgment to use it with an individual for therapeutic purposes. An OT practitioner teaching macramé to a patient assesses, reassesses, and modifies as necessary throughout the process. This requires ongoing skill and judgment. An OT aide may "perform delegated, selected. skilled tasks in specific situations under the intense close supervision of an OT practitioner." Individual state laws, which would supersede the AOTA position paper, may further restrict the use of aides. Answers A, C, and D do not require the skill and judgment of an OT practitioner. See reference: AOTA: Position paper: Use of occupational therapy aides in occupational therapy practice.

188. (B) treat the area as if an infectious spill had occurred. Even though urine is not listed as an infectious fluid, the darkness of the urine may be indicative of the presence of blood. Therefore, the area should be treated as if an infectious spill occurred. The first actions to be taken when a spill occurs are to contain the area, clean up the spill, and disinfect the area of the spill. Answers A and D do not recognize the fact that an infectious spill may have occurred. Answers C and D are incorrect because they risk the safety and welfare of the patient. See reference: Occupational Safety and Health Administration.

189. (A) At entry level. COTAs may collect factual information for screening patient referrals under the supervision of an OTR. This information is often collected through chart reviews or discussions with other medical professionals and the patient or family members. The OT Roles document indicates performance of this task is appropriate at the entry level. See reference: AOTA: Occupational therapy roles.

190. (A) The section of the note that contains subjective information. Both statements in statement A reflect information that may be obtained from the patient chart or interviews with the patient, family, or other personnel. These statements are viewed as subjective in that they cannot be measured. Objective patient data (answer B) includes the standardized measurements that a COTA would contribute to the discharge evaluation. Assessment (answer C) usually includes an analysis of the objective findings. The plan and recommendations section (answer D) reviews the patient's discharge disposition and recommends follow-up services. See reference: Hopkins and Smith (eds): Perinchief, JM: Service management.

191. (B) The objective portion. Objective data include measurable data such as that included in statement F. The subjective section contains statements made by the patient, the family, or the patient's significant other. The assessment section includes judgments based on the patient's performance. The plan would include recommendations for discharge planning. See reference: Hopkins and Smith (eds): Perinchief, JM: Service management.

192. (B) Statements C, E and G. These statements represent a specific plan of action to be followed while discharging the patient. One statement indicates the setting to which the patient is to be discharged. The second statement lists equipment needs upon discharge. The final statement indicates further services that will be needed by the patient. Answers A, B, and D include statements that would be included in the subjective, objective, or assessment areas of the SOAP note. See reference: Hopkins and Smith (eds): Perinchief, JM: Service management.

193. (D) Statement G. Answers A, B, and C are statements regarding Janie M.'s discharge. Only statement G includes a recommendation for continued OT services. See reference: Hopkins and Smith (eds): Perinchief, JM: Service management.

194. (D) statement D. This is the only statement that includes objective measurements. Statements A, B, and C include subjective statements by the patient or her family. Statement C belongs in the Plan section of the note. See reference: Hopkins and Smith (eds): Perinchief, JM: Service management.

195. (C) supervision of noncertified personnel. Under the supervision of a registered occupational therapist, COTAs often participate in orienting, training, and evaluating the performance of unlicensed or noncertified personnel. Quality-assurance programs (answer A) should be established by team members and not independently. COTAs may supervise other COTAs (under the supervision of an OTR), but supervision of OTRs must be carried out by OTRs (answer B). Management responsibilities (answer D) are also within the scope of practice of the OTR. See reference: AOTA: Occupational therapy code of ethics.

196. (A) The OT department will provide inservices on relevant information on a regular basis. A policy provides information about actions that need to be taken. The steps involved in enacting a policy are the procedure. Procedures state how a policy is carried out, in what sequence, and by whom. Answers B, C, and D are all examples of procedure. See reference: Hopkins and Smith (eds): Perinchief, JM: Service management.

197. (B) Tip the wheelchair backward and guide it down the ramp forwards. This is the recommended technique for going down a steep ramp. The individual sitting in the wheelchair can also help to control the wheels, if capable of doing so, by grasping the hand rims. It would be difficult for the person guiding a wheelchair backwards down a ramp (answer A) to see where he or she is going. Only very strong individuals can propel themselves independently down a steep ramp (answer C). Using two people to move a wheelchair down a steep ramp could be awkward and dangerous (answer D). See reference: Pedretti (ed): Adler, C, and Tipton-Burton, M: Wheelchair assessment and transfers.

198. (A) incident report. Facilities use incident reports to document accidents such as this. Although the incident may be referred to in a daily progress note (answer B), an incident report must also be filed. An incident report form includes a level of detail that may not be achieved in a letter (answer C), and a verbal report (answer D) is not a form of documentation. See reference: Ryan (ed): Jones, RA: Service operations. *Practice Issues in Occupational Therapy*.

199. (B) hot-water pans for splinting, hot-air guns, and power tools. Many facilities require electrical checks to be performed on all electrically powered equipment on an annual or semiannual basis. The rehabilitation department often performs maintenance on its own wheelchairs, even though the maintenance department handles wheelchairs belonging to the rest of the facility (answer A). The OT department is usually responsible for its adaptive equipment inventory (answer C) and for determining the status and location of flammable liquids (answer D). See reference: Ryan (ed): Jones, RA: Service operations. *Practice Issues in Occupational Therapy*.

200. (A) close. Close supervision is direct daily contact between the supervisor and the employee. This form of supervision is recommended for entry-level COTAs or COTAs entering a new practice setting. Routine supervision (answer B) is appropriate for intermediate-level COTAs. General supervision (answer C) is appropriate for advanced-level COTAs. Minimal supervision (answer D) is appropriate only for OTRs. See reference: AOTA: Occupational therapy roles.

SIMULATION EXAMINATION 5

Directions: Circle the correct answer to the following questions. When you have completed this examination, check your answers against the answer key that follows. As you will see, an explanation is given for each answer along with a reference for further study; the book author is listed as well as the chapter author. See the bibliography for complete references.

1. To help determine a third grader's readiness for discharge from direct OT as a related service, what criteria should the COTA focus on?

A. Whether the disability interferes with the child's education.
B. The degree of functional skills.
C. Independence in ADLs.
D. Accessibility of the learning environment.

2. Kathleen is about to be discharged from occupational therapy following rehabilitation for a hand injury. She has not been able to work for 3 months, and remains unable to perform her job as a sales manager in a clothing store. What should the OTR/COTA team recommend concerning occupational therapy services?

A. Kathleen should continue to perform her home program.
B. Home health OT.
C. A work hardening program.
D. Discontinuation of OT services.

3. During a routine transfer, Mr. M.'s legs buckle, causing him and the COTA to fall to the floor. The most appropriate way for the COTA to document this incident is in a(n):

A. incident report.
B. daily progress note.
C. letter to the department head.
D. verbal report to the department head.

4. Direct OT services are being discontinued for a student with attention deficit disorder, but consultation will be provided to help her adjust to the new classroom. Which of the following recommendations can the COTA make to help the teacher adapt the environment to promote optimal learning conditions without affecting the girl's classmates?

A. Use dim lighting and reduce glare by turning down lights.
B. Remove all posters and visual aids to reduce visual distractions.
C. Provide a screen to reduce peripheral visual stimuli.
D. Restructure classroom activities into a series of short-term tasks.

5. An OTR/COTA team needs to report discharge information and document the information in the patient's chart. At what level does the COTA participate in making discharge recommendations?

A. An entry-level COTA may perform the task independently.
B. An intermediate-level COTA may perform the task independently.
C. A COTA contributes to the process but does not complete the task independently.
D. A COTA cannot perform the task.

6. The COTA is working on sequencing skills with a young woman who is s/p TBI. The activity that would BEST address this goal is:

A. leather stamping using tools in a random design.
B. stringing beads for a necklace, following a pattern.
C. putting together a 20-piece puzzle.
D. playing "Concentration," a card-matching game.

7. The BEST way to adapt a chair in order to inhibit extensor tone and make sitting possible is to use a:

A. lateral trunk support.
B. seatbelt at the hips and ankle straps.
C. wedge-shaped seat insert that is higher in front.
D. lap board fastened to the arm rests of the chair.

8. A COTA providing home-based care to an individual with AIDS learns from his care giver that he has become too weak to turn himself in bed. What is the MOST important modification to the treatment plan for the COTA to recommend?

A. To begin a strengthening program.

due on alternating Thursday afternoons. Knowing she will see the client the next day (11/15/96), and reluctant to wait another 2 weeks to submit for payment, she bills for treatment using the 11/14/96 date. This COTA's action is:

A. acceptable, because treatment has been scheduled for the next day.
B. acceptable if the agency she works for allows it.
C. unacceptable, because it violates the Code of Ethics.
D. unacceptable, because if the patient is still ill and unable to participate in therapy on 11/15/96, a delay of more than 1 day is unacceptable for billing purposes.

30. A COTA has just begun working in an early intervention program after working on an adult rehab unit for 5 years. The level of supervision this COTA should receive is:

A. close.
B. routine.
C. general.
D. minimal.

31. The COTA may do an informal assessment of visual form perception in an 8-year-old child by having him or her:

A. play a game of marbles.
B. match picture dominoes.
C. play a matching-by-memory game such as "Memory."
D. assemble a 16-piece puzzle.

32. A COTA practicing in a school-based setting is interested in training students in Level II fieldwork. Before accepting Level II students, the COTA should have at least:

A. 6 months experience.
B. 1 year experience.
C. 2 years experience.
D. 3 years experience.

33. The COTA is working with developmentally disabled clients in a sheltered workshop. She realizes that a worker is having difficulty learning the assembly sequence for a knife-fork-spoon package. The COTA decides to use backward chaining. In this case, backward chaining involves:

A. encouraging the individual to reverse the packaging sequence.
B. asking the client only to put the last piece into the package.
C. praising the client for close approximations (such as including a knife, fork, and two spoons).
D. demonstration and repetition by the COTA of the correct sequence before each of the worker's attempts.

34. Ken is a 57-year-old man experiencing progressive weakness. A long-term goal is for the family to carry out his feeding program. They have achieved the short-term goal of understanding how Ken's disability affects his ability to feed himself. Which statement is the BEST example of a revised short-term goal?

A. "Pt. will participate in feeding program."
B. "Pt. will feed himself with moderate assistance."
C. "Family will feed pt. safely and independently 100 percent of the time."
D. "Family will demonstrate independence in positioning pt. correctly for feeding so that he can swallow safely."

35. A basic request for occupational therapy services that may come from a nurse, social worker, or teacher is referred to as a(n):

A. recommendation
B. plan of treatment
C. intervention strategy
D. referral

36. A COTA works with a 16-year old boy with C5 quadriplegia at lunchtime each day to develop independence in feeding. Which type of equipment would be MOST appropriate for this individual?

A. A wrist-driven flexor hinge splint.
B. A mobile arm support.
C. An electric self-feeder.
D. Utensils with built-up handles.

37. The primary role of the COTA when treating an individual who has recently been diagnosed with rheumatoid arthritis (RA) is to:

A. increase strength with resistive exercises.
B. provide positioning and/or adaptive equipment.
C. provide emotional support.
D. prepare the patient for surgical intervention.

38. Which of the following devices would help a person who uses a mouth stick to work on a computer by keeping the mouth stick from striking other keys accidentally?

A. A moisture guard.
B. A key guard.
C. An auto-repeat defeat.
D. One-finger-access software.

39. When reporting data collected to the OTR, it is important for the COTA to:

A. observe everything the patient said and did during the interview and provide extensive notes for the OTR to read.
B. provide the OTR with a comprehensive treatment plan based on the results of the evaluation.
C. provide a summary of observations of the patient's behavior, including what the patient said and did during the interview.
D. provide an interpretation of how the patient behaved during the interview.

40. A patient gives the COTA $50.00 as a token of his appreciation after 3 weeks of intensive rehabilitation. Which of the following responses is MOST consistent with the Occupational Therapy Code of Ethics?
A. Accept the gift and use it to buy a new radio.
B. Decline the gift but accept it if the patient is insistent.
C. Decline the gift and explain that a COTA cannot accept gifts from patients.
D. Accept the gift and use it to buy a textbook for the department.

41. A COTA is working on keyboarding activities with a man with asymmetrical muscle tone who keeps falling to the side while sitting in his wheelchair. The wheelchair adaptation that would BEST stabilize his upper body in a midline position would be a(n):
A. reclining wheelchair.
B. arm trough.
C. lateral trunk support.
D. lateral pelvic support.

42. The COTA is performing passive range-of-motion exercises with a patient with quadriplegia. In order to encourage the development of tenodesis, the COTA must be sure to position the patient's wrist in:
A. neutral position during finger flexion and extension.
B. flexion during finger flexion and extension.
C. extension during finger flexion and flexion during finger extension.
D. flexion during finger flexion and extension during finger extension.

43. A COTA on a rehabilitation unit is working on LE dressing with a 23-year-old man with a spinal cord injury. As the client tries to put on his underwear, he notices an erection and asks the COTA how it is possible for him to have an erection and if he will be able to have sex. The COTA is slightly embarrassed and uncomfortable with the question. The BEST action for the COTA to take is to:
A. tell him she will find out the answers to his questions and get back to him with an answer by the next morning.
B. answer his questions to the best of her ability and quickly return to the LE dressing program.
C. refer him to his physiatrist.
D. refer him to her OTR supervisor, who has attended a workshop on sexuality and spinal cord injury.

44. A person with a spinal-cord injury at the C8 level will be able to perform self-feeding independently using:
A. a mobile arm support.
B. a universal cuff.
C. built-up utensils.
D. no adaptive equipment.

45. OT practitioners should wear gloves when working with:
A. individuals with open wounds who have been diagnosed with HIV.
B. individuals with third-degree burns.
C. individuals with open wounds who have been diagnosed with hepatitis.
D. all individuals with open wounds.

Questions 46–48 pertains to this case study:

Mrs. B is a 79-year-old woman with RA. The COTA is contributing to the initial evaluation by performing a functional assessment of her upper extremities.

46. The COTA observes that Mrs. B has limited internal rotation when she is unable to touch:
A. the back of her neck.
B. the top of her head.
C. her lower back.
D. her opposite shoulder.

47. Mrs. B also demonstrates functional limitations in shoulder abduction and external rotation. She is MOST likely to have difficulty with:
A. buttoning her shirt.
B. combing her hair.
C. tucking in her shirt in the back.
D. tying shoelaces.

48. The COTA notes AROM is limited to slightly less than 90 degrees of shoulder flexion. While in this position, Mrs. B is able to tolerate moderate resistance. The COTA observes PROM to be the same as AROM. The patient's manual muscle test score would be:
A. normal (5).
B. good (4).
C. fair (3).
D. fair minus (3-).

49. The COTA observes a 4-year-old with autism waving his hand in front of his eyes repeatedly in an apparent purposeless manner. The most relevant observation to be reported to the supervising therapist is:
A. the ability of eyes to focus at close range.
B. the degree of wrist mobility.
C. the hand preference.
D. the presence of self-stimulatory behavior.

50. An entry-level COTA is completing designated areas of the discharge report. The section that the COTA would MOST likely leave to be completed by the OTR is the:
A. discharge recommendations.
B. patient's current level of independence in activities of daily living.
C. patient's most recent strength and coordination measurements.

D. patient's discharge disposition.

51. A 12-year-old girl is hospitalized with anorexia nervosa. The COTA has been assigned to collect data on her family background, education, and habits via chart review. The COTA would find this information in the :
A. nurse's notes.
B. doctor's notes.
C. social worker's notes.
D. admitting note.

52. When interviewing the parents of a 1-year-old client, the COTA obtains information by asking a certain number of prepared questions, which she adheres to closely. This type of interview is called:
A. semistructured.
B. structured.
C. criterion-referenced.
D. open-ended.

53. The COTA is working with a 7-year-old boy who exhibits tactile defensiveness. Which area of the child's occupational performance is MOST likely to be affected?
A. reading skills.
B. dressing habits.
C. friendships.
D. hobbies.

54. The *BEST* activity to develop "position in space" skills in a 6-year-old child is:
A. identifying letters on a distracting page.
B. finding geometric shapes scattered in a box.
C. following directions about objects located in front, back, and to the side.
D. making judgments about moving through space.

55. COTAs employed by home-health agencies primarily see patients who:
A. require a wheelchair for mobility.
B. are not able to drive to an outpatient treatment center.
C. are homebound.
D. require moderate assistance for ambulation.

56. A child diagnosed with arthrogryposis has been referred for an occupational therapy evaluation. The COTA will focus on ADL training knowing that the child will have ongoing problems with:
A. obstetric paralysis.
B. hip dislocation.
C. joint inflammation.
D. joint contractures.

57. Matthew is in the late stages of AIDS and bedridden. Flexion contractures have begun to develop in his right hand and he has been referred to OT for splinting. The MOST appropriate splint for the COTA to fabricate is a:
A. dorsal wrist splint.
B. functional-position resting splint.
C. volar wrist-cock-up splint.
D. dynamic finger-extension splint.

58. Shima has athetoid cerebral palsy and is working on self-feeding skills. She is able to grasp a utensil, but the food keeps sliding off her plate when she attempts to pick it up with a fork or spoon. The MOST appropriate piece of equipment for the COTA to recommend is a:
A. swivel spoon.
B. nonslip mat.
C. mobile arm support.
D. scoop dish.

59. Julian is 3 years old and has feeding difficulties due to reduced oral-motor control and oral defensiveness. His parents would like him to be able to eat family meals with them, including such foods as meats (cut up), sandwiches, and vegetables. The COTA explains that the parents can start to introduce these foods when Julian is able to handle the following foods:
A. apple sauce and mashed bananas.
B. dry cereals with milk.
C. strained fruits and vegetables.
D. scrambled eggs.

60. The program that ensures that disabled children receive educational services in the LEAST restrictive environment is:
A. the Americans with Disabilities Act.
B. the Education for All Handicapped Children Act.
C. Children's Protective Services.
D. Medicare.

61. Connie is 13-years old and has a diagnosis of athetoid cerebral palsy. She would like to be able to dress herself independently. The COTA recommends looking for the following features when Connie selects clothing:
A. Mini Tees made of elasticized fabric.
B. dresses with side zippers and zipper pulls.
C. oversized tee shirts and elastic-top pants.
D. shirts with front closures, such as snaps or large buttons.

62. What type of wheelchair seat is best for providing postural support for a child with abnormal muscle tone?
A. Hard and firm.
B. Soft cushion.
C. Sling seat.
D. Gel cushion.

63. During a coloring activity, the COTA observes a preschooler stabilizing his crayon between thumb and fingertips. The COTA documents this grasp correctly as:
A. pincer grasp.
B. radial-digital grasp.

C. palmar grasp.
D. lateral pinch.

64. An 8-year-old girl has achieved her goal of using a "dynamic tripod grasp" for writing with a pencil. When reassessing the child's performance, the COTA will indicate that:
A. the child's pencil skills continue to be delayed.
B. treatment for this problem may be discontinued.
C. treatment for this problem should continue.
D. other children her age have also just developed this pencil grasp.

65. A COTA with several years of experience receives general supervision from an OTR supervisor. This COTA has contact with her supervisor:
A. once a day.
B. every 2 weeks.
C. once a month.
D. as needed.

66. A 1-year-old girl with cerebral palsy demonstrates poor head control. In order to improve the child's ability to be fed and to eat, what aspect of postural control should be addressed FIRST?
A. Shoulder.
B. Head.
C. Trunk.
D. Hand.

67. The owner of the out-patient facility where a COTA is employed announces that they are expecting a visit from an accrediting agency which surveys inpatient and comprehensive outpatient rehabilitation programs. The agency referred to is:
A. AOTA.
B. JCAHO.
C. CARF.
B. NBCOT.

68. An individual with carpal tunnel syndrome has been fitted with a splint. Her long-term goal is to return to work as a secretary. A related short-term goal is:
A. "Pt. will demonstrate an understanding of work simplification techniques."
B. "Pt. will demonstrate ability to don and doff splint correctly."
C. "Pt. will demonstrate ability to type for 10 minutes with wrists in 10 degrees of flexion."
D. "Pt. will use lightweight cookware for meal preparation."

69. A COTA is working on morning ADLs with a man who is s/p TBI. He requires prompting to apply shaving cream to his face and to pick up the razor. He is then able to complete the activity without further prompting. This is likely to be documented as a deficit in which of the following performance components?
A. Impulsivity.
B. Initiation.
C. Memory.
D. Attention.

70. Which statement best exemplifies a policy?
A. The OT department will provide inservices on relevant information on a regular basis.
B. Inservice presentation will rotate among OT practitioners within the department.
C. Individuals presenting inservices must sign up for the conference room at least 2 weeks in advance.
D. Inservice content should be approved by the Director of Occupational Therapy 2 weeks before the presentation.

71. The COTA is working with a 75-year-old woman diagnosed with an organic mental disorder, admitted after accidentally setting fire to her kitchen. The MOST appropriate approach to use with her in addressing homemaking skills would be:
A. teach her how to safely use kitchen appliances.
B. instruct her in organizational time management skills so that she is able to shop for and prepare 2-3 meals a day for herself.
C. discuss with her using a meals-on-wheels service.
D. emphasize the need for her to resume her previous life roles, such as that of independent homemaker.

72. COTAs working in psychosocial settings are responsible for establishing and maintaining a safe environment in craft areas. The BEST way for the COTA to account for all tools at the start and close of groups is to:
A. keep track of the keys to storage cabinets and unit doors.
B. have all materials and supplies ready before the group begins.
C. allow only clients who have no behavioral risk precautions to attend groups.
D. use a tool-storage area, painted with tool shadows or outlines, that can be locked.

73. A COTA is about to begin working with a 2-year-old child with hypotonia and extremely poor head control who is unable to maintain a sitting position. The first pre-sitting activity the COTA should plan is:
A. forward and backward movement on a ball with the child in prone position
B. forward and side-to-side movement with the child sitting on a ball.
C. forward and side-to side movement on a tilting board with the child in quadruped position.
D. place the child supine on a mat and pull him or her into sitting position.

74. While working with a 9-year-old boy in his class-

room, the COTA notices that the boy is demonstrating a hypertonic extension pattern. The wheelchair adjustment that will correct this problem is:

A. lengthening back support.
B. use of a hip trap.
C. use of a shoulder harness.
D. increased angle of flexion at the hip.

75. A new employee is becoming acquainted with the OT department's policy and procedure manual during her first week on the job. Which of the following is the BEST example of a statement that would be found in the "Procedures" section of the manual?

A. "The OT department will provide inservices on relevant information on a regular basis."
B. "All OT personnel are required to participate in continuing education at least annually."
C. "Individuals presenting inservices must sign up for the conference room at least 2 weeks in advance."
D. "Employees are entitled to 1 continuing education day per year."

76. When teaching children with moderate mental retardation to feed, groom, and dress themselves, the following method is the MOST effective:

A. forward and backward chaining.
B. practice and repetition.
C. demonstration.
D. role-modeling.

77. An advanced-level COTA who has worked at an independent living center for the past 7 years has been offered the position of Director of the program. There are no funds to pay for OTR supervision. According to the AOTA, can the COTA accept the position?

A. Only if the COTA can find some way to fund OTR supervision.
B. Yes, as long as state regulations allow autonomous practice and the COTA recognizes situations that require consultation with or referral to an OTR.
C. No. The COTA cannot work in this practice setting without OTR supervision.
D. Only if the COTA relinquishes use of the credentials "COTA."

78. Health care coverage for disabled individuals, people with end stage renal disease, or those over 65 is MOST likely paid for by:

A. Medicare.
B. Medicaid.
C. third-party payers.
D. Private pay.

79. The MOST severe sanction that the National Board for Certification in Occupational Therapy (NBCOT) may apply against a COTA who has demonstrated misconduct is:

A. a reprimand.
B. a censure.
C. probation.
D. revocation.

80. National Board for Certification in Occupational Therapy (NBCOT) regulations and state licensure laws regulate the provision of occupational therapy services. The relationship between the two is such that:

A. state licensure laws supersede NBCOT regulations regarding the practice of occupational therapy.
B. NBCOT regulations supersede individual state licensure laws regarding the practice of occupational therapy.
C. NBCOT regulations and state licensure laws are viewed equally and enforced equally.
D. NBCOT regulations are recommended but are not enforceable. However, state licensure laws are enforceable.

81. The COTA is monitoring use of a static wrist splint for a 12-year-old girl with juvenile rheumatoid arthritis. The PRIMARY purpose of the splint is to:

A. inhibit hypertonus.
B. increase range of motion.
C. prevent deformity.
D. correct deformity.

82. Which of the following is the BEST example of the "Plan" section of a discharge summary using a SOAP note format?

A. "Pt. reports he will continue to practice proper body mechanics at work."
B. "Pt. demonstrates independence in his home exercise program."
C. "Pt. has expressed his desire to return to work but does not yet demonstrate the capacity for sitting tolerance required."
D. "Pt. has been provided with a lumbar support and a written copy of his home program."

83. The majority of occupational therapy practitioners working in mental health provide services to individuals with:

A. chronic mental illness.
B. substance abuse disorders.
C. mild mental retardation
D. eating disorders.

84. A COTA is working with an individual who demonstrates poor handwriting skills as a result of muscle weakness. The activity that represents a compensatory strategy is:

A. learning to type.
B. practicing fine motor coordination exercises.
C. practicing letter or shape formations.
D. strengthening the finger flexors and extensors.

85. COTAs are MOST frequently found working with which age group?
A. up to 3 years of age.
B. 6–12 years of age.
C. 19–64 years of age.
D. 75–84 years of age.

86. A COTA may independently administer standardized tests:
A. as a level II student.
B. once service competency has been established.
C. once licensure has been received.
D. when NBCOT certification is received.

87. A COTA is responsible for supervising volunteers in an occupational therapy department. The MOST appropriate task for a volunteer is:
A. transporting patients to and from therapy.
B. working with a patient once the OT practitioner has set up the activity.
C. assisting with stock and inventory control.
D. completing chart reviews.

88. A COTA performs a kitchen check-out with an elderly woman before discharge and documents that it will be safe for her to cook small meals in the kitchen. The supervising OTR cosigns the COTA's note. The COTA is named in a lawsuit months later by the family of the woman, who was severely burned while cooking her own dinner. Which professional(s) could be held accountable?
A. Only the OTR could be held accountable.
B. Only the COTA could be held accountable.
C. Both the COTA and OTR could be held accountable.
D. Neither the COTA or OTR could be held accountable.

89. The Standards of Practice for Occupational Therapy (SOP) states that a COTA "may contribute to the assessment process under the supervision of a registered occupational therapist." This should be interpreted to mean that a COTA:
A. must contribute to the assessment process.
B. should contribute to the assessment process.
C. may perform up to 50 percent of the assessment process.
D. may perform variable portions of the assessment process.

90. At what level should COTAs MINIMALLY participate in the research process?
A. COTAs are not required to participate in research.
B. COTAs should read, interpret and apply OT research.
C. COTAs should participate in the data collection process.
D. COTAs should contribute to the development of a research question.

91. Shira is 8 years old and has multiple handicaps. She is beginning to develop some controlled movement in her upper extremities. The COTA should discuss the introduction of switch-operated assistive technology with the OTR when Shira:
A. develops tolerance of an upright sitting posture.
B. can reach and point with accuracy.
C. demonstrates any reliable, controlled movement.
D. develops isolated finger control.

92. The COTA is leading a grooming group for female clients in a psychosocial treatment setting. In order to comply with universal precautions, the COTA should:
A. use disposable cotton swabs and have clients bring their own cosmetics.
B. use disposable gloves when combing client's hair.
C. wash and dry makeup brushes between uses.
D. avoid bringing cosmetics with glass containers to the group.

93. After one session with a new patient in a psychosocial treatment setting, it has become apparent to the COTA that the woman is highly distractible and cannot complete a magazine collage when in a group. The best approach for the COTA to use is to:
A. speak slowly and softly to the patient.
B. coax and praise the patient until she completes the task.
C. ask the rest of the group members to stop talking.
D. position the patient so she is facing a blank wall.

94. An individual who is HIV-positive cuts his finger while working on a copper tooling project. According to universal precautions, the COTA should:
A. throw the piece of copper tooling into the trash can and get the individual a new piece of copper to use.
B. get out the clinic's first aid kit and put a band-aid on the individual's cut finger.
C. locate a puncture resistant container that the copper piece could be placed into before disposing of it.
D. wipe up any blood that is on the countertop with a paper towel.

95. The COTA has planned a community outing that involves walking outdoors from the bus stop to the bank, the utility company, and the grocery store on a hot summer day. Several individuals in the group take neuroleptic medications. The COTA will need to take precautions for which of the following possible side effects?
A. Hypotension.
B. Photosensitivity.
C. Excessive perspiration.

D. Weight gain.

96. Leroy has difficulty self-feeding, as a result of abnormal muscle tone. When discussing mealtime with his parents the COTA should address which issue first?
A. The type of chair he should sit in.
B. The foods he should be served.
C. The utensils he should use.
D. The place where his meals should be served.

97. A COTA with 10 years of experience is working in a rehabilitation unit. This individual has refined her skills and is able to contribute knowledge to others as well as act a resource person. This person will most likely be functioning at a level of:
A. advanced, with general supervision.
B. intermediate, with routine or general supervision.
C. entry level, with close supervision.
D. advanced, with minimal supervision.

98. A COTA is preparing a 30-year-old man with paraplegia for discharge. She presents to him the rights of individuals with physical or mental disabilities concerning employment, housing, public accommodations, and transportation. The law guaranteeing these rights is the:
A. Architectural Barriers Act of 1969.
B. Federal Rehabilitation Act of 1973.
C. Fair Housing Amendment Act of 1988.
D. Americans with Disabilities Act of 1990.

99. One week after an experienced COTA begins a new job in a nursing home, her supervising OTR resigns. There is not another OTR on staff. The nursing home administrator advises the COTA to continue treating patients, and promises to hire an OTR within a week. The MOST acceptable action for the COTA to take is to:
A. refuse to provide OT services to patients until an OTR has been hired to supervise her.
B. agree to provide OT services to patients for the first week, but not beyond that.
C. provide OT services only to patients who will suffer if they don't receive OT services.
D. report the nursing home to the AOTA.

100. An OTR and an entry-level COTA both work on an inpatient psychiatric unit. They each work 4 days a week, overlapping schedules only on Mondays. Which of the following tasks would be inappropriate for the OTR to ask the COTA to perform?
A. Lead the daily craft group.
B. Begin the assessment process when individuals are admitted on the weekends. The OTR will finish the assessment on Monday.
C. Work with individuals requiring ADL training on Saturday and Sunday mornings.
D. Carry out a leisure-planning group on Saturday afternoon.

101. An 18-year-old student with mental retardation is being discharged from an occupational therapy program in a large metropolitan school to a community sheltered workshop. The MOST important information for the COTA to communicate to the workshop manager is the student's:
A. leisure interests.
B. ability to follow rules/instructions.
C. preferred grasp patterns.
D. level of reflex integration.

102. The COTA responds to an individual by paraphrasing in order to:
A. refocus or redirect the individual's comments.
B. show acceptance and understanding to the individual.
C. force the individual to make a choice.
D. elicit additional information from an individual.

103. A COTA is recommending community resources to an individual with multiple sclerosis (MS) who is about to be discharged. All of the following are appropriate EXCEPT a(n):
A. aquatic therapy program led by an OTR in a warm-water pool (bathtub temperature).
B. ROM dance program provided by a COTA through the hospital's outpatient center.
C. list of local restaurants that are wheelchair accessible.
D. nonaerobic exercise program provided by a PT at a local community center.

104. Wendy is participating in an assertiveness training group. The expected outcome of this intervention is that Wendy will improve her ability to:
A. engage in relevant conversations with her coworkers.
B. use appropriate facial expressions when disagreeing with her coworkers.
C. express disagreement with her coworkers in a productive manner.
D. use courteous behavior when disagreeing with her coworkers.

105. The outcome that should be expected after an individual has implemented an energy conservation program is the ability to:
A. get dressed without becoming fatigued.
B. lift heavy cookware without pain.
C. do handicrafts without damaging joints.
D. dust and vacuum more quickly.

106. When dressing a child with strong extensor tone in the lower extremities, which position would make donning shoes and socks easier?
A. Extend the child's hips and knees.
B. Flex the child's hips and knees.
C. Extend the child's shoulders.
D. Dorsiflex the child's ankles.

107. The COTA is teaching a client with chronic obstructive pulmonary disease how to modify his bathing techniques when he goes home from the hospital. What is the best method?
A. A tub bath using hot water.
B. A hot shower using a bath chair.
C. A lukewarm shower using a bath chair.
D. A tub bath using lukewarm water.

108. Limit setting concerning impulsivity would be MOST important with which of the following diagnoses in an inpatient setting:
A. Depression and anxiety.
B. Alcoholism and anorexia nervosa.
C. Mania and borderline personality disorder.
D. Delirium and dementia.

109. COTAs most frequently work with patients diagnosed with:
A. CVA.
B. cerebral palsy.
C. developmental delay.
D. fractures.

110. An OT supervisor observes a COTA in a local establishment listening to a band after work one day. The supervisor observes the COTA being intimate with a gentleman who is currently being treated on an outpatient basis by the COTA he is with. The response which is MOST consistent with the occupational therapy code of ethics is for the supervisor to:
A. indicate to the COTA that she may maintain the relationship as long as it does not impair the patient's treatment.
B. notify the state licensure board and terminate the employee.
C. notify the NBCOT of the situation and reassign the patient to a different OT practitioner.
D. discipline the employee and refer the patient to another outpatient center.

111. The COTA is preparing for the discharge of a 9-year-old with limited upper-extremity range of motion. The most important home adaptation to recommend concerning use of the toilet is:
A. installation of safety bars next to the toilet seat.
B. mounting of a wide-base toilet seat.
C. placement of a skidproof stepping stool next to the toilet.
D. installation of a bidet with a spray wash and air-drying mechanism.

112. A COTA has been assigned a patient who was diagnosed with lung cancer that has metastasized to his brain. The COTA spends 15 minutes reviewing the patient's chart and talking with his nurse, who indicates that the patient is preoccupied with finances. As the COTA enters the room, the man states that he does not want to be seen for occupational therapy because his insurance has run out and he cannot afford to pay for the treatment. What is the BEST response for the COTA?
A. Treat the patient according to the physician's order and notify the nurse that the man's preoccupation with finances continues.
B. Do not treat the patient, because of his refusal, and document the interaction in the chart.
C. Treat the patient but do not charge for or document the services.
D. Do not treat the patient but charge for the time spent completing the chart review.

113. A COTA working in a long-term care facility has her notes cosigned weekly by her supervising OTR. Which of the following is NOT a valid reason for this requirement?
A. The AOTA requires the cosignature of the supervising OTR.
B. Cosigning may be required for reimbursement.
C. The employer may require cosigning.
D. Cosigning may be required by the state regulatory act.

114. The most appropriate ADL assessment instrument for an adult in an acute care psychosocial setting is the:
A. Kohlman Evaluation of Living Skills (KELS).
B. Milwaukee Evaluation of Daily Living Skills (MEDLS).
C. Occupational History Interview
D. Routine Task Inventory

115. When a new patient is referred for psychiatric services, the COTA and OTR both review the chart. Then the OTR completes performance measures, and the COTA performs an interview. The COTA/OTR team will rely on the interview part of this assessment to address the individual's:
A. diagnosis.
B. current medications.
C. ability to concentrate and solve problems.
D. view of the problem and an overall goal.

116. The COTA is leading a stress management group which includes a woman who is schizophrenic and actively hallucinating. The following stress management technique is CONTRAINDICATED for this individual:
A. aerobic exercise.
B. communication skill training.
C. mental imagery.
D. deep breathing.

117. In carrying out inpatient treatment groups for individuals with schizophrenia, the COTA should routinely:
A. use projective media such as clay to facilitate expression of feelings.
B. allow individuals to work in isolated areas away from the group.
C. use simple, highly structured activities.
D. discuss the individuals' delusions with them.

118. The COTA is planning a community-living program for patients who are to be discharged following an average of 25–30 years of hospitalization. One of the goals of this program is to train the patients to manage their money. Which of the following activities should be INITIALLY used to address this goal?
A. Providing each patient with 25 dollars to spend during a group trip to the local shopping center.
B. Providing samples of coins and paper money.
C. Using a board game to introduce the concept of receiving and spending money.
D. Establishing a hospital based community store where the patients could buy clothing.

119. The COTA is working with an adult with schizophrenia who has tactile defensiveness. The aspect of ceramics that would be MOST intolerable for this client would be:
A. wedging the clay.
B. imprinting a design using a rolling pin.
C. glazing.
D. firing.

120. A child with deficits in sensory integration demonstrates hypersensitivity to movement activities by becoming nauseated and dizzy. The most appropriate movement to use with the large therapy ball for this child is:
A. movement in any position or direction.
B. no movement.
C. slow and predictable movement.
D. quick and unpredictable movement.

121. The COTA is participating in an evaluation of an older adult in the early stage of Alzheimer's Disease. The functional deficit most likely to be evident is:
A. aphasia
B. incontinence.
C. memory impairment
D. inability to dress and undress.

122. The COTA needs to evaluate how a client uses her time and how she feels about the activities she performs in a typical week. The BEST evaluation for the COTA to use is the:
A. Lower Cognitive Level.
B. Allen Cognitive Level.
C. Leisure Activity Profile.
D. Activity Configuration.

123. Asking a middle-aged individual about the grade school he or she attended is one way of obtaining data about the individual's:
A. comprehension.
B. orientation.
C. long-term memory.
D. short-term memory.

124. The COTA is working with an elderly client who has been taking antipsychotic medications for many years. The side effects experienced by this individual include impaired swallowing and involuntary, jerky arm and leg movements. These behaviors are best described as:
A. Parkinsonian syndrome.
B. antipsychotic medication overdose.
C. tardive dyskinesia.
D. lithium toxicity.

125. Which of the following is a nonstandardized test used by occupational therapy practitioners in a physical disabilities setting?
A. The Motor Free Visual Perceptual Test.
B. The Minnesota Rate of Manipulation Test.
C. The Manual Muscle Test
D. The Purdue Pegboard Evaluation.

126. A 12-year-old boy with limited fine motor control wants to play checkers with his brother. To allow him to participate using only palmar grasp, the COTA makes the following adaptation:
A. attaching Velcro to the playing board and markers.
B. mounting half-inch-diameter dowels vertically on the markers.
C. placing a magnetic playing board upright.
D. replacing markers with lightweight playing pieces.

127. During the interview with the parents of a 3-year-old child with mild cerebral palsy, the COTA learns that the child is regularly fed by his grandmother and does not have any independent feeding skills. The COTA should first address the following issue:
A. the degree of abnormal muscle tone in the UEs.
B. the possibility of developmental delay.
C. the cultural context and family interaction patterns.
D. the need for adapted equipment.

128. The goal for a 12-year-old girl with limited grip strength is to become independent in self-care. To work toward this goal, which is the BEST method to gradually develop hair care skills?
A. Have the client use a weighted brush and gradually decrease the weight.
B. Color-code combs and brushes, beginning with bright colors, and gradually reduce the intensity of the color cues.
C. Have the client use a brush with a thick handle, and gradually decrease the thickness.
D. Give the client physical cues to begin with, then change to gestural cues and finally to verbal cues.

129. The husband of a woman being treated for bipolar disorder describes his frustration with the ups and downs of his wife's condition. The BEST support group to refer this man to is:
A. Al-Anon.
B. family therapy.
C. National Alliance for the Mentally Ill.

D. Recovery, Inc.

130. Although her lower extremities are correctly positioned, Kim, a child with cerebral palsy, tends to flex forward while riding her adapted tricycle. The adaptation that would BEST enable her to maintain a more upright position is:
A. raising the seat height.
B. raising the handlebars.
C. lowering the seat height.
D. lowering the handlebars.

131. A newly graduated COTA and an OTR have been hired as part of a treatment team on an inpatient rehabilitation unit. The entire rehabilitation team includes a physician, a physical therapist, a rehab nurse, a therapeutic recreation specialist and a neuro-psychologist. A patient has just been admitted to the rehabilitation unit with a primary diagnosis of complicated hip fracture and a secondary diagnosis of rheumatoid arthritis. For assessment purposes, the MOST appropriate role delineation would be for the COTA to assess:
A. weight bearing status for ADLs, and the OTR to assess cognition.
B. cognition, and the OTR to assess weight bearing status for ADLs.
C. dynametric grip strength, and the OTR to assess weight bearing status for ADLs.
D. leisure interest, and the OTR to assess weight bearing status for ADLs.

132. During manual muscle testing of shoulder flexion, the individual is able to move the arm through the full range of motion but can tolerate only minimal resistance against gravity. The strength according to the manual muscle test (MMT) is:
A. fair minus.
B. fair.
C. fair plus.
D. good minus.

133. An OTA student needs to design an adaptation in order to complete his level II fieldwork experience. He decides to focus on gardening for a client with a low-back injury. The MOST appropriate adaptation for him to design would be:
A. ergonomically correct hand tools.
B. a wheelbarrow with elongated handles.
C. a 12-inch-high seat with tool holders.
D. a raised-bed garden.

134. The COTA is planning a meal preparation activity for a 42-year-old woman with attentional and organizational deficits secondary to alcohol abuse. The treatment goals address her difficulties in properly sequencing tasks. The MOST appropriate activity to use initially is:
A. setting the table.
B. planning an entire meal.
C. baking cookies using a recipe.
D. preparing a shopping list.

135. A COTA provides a leather-working activity to a man with a C7 spinal cord injury. The aspect of the activity that requires the GREATEST degree of fine motor coordination is:
A. lacing with a whipstitch.
B. punching holes for lacing with a rotary hole-punch.
C. lacing with a double cordovan stitch.
D. measuring and cutting the exact length of leather lacing.

136. A 10-year-old boy demonstrates aggressive and disruptive behavior in school, which is a result of his low sensory threshold. For the upcoming class trip by bus to the zoo, the COTA should advise the teacher to:
A. review the bus rules with the boy and apply consequences consistently.
B. let the boy sit at the front of the bus and use his tape player and earphones.
C. give the boy the responsibility of monitoring his peers as "bus patrol."
D. let the boy set the criteria for a successful trip and reward him if the criteria are met.

137. The activity for which good ventilation is MOST important is:
A. painting with acrylic paints.
B. leather tooling.
C. painting ceramics.
D. copper tooling.

138. Mr. G. has Parkinson's disease and is at risk for aspiration. When instructing his caregivers in proper positioning during feeding, the COTA should recommend:
A. feeding Mr. G. in bed in a supine position.
B. seating Mr. G. upright on a firm surface with his chin slightly tucked.
C. positioning Mr. G. in a semi-reclined position in a reclining chair.
D. feeding Mr. G. in bed in a side-lying position.

139. The COTA is considering possible topics for a discharge planning group for individuals treated in an inpatient psychiatric unit. The MOST important topic to address, because of its significance in reducing rehospitalization, is:
A. managing family conflicts.
B. living skills needed for keeping after-care appointments.
C. coping strategies for continuing medication compliance.
D. education about problems with alcohol and substance use.

140. After the OTR has fabricated a splint for an individual with a hand injury, he asks the COTA to monitor the patient's splint use. It is MOST important for the COTA to make certain that:

A. the individual's fingers are flexed in a functional position.
B. the individual's thumb is opposed and abducted.
C. the splint is being worn at all times.
D. pressure marks or redness disappear after 20 minutes.

141. The COTA is beginning training in meal preparation with a 35-year-old homemaker following a TBI. The activity that should be introduced FIRST is:
A. making a peanut butter and jelly sandwich.
B. preparing a hot cup of tea with sugar.
C. pouring a glass of orange juice.
D. cooking a grilled ham and cheese sandwich.

142. Observing Mrs. S. during the evaluation, the COTA notes that her right arm lays limply by her side. In documenting this observation, the COTA would use the term:
A. paralysis.
B. flaccidity.
C. subluxation.
D. spasticity.

143. The COTA plans to use a "no-bake" cookie activity with a group of young adults in a psychosocial treatment setting. The activity will take about 20 minutes. The COTA will gently encourage members to rely on others in the group and reinforce positive behaviors. This activity is representative of which of the following group levels?
A. project group.
B. egocentric-cooperative group.
C. cooperative group.
D. mature group.

144. Cesar is 6 years old and has a diagnosis of attention deficit disorder - hyperactivity type. In order to work on increasing his attention span, his COTA introduced a construction activity. When the blocks were placed in front of Cesar, he swept most of them onto the floor and started throwing the remaining ones around the room. How can the COTA restructure the activity for more success?
A. Use soft foam blocks.
B. Provide blocks of one color only.
C. Use interlocking blocks.
D. Present only a few blocks at a time.

145. A 4-year-old child with athetoid cerebral palsy is about to be discharged from a rehabilitation setting to home. The COTA is instructing the family how to use correct jaw control when feeding the child from the side. The best instructions are, "Control jaw opening and closing with your:
A. index and middle fingers; place your thumb on the child's cheek."
B. index and middle fingers; place your thumb on the child's larynx for stability."
C. whole hand on the child's jaw."
D. index and middle fingers; place your thumb on the child's ear for stability."

146. A 12-year-old girl with juvenile rheumatoid arthritis demonstrates hand weakness. Which of the following pieces of adaptive equipment would be MOST effective in preventing hand fatigue?
A. Reacher.
B. Jar opener.
C. Pencil gripper.
D. Plate guard.

147. The COTA wants to use a drawing activity with adolescent girls diagnosed with eating disorders. Which of the following would be the MOST appropriate activity?
A. The COTA asks a group member to lean against a wall where a large piece of paper had been posted. She then outlines the girl's body shape with a marker. She then asks the other group members to draw clothes and accessories on the silhouette.
B. The COTA asks members of a small group to draw pictures of themselves on a piece of paper. The COTA then leads a discussion about body-image concerns and links the discussion to the groups members' drawings.
C. The COTA asks all group participants to draw pictures of their current families. The COTA leads a discussion that focuses on the underlying family dynamics symbolized in the drawings.
D. The COTA meets separately with each girl and asks her to draw a picture of a person doing an activity. After the girl draws the picture, the COTA asks the girl to describe what the person in the drawing is doing; the COTA also asks the girl what skills she used while drawing this picture.

148. A COTA in a work-hardening program needs background information about an individual's work history. The best method for obtaining detailed information about the individual's job requirements is:
A. interviewing the individual.
B. examining an analysis of the individual's job.
C. looking up the individual's job in the Dictionary of Occupational Titles.
D. requesting information from the referring physician.

149. In the middle of a wheelchair-to-bed transfer, an obese patient begins to slip from the grasp of an average-size COTA. The BEST action for the COTA to take is to:
A. ease the patient onto the floor, cushioning his fall.
B. reverse the transfer, getting the patient back in the wheelchair.
C. continue the transfer, attempting to get the

patient to the bed.
D. call next door for assistance.

150. A COTA has provided a Nosey Cup to an individual with dysphagia. She explains to family members that the purpose of the cut-out in the Nosey Cup is to:
A. slow the drinking process.
B. allow the chin to remain tucked when drinking.
C. allow the caregiver to control the flow of liquid.
D. minimize biting reflexes when the cup is placed in the mouth.

151. An individual is about to be discharged to home following a hip arthroplasty. He is able to ambulate with a quad cane, but his balance remains slightly impaired. When preparing a home evaluation, which is the most important safety recommendation for the COTA make?
A. Remove all throw or scatter rugs.
B. Place lever handles on faucets.
C. Install a ramp where there are steps.
D. Install a handheld shower.

152. A COTA must demonstrate service competency in performing the manual muscle test before performing manual muscle testing on patients. One way for the COTA to demonstrate service competency is to:
A. consistently obtain the same results as a competent OT practitioner performing the same procedure.
B. pass the NBCOT exam.
C. attain a minimum number of continuing education credits related to manual muscle testing.
D. practice for a minimum of 1 year.

153. The COTA is planning to use remedial strategies to prepare individuals treated in a psychosocial setting for job hunting. The activity MOST consistent with this approach is:
A. reviewing the NPI Interest Checklist.
B. a class about job-seeking strategies.
C. modification of the work environment to reduce stress.
D. an expressive group magazine collage using pictures of different types of workers.

154. A child with a poor postural stability is developmentally ready for toileting. The element of the treatment plan that should be considered FIRST is:
A. training in management of fasteners.
B. provision of foot support.
C. provision of a seatbelt.
D. training in climbing onto the toilet.

155. An individual with left hemiparesis and impaired balance wishes to vacuum the floors upon return home. The BEST type of vacuum cleaner for the COTA to recommend is a(n):
A. canister vacuum cleaner.
B. upright vacuum cleaner.
C. self-propelled vacuum cleaner.
D. handheld cordless vacuum cleaner.

156. A man who works as a cashier needs to improve standing tolerance from 10 minutes to 2 hours. To grade activities that will improve his standing tolerance, the COTA should:
A. have him simulate bagging groceries, beginning with lightweight objects and progressing to heavier objects.
B. have him carry a bag of groceries around the gym, increasing the number of trips around the gym each day.
C. stand at a high table while working on a puzzle for increasing amounts of time each day.
D. perform theraband exercises that emphasize gluteal, hamstring, and quadriceps strengthening, gradually increasing the resistance of the Theraband.

157. The subjective section of the SOAP format includes:
A. measurement results.
B. analysis of measurements recorded.
C. speculative information.
D. quotes from the individual.

158. Most COTAs are employed in:
A. rehabilitation hospitals.
B. school systems.
C. skilled nursing facilities.
D. psychiatric hospitals.

159. The COTA is a member of a treatment team reviewing treatment options for an individual who is experiencing acute psychiatric symptoms but is not suicidal. This individual has been living with family members. The BEST treatment environment for this individual to receive occupational therapy services would be:
A. partial hospitalization.
B. day care.
C. day treatment.
D. community mental health center.

160. The primary diagnosis most frequently treated by COTAs is:
A. learning disabilities.
B. developmental delay.
C. CVA/hemiplegia.
D. fracture.

161. In order for a school-aged child to receive occupational therapy services in a school system, which one of the following forms must be completed?
A. UB-82
B. FIM
C. IEP
D. HCFA-1500

162. A COTA in a work-hardening program is working with a man with an excessive anterior pelvic tilt. Instruction in proper body mechanics should emphasize correction of:
A. stenosis.
B. scoliosis.
C. kyphosis.
D. lordosis.

163. The COTA who uses pictures, music, and discussion questions with a group of elderly clients to encourage them to verbalize their thoughts and feelings about their first ride in a car is using:
A. remotivation
B. reality orientation
C. compensatory strategies
D. environmental modification

164. A 3-year-old child with a diagnosis of mental retardation is dependent in all areas of dressing. If the COTA uses a developmental approach with this child, which skill will he or she address FIRST?
A. Donning garments with the front and back correctly placed.
B. Donning a T-shirt.
C. Doffing socks.
D. Buttoning and tying bows.

165. A physician's referral for occupational therapy services may be required by:
A. AOTA, federal, and state governmental agencies.
B. federal and state governmental agencies, and third-party payers.
C. third-party payers, individual facilities, and AOTA.
D. AOTA, third-party payers and state governmental agencies.

166. The COTA is selecting an activity to use with a woman with paranoid schizophrenia. Which of the following activities is contraindicated for this client?
A. Playing "Whisper Down the Lane."
B. Making jewelry out of paper clips and contact paper.
C. Putting together puzzles of geometric designs.
D. Organizing files for the OT department.

167. An individual is unable to bring her hand to her mouth for feeding because of weakness in supination. The MOST helpful adapted utensil for her would be a:
A. spoon with an elongated handle.
B. spork.
C. spoon with a built-up handle.
D. swivel spoon.

168. A good way for an individual with arthritis to maintain range of motion while performing housework is:
A. use short strokes with the vacuum cleaner.
B. keep elbow flexed when ironing.
C. keep lightweight objects on low shelves.
D. use dust mitt to keep fingers fully extended.

169. Magdelena has difficulty attending to tasks. The COTA should recommend to the supervising OTR that OT services be discontinued when:
A. her goals have been met, and she can no longer benefit from OT services.
B. her goals have not been met, but she could benefit from continued services.
C. her goals have been met, but she could benefit from continued services.
D. Magdelena feels that she has not made gains despite objective measures to the contrary.

170. The COTA is working on a copper tooling project with an individual on an inpatient psychiatric setting who is HIV positive. While placing the piece of copper over the template, the patient cuts his finger on the edge of the copper. The COTA should immediately follow:
A. suicidal precautions.
B. universal precautions.
C. escape from unit precautions.
D. medical precautions.

171. While running a nutrition awareness group, the COTA observes that one member tends to monopolize the discussion. Which intervention would be BEST to implement after other, more conservative, approaches have been unsuccessful?
A. Sit beside the person who is monopolizing and touch his or her hand or arm as a reminder not to interrupt others who are talking.
B. Confront the individual's behavior: "Are you aware that your frequent interruptions prevent others from having a chance to contribute?"
C. Redirect the individual: "Now, let's hear what others have to say about this."
D. Restructure the task: select a group activity that requires sequential turn taking.

172. The following treatment program format emphasizes discharge planning for individuals with mental health problems:
A. Club house.
B. Community mental health center.
C. Acute care hospitalization.
D. Quarterway house.

173. The COTA is working with a man with impaired memory. When the client is unable to follow verbal instructions, the COTA changes her approach to demonstration. This is an example of:
A. activity analysis.
B. activity adaptation.
C. grading the activity.
D. clinical reasoning.

174. An ultralight wheelchair would be appropriate for a child with the following functional needs:
A. sliding transfers.
B. desk work.
C. wheeling efficiency.
D. work surface height adjustment.

175. The COTA is planning a group where he will involve group members in a game of chance. The only game listed that is a game of chance is:
A. baseball card collecting.
B. bingo.
C. charades.
D. balloon volleyball.

176. Most of the clients of a COTA working in an outpatient setting are enrolled in HMOs. The term used to describe the preestablished rate of payment per diagnosis is:
A. fee for service.
B. capitation.
C. cost shifting.
D. cost control.

177. A woman who is s/p hip arthroplasty needs to be independent in kitchen activities. Initially, she is only able to prepare a peanut butter and jelly sandwich. The appropriate grading sequence would be:
A. prepare a tossed salad, make garlic bread, make spaghetti sauce and meatballs.
B. prepare a can of soup, make a grilled cheese sandwich, make instant pudding.
C. broil a steak, bake a potato, steam asparagus.
D. scramble eggs, toast bread, prepare a bowl of cereal and milk.

Question 178 pertain to this case study:

James is a 21-year-old man with complete T8 paraplegia resulting from a gunshot wound.

178. The COTA can predict that James will PROBABLY achieve the following level of independence in bathing, dressing and transfers:
A. Complete independence with self-care and transfers.
B. Independence with self-care and minimal assistance with transfers.
C. Minimal assistance with self-care and moderate assistance with transfers.
D. Dependence with both self-care and transfers.

179. The COTA is working with a man with impaired memory. When he is unable to follow verbal instructions, the COTA contemplates the individual's strengths and weaknesses, goals, and alternative methods for reaching those goals. This is an example of:
A. activity analysis.
B. activity adaptation.
C. grading the activity.
D. clinical reasoning.

180. The COTA is working with a young adult with a behavior disorder. When selecting computer software to use with the client, the most important consideration is:
A. whether the program offers simulations of social skills.
B. whether the program allows the "teacher," i.e., the COTA, to adjust the number, type, and frequency of attempts the individual can make to use the program.
C. whether, if it is game software, the game requires the cooperative efforts of two or more persons to achieve a successful outcome.
D. whether, in the case of game software, the games are noncompetitive in nature.

181. The COTA is instructing a 41-year-old woman who has had a myocardial infarction in energy conservation techniques. The BEST example of limiting the amount of work needed for a task is:
A. using a side-loading washer.
B. wearing permanent press clothing.
C. using an extended-handle dustpan.
D. using good body mechanics.

182. In planning a therapeutic dressing program for a 5-year-old child who is mentally retarded, the COTA's FIRST consideration should be the need for:
A. adaptive equipment.
B. adaptive clothing.
C. proper positioning.
D. adapted teaching techniques.

183. Carolyn is s/p TBI and exhibits good strength with ataxia in both upper extremities. The writing adaptation that would be MOST appropriate for her is:
A. a keyboard.
B. a universal cuff with pencil-holder attachment.
C. a balanced forearm orthosis with built-up felt-tip pen.
D. a weighted pen and weighted wrists.

184. The COTA is working on transfer training activities with a woman with hemiplegia and her family. The COTA will teach them to perform transfers:
A. only to her unaffected side of the body.
B. only to her affected side of the body.
C. to both sides of her body.
D. only to the side from which the commode will be approached.

185. An individual has demonstrated competence in heating canned soup. The COTA recommends to the supervising OTR modifying the treatment plan and upgrading the cooking activity to:
A. baking brownies.

B. making an apple pie.
C. making toast.
D. making a fresh fruit salad.

186. The COTA is evaluating two-point discrimination in an individual with a median nerve injury. The COTA should:
A. apply the stimuli beginning at an area distal to the lesion progressing proximally.
B. test the involved area first, then the uninvolved area.
C. present test stimuli in an organized pattern to improve reliability during retesting.
D. allow the individual unlimited time to respond.

187. While in occupational therapy, an individual with C6 quadriplegia complains of a headache, chills, and sweating. The COTA should immediately:
A. tip the individual's chair backwards to increase his/her blood pressure.
B. take the individual's heart rate and blood pressure.
C. give the individual fruit juice to increase his blood sugar levels.
D. unclamp the individual's catheter and tap over the bladder.

188. An individual with a C6 spinal cord injury is unable to button his shirt. The MOST appropriate piece of adaptive equipment for the COTA to provide him with is a buttonhook:
A. with an extra-long, flexible handle.
B. with a knob handle.
C. on a ½-inch diameter, 5-inch long wooden handle.
D. attached to a cuff that fits around his palm.

189. A new COTA works in a busy rehabilitation department. Half of the department's OT staff is out with the flu, including her supervisor. The COTA observes an aide carrying out a morning ADL session with the patient who is scheduled for discharge the next day. The most responsible action for the COTA to take is to:
A. allow the aide to finish so the patient will be prepared for discharge.
B. excuse the aide and complete the session herself.
C. bring the issue to the attention of the facility administrator.
D. discuss her concerns with an OTR who is present.

190. A COTA is supervising an occupational therapy aide. Duties that the COTA may assign to the aide include:
A. setting up or cleaning up treatment activities.
B. instructing a patient in an active range-of-motion exercise program.
C. completing ADL training with a patient.
D. selecting adaptive equipment from a catalog.

191. A patient with C4 quadriplegia informs his COTA that he will commit suicide if he is never able to walk again. The BEST response for the COTA to give is:
A. "Don't worry, you never know how things might turn out."
B. "You'll feel better if you start to talk with some of the other patients on your unit."
C. "You sound like things are looking pretty bad to you right now."
D. "Most individuals with quadriplegia can lead very fulfilling lives."

192. The COTA is working on sitting balance with an individual with C6 quadriplegia. The BEST position for the individual's hands to be in when using them for support is with the fingers:
A. extended and adducted.
B. flexed at all joints.
C. extended and abducted.
D. adducted and flexed only at the metacarpal-phalangeal joints.

193. Which features are necessary when ordering a wheelchair for an individual who will be performing a sliding board transfer with assistance of the family upon discharge?
A. Lightweight frame, swing-away leg rests.
B. Reclining back rest, elevating leg rests.
C. Swing-away leg rests, removable arm rests.
D. Elevating leg rests, removable arm rests.

194. The treatment plan for a child with a visual discrimination problem should include the following adaptation of visual materials:
A. low contrast and defined borders.
B. high contrast and defined borders.
C. high contrast and ambiguous borders.
D. low contrast and ambiguous borders

195. The COTA is working with a group of individuals with substance-abuse disorders. He wants to use an activity that will allow the individuals both to experience success after making a mess and to delay gratification. The activity process that BEST provides this experience is:
A. working in a group with three other individuals.
B. selecting the design pattern for a tile trivet.
C. applying grout to a tile trivet and waiting for it to dry.
D. cleaning off the table at the end of the group.

196. An individual with a weak grasp has difficulty holding a fork. The COTA wants to assess whether providing a fork with a built-up handle would be beneficial to this individual. The BEST way for the COTA to fabricate the equipment needed is to:
A. slip a piece of cylindrical foam onto the fork handle.
B. fabricate a built-up handle out of a thermoplastic material.

C. wrap the fork handle with adhesive-backed foam.
D. use a plastic fork and wrap a washcloth around the handle.

197. The first and most effective method occupational therapy practitioners should use to prevent the spread of disease is:
A. wearing gloves.
B. wearing a mask.
C. frequent handwashing.
D. wearing a gown over work clothes.

198. A COTA is evaluating an individual's ability to transfer from a wheelchair to a tub bench. During the evaluation, the COTA has to cue the individual to lock his wheelchair brakes and help him lift his legs from the wheelchair into and out of the tub. He is able to scoot himself from the wheelchair to the tub bench with occasional loss of balance. How would the COTA rate his performance?
A. Dependent.
B. Requiring minimal assistance.
C. Requiring moderate assistance.
D. Requiring maximal assistance.

199. The OTR has asked the COTA to identify how the patient spends his leisure time, which leisure activities he especially enjoys, and which others he has participated in that he would be interested in renewing. The MOST appropriate tool for the COTA to use is the:
A. Kohlman Evaluation of Living Skills (KELS).
B. NPI Interest Checklist.
C. Activity Configuration.
D. Scorable Self-Care Evaluation.

200. A 12-year-old girl with behavior problems has difficulty with peer interactions. The MOST important factor to incorporate into her treatment plan is:
A. provide activities in an authoritarian environment.
B. allow her the opportunity to develop basic social skills on her own.
C. provide enjoyable activities in a safe and accepting environment.
D. establish rules for group play.

ANSWERS FOR SIMULATION EXAMINATION 5

1. (A) Whether the disability interferes with the child's education. Related services are defined as services needed to help a student benefit from education. If the student's disability no longer interferes with education, OT as a related service can be discontinued. Functional skills (answer B) and ADLs (answer C) may be ongoing goals in therapy as provided in a rehab setting or hospitals but would not be provided as a related service in the schools. Accessibility of the learning environment (answer D) is an important concern, but it would be covered in consultation with the school or teacher, not through direct service provision. See reference: Case-Smith, Allen, and Pratt (eds): Johnson, J: School-based occupational therapy.

2. (C) A work hardening program. Work hardening programs are designed to "move the injured worker from a submaximum level of performance to a level of functioning adequate for entry or reentry into the competitive work force. Practitioners use graded activities and exercises to increase endurance, strength and positional tolerance for ... activity needed by the worker to perform the job." Continuing to perform her home program (answers A and D) or discontinuing OT services would probably not enable Kathleen to return to the work force after a three month absence. Home health OT (answer B) is appropriate for individuals who are unable to leave their homes to attend outpatient therapy. See reference: Ryan (ed): Engh, J and Taylor, S: Work hardening. *Practice Issues in Occupational Therapy.*

3. (A) incident report. Facilities use incident reports to document accidents such as this. Although the incident may be referred to in a daily progress note (answer B), an incident report must also be filed. An incident report form includes a level of detail that may not be achieved in a letter (answer C), and a verbal report (answer D) is not a form of documentation. See reference: Ryan (ed): Jones, RA: Service operations. *Practice Issues in Occupational Therapy.*

4. (C) Provide a screen to reduce peripheral visual stimuli. Although all the answers describe techniques that could assist the student, the use of a carrel is most appropriate in a mainstreamed classroom, because the other methods or adaptations (answers A, B, and D) could have a negative impact on the other children's ability to learn. See reference: Case-Smith, Allen, and Pratt (eds): Schneck, CM: Visual perception.

5. (C) A COTA contributes to the process but does not complete the task independently. The COTA participates in this process by providing factual information to the OTR and collaboratively identifying discharge needs. However, because of the analytical nature of discharge recommendations, the COTA does not complete this activity independently. Answers A and B are incorrect because they do not take into account the analytical nature of the task. Answer D is incorrect because it does not allow for the input of data from the COTA. See reference: AOTA: Occupational therapy roles.

6. (B) stringing beads for a necklace, following a pattern. This is the only activity of those listed that requires the woman to follow a sequence in order to achieve the desired outcome. Leather stamping in a random design (answer A) does not require sequencing skills but does require coordination, visual-motor integration, and strength. Putting together a puzzle (answer C) requires perception of spatial relations. Playing "Concentration" (answer D) requires memory and attention span. See reference: AOTA: Uniform Terminology for Occupational Therapy, third edition.

7. (C) wedge-shaped seat insert that is higher in front. A wedge-shaped seat insert will increase hip flexion to more than 90 degrees, which is inhibitory to an extensor pattern. Answer A is incorrect, because lateral trunk supports will only prevent the trunk from falling to the side. Answer B is incorrect, because a seatbelt at the hips and ankle straps will hold a child in a chair but cannot inhibit an extension pattern. Answer D is incorrect, because although a lap board fastened to the arm rests may contribute to holding a child in a chair, it does not affect the angle of the hip joint, which is necessary to decrease extensor tone in sitting. See reference: Case-Smith, Allen, and Pratt (eds): Shepherd, J, Procter, SA, and Coley, IL: Self-care and adaptations for independent living.

8. (C) To teach the caregiver how to lift and turn the client safely. Individuals unable to move themselves and those with sensory loss are susceptible to the development of decubiti. Skin damage results from pressure on the skin over a prolonged period of time. The skin over bony prominences is particularly prone to the development of decubitous ulcers. Frequent position changes are essential for these individuals to prevent skin breakdown and the risk of serious infection. If the patient were already involved in a strengthening program (answer A), it may be appropriate to change it to a maintenance program at this point. A bed-mobility program (answer B) and an environmental control unit (answer D) would be appropriate if the individual has potential in these areas, but instructing the care giver in how to reposition the patient is the highest priority modification. See reference: Trombly (ed): Bentzel, K: Remediating sensory impairment.

9. (A) Infection Control plan. An infection control plan will most likely include appropriate techniques and procedures for storing and handling foods within the occupational therapy department. Such plans specify the shelf-life of certain foods, standards for food storage, use of hair nets, and cooking temperatures and times. A risk management plan (answer B) addresses the issue of liability in reference to negligence and malpractice issues. Emergency procedures (answer C) specify the procedures and techniques to be used in a critical situation (i.e., fire, code blue, severe weather alert, etc.). An environmental survey (answer D) is a plan that inspects a service area for potential hazards and dangers and corrects the situation. See reference: Ryan (ed): Jones, RA: Service operations. *Practice Issues in Occupational Therapy.*

10. (A) Physical agent modalities are not within the scope of practice of COTAs. "Physical agent modalities may be used by occupational therapy practitioners when used as an adjunct to or in preparation for purposeful activity by a practitioner who has demonstrated service competency." Service competency in this area involves possessing the theoretical background and technical skills for the safe and effective use of the modality. Therefore, a COTA who has demonstrated service competency in this area may use physical agent modalities as part of OT intervention. Avoiding harm (answer B), possessing competence (answer C), and referral to appropriate providers when necessary (answer D) are all required by the OT Code of Ethics. See reference: AOTA: Occupational Therapy Code of Ethics. Also AOTA: Policy: Registered occupational therapists and certified occupational therapy assistants and modalities.

11. (D) ability to relate to others. "Autism is a pervasive developmental disorder characterized by severe permanent behavioral and cognitive disabilities. . . particularly associated with autism are the inability to relate to others and the display of ritualistic, repetitive behaviors." The degree of the child's ability to relate is directly related to function. Answers A, B, and C may be normal in a child with autism, but because of his inability to relate, these skills may be nonfunctional splinter skills. See reference: Case-Smith, Allen, and Pratt (eds): Gordon, CY, Schanzenbacher, KE, Case-Smith, J, and Carrasco, R: Diagnostic problems in pediatrics.

12. (C) Making a wooden birdhouse. Individuals with diabetes often experience loss of the sense of touch and pain, as well as impaired circulation, which can affect their ability to heal. An unnoticed splinter could result in infection, even amputation. Therefore, a project such as woodworking that would expose Antonio to the risk of splinters would be contraindicated. Baking (answer B) and making latch hook rugs (answer D) could be structured to address standing balance and tolerance, but may be seen as feminine activities by some men. Gender association in itself is not a contraindication, but these activities could be considered poor choices if not meaningful to the individual. A group ball-toss activity (answer A) can also be structured to address standing balance and tolerance. See reference: Drake: Woodworking.

13. (D) Recommend hospice OT. Occupational therapy in hospice care focuses on role performance, quality of life, locus of control, and adaptation. This type of intervention may bring quality and meaning to Alma's remaining days. It is unlikely that Alma, who is depressed about a terminal illness, will actually carry out a home program (answer A). Not all home health OT practitioners (answer B) have the expertise to work with terminally ill patients using a hospice approach. Discontinuing OT services altogether (answer C) would not facilitate continuation of Alma's role performance. See reference: Hopkins and Smith (eds): Pizzi, M: Environments of care: Hospice.

14. (C) During discussion at lunch in the cafeteria. Confidential information about an individual must be respected by OT practitioners and should not be discussed in public places. Phone calls (answer A), written reports (answer B), and discussion in the OT office (answer D) are all acceptable ways for a COTA to communicate with a supervising OTR. See reference: Early: Data gathering and evaluation; also AOTA: Occupational therapy code of ethics.

15. (D) take a few days to teach himself the activity before leading the group. This action demonstrates such important professional behaviors as initiative, problem solving, and respect for his supervisor's time. Answer A requires the supervisor to take time out of his or her schedule. Answer B could be an appropriate action, but the COTA would need to discuss the change in treatment plan with the OTR before implementing it. In addition, taking the initiative to learn a new intervention and add to his repertoire is an example of professional behavior. *No* COTA should engage in an activity that he or she is not competent in, but refusing to lead the quilting group (answer D) is the least professional way of responding. The other answers are better alternatives. See reference: Early: Supervision.

16. (A) the same results in three successive treatment trials. Service competency is established when two occupational therapy practitioners obtain the same results on three successive trials. It is in this manner that the two professionals may identify if they are completing the procedure in the same manner. Answers B, C, and D either do not allow for enough successive trials or require that the occupational therapy practitioners have identical results. See reference: AOTA: Occupational therapy roles.

17. (C) Pin the Tail on the Donkey. For the defensive child, tactile stimuli may be perceived as extremely threatening if the child cannot anticipate them. Any game that requires blindfolds or other means of occluding vision, therefore, serves to heighten defensiveness and will interfere with Jennifer's socialization and participation in the game. Answers A, B and D are played using vision. While there may be touch involved, the stimulus can be anticipated and actively controlled by the child; therefore, Jennifer could participate more successfully. See reference: Case-Smith, Allen, and Pratt (eds): Parham, LD and Mailloux, Z: Sensory integration.

18. (B) NOT occurred so she does not need to use universal precautions. OSHA has identified materials that require universal precautions to be blood, semen, vaginal secretions, cerebrospinal fluid, synovial fluid, pleural fluid, pericardial fluid, peritoneal fluid, amniotic fluid, any body fluid with visible blood, any unidentifiable body fluid, and saliva from dental procedures. Since the urine did not have visible blood in it, it would not be considered an exposure. Answers A and C are incorrect because they indicate that an exposure has occurred. Answer D is incorrect because it is not necessary to use universal precautions unless exposure has occurred. In addition, it should be noted that items OSHA has identified as not needing universal precautions are feces, nasal secretions, sputum, sweat, tears, urine, and vomitus. See reference: Occupational Safety and Health Administration.

19. (B) copper tooling. Liver of sulfate, used to antique the copper design, is toxic. Wood burning (answer A) may create smoke and odor noxious to individuals with respiratory disease. Dough art (answer C) contains salt and is very drying to the skin. Papier mache (answer D) is very messy but uses flour and water, which are nontoxic. See reference: Johnson, C, Lobdell, K, Nesbitt, J, and Clare, M: Therapeutic crafts.

20. (B) Reviewing charts to elicit relevant information. The five steps involved in a quality-assurance plan are: (1) identifying the indicators of quality care; (2) collecting measurable data, often by chart review; (3) determining the cause of a problem; (4) implementing remedial action; and (5) performing the measurement process again to see if the problem has been solved. The most appropriate steps for the COTA to perform are chart review (answer B) and implementing remedial action as appropriate. OTRs and COTAs in an OT department often work together to determine the design and analysis of the quality improvement plan (answers A and C). The department head is usually responsible for writing a report (answer D). See reference: Hopkins and Smith (eds): Perinchief, JM: Service management.

21. (A) up and the collar toward her body. Answers B, C, and D are incorrect placements and would result in failure to perform the activity successfully. See reference: Pedretti (ed): Foti, D, Pedretti, LW, and Lillie, S: Activities of daily living.

22. (B) outpatient OT. "It is no longer expected that patients discharged to home will be totally independent. . . These patients are frequently capable of achieving further gains and could appropriately be followed . . . in an outpatient setting." A patient with such high levels of function is not an appropriate candidate for a home health referral (answer A). Work-hardening programs (answer C) are for individuals who are severely deconditioned as a result of disease or injury or those who have significant discrepancies between their symptoms and objective findings. If Sam has potential for further functional improvement, continuation—not discontinuation (answer D)—of services is indicated. See reference: Trombly (ed): Woodson, AM: Stroke.

23. (B) Ask Ruby to try some lacing on her own and praise her for what she has been able to do. All of the responses are increments of approaches used for decreasing dependency needs, but answer B is the best next step in this case because it allows the patient to attempt some lacing in the presence of the COTA, who in turn offers reassurance that the patient is actually able to do the activity. The step in answer B would be followed by the step in answer D. Here the patient is required to attempt some lacing without benefit of the COTA at her side; the COTA is nearby, but working with another patient. As the patient is able to do more of the activity independently, written instructions (answer A) replace the COTA as instructor. Finally, when the patient is feeling comfortable with self-instruction, asking her to work on the project out of the presence of the COTA (answer C) heightens the level of self-responsibility. See reference: Early: Analyzing, adapting, and grading activities.

24. (C) Assessment. The Assessment part of a SOAP note addresses the effectiveness of treatment and any changes needed, the status of the goals, and justification for continuing occupational therapy treatment. The Subjective portion of a SOAP note (answer A) includes what the patient reports or comments about the treatment. The Objective portion of the SOAP note (answer B) focuses on measurable and/or observable data obtained by the OT practitioner through specific evaluations, observations, or the use of therapeutic activities. The Plan section of a SOAP note includes statements related to continuing treatment, the frequency and duration of the treatment, suggestions for additional activities or treatment techniques, the need for further evaluations, and recommendations for new goals as needed. See reference: Ryan (ed): Backhaus, H: Documentation. *Practice Issues in Occupational Therapy*.

25. (D) lightweight wheelchair and hospital bed.

Durable medical equipment is defined by Medicare as "that which can withstand repeated use, is primarily and customarily used to serve a medical purpose, and generally is not useful to a person in the absence of illness or injury." Answers A, B, and C are incorrect because they include items such as reachers, shower chair, handheld shower and long-handled sponge, which are not considered as serving a "medical purpose." Depending on the patient's medical condition, a bedside commode may be covered. See reference: Bair and Gray (eds): Scott, S, and Somers, FP: Payment for occupational therapy services.

26. (B) give praise for completed dressing; do not help him get dressed. Since Ross has achieved dressing independence, he does not need assistance (answer A), clothing adaptations (answer C), or verbal prompts (answer D) to complete the task. In fact, assisting him now may cause him to lose his independence and regress to relying on his parents again. See reference: Ryan (ed): McFadden, SA: The child with mental retardation. *Practice Issues in Occupational Therapy.*

27. (D) wind-up toys. Wind-up toys give mostly visual stimulation and "do things" on their own, without requiring active exploratory play. Answers A and B lend themselves to active tactile exploration, and answer C provides auditory feedback, encouraging continued involvement. See reference: Logigian and Ward (eds): Logigian, MK: Physical disorders.

28. (B) adult day care. This environment provides programming for the elderly that is psychosocial in nature and focuses on avocational skills and social activities. Partial hospitalization (answer A) is a type of outpatient program that serves as a transition to community living. It offers most of the structure and services available on an inpatient unit while allowing individuals to live in the community and to receive services by visiting the program. Home health care (answer C) provides treatment services to individuals in their own homes who have chronic or debilitating illnesses, in order to increase their functional independence. While most individuals who receive home health services have disabilities that are primarily physical, secondary psychiatric disorders are quite common. Psychosocial rehabilitation centers (answer D) focus on the social rather than the medical aspects of mental illness. The psychosocial club or rehabilitation center provides socialization programs, daily living skills counseling, pre-vocational rehabilitation, and transitional employment. See reference: Early: Treatment settings.

29. (C) unacceptable, because it violates the Code of Ethics. Whether or not an alternate date has been arranged (answer A) or the agency the COTA works for allows it (answer B), stating services were provided on a day when they, in actuality, were not, is falsification of documentation and violates the OT Code of Ethics. The client's inability to participate in therapy the next day due to illness (answer D) would only serve to further complicate an already compromised situation; however, this is not the reason why the action is unacceptable. See reference: Hopkins and Smith (eds): Hansen, RA: Ethics in occupational therapy.

30. (A) close. Close supervision is direct daily contact between the supervisor and the employee. This form of supervision is recommended for entry-level COTAs or COTAs entering a new practice setting. Routine supervision (answer B) is appropriate for intermediate-level COTAs. General supervision (answer C) is appropriate for advanced-level COTAs. Minimal supervision (answer D) is appropriate only for OTRs. See reference: AOTA: Occupational therapy roles.

31. (B) match picture dominoes. A game of matching dominoes involves visual form perception defined as "matching one design with another." Playing marbles (answer A) and assembling a puzzle (answer D) address spatial perception skills. Playing "Memory" (answer C) requires visual memory in addition to form-perception skills. See reference: Case-Smith, Allen, and Pratt (eds): Schneck, CM: Visual perception.

32. (B) 1 year experience. Fieldwork educators, or supervisors, may be COTAs or OTRs with a minimum of 1 year of experience. These individuals should be competent and knowledgeable and able to function as good role models. There is no guideline indicating the amount of experience needed to supervise Level I students. See reference: Hopkins and Smith (eds): Cohn, EN: Fieldwork education: Professional socialization. Also AOTA: Essentials and guidelines for an accredited educational program for the occupational therapy assistant.

33. (B) asking the client only to put the last piece into the package. "Working backwards" from the last (successful) step of a sequence is known as backward chaining. Answer A is the *opposite* of what backward chaining means. Answer C is more descriptive of shaping behaviors, and answer D is more descriptive of modeling behaviors. See reference: Early: Models of mental health and illness.

34. (D) "Family will demonstrate independence in positioning pt. correctly for feeding so that he can swallow safely." Goals should be functional, measurable, and objective. In addition, short-term goals must relate to the long-term goal being addressed. This answer meets those criteria. Answer A does not provide measurable criteria, nor does it directly relate to the long-term goal of family training. Answer B, while measurable, does not relate to the long-term goal. Answer C describes the long-term goal of family independence in the feeding program. See reference: AOTA: Writing functional goals. *Effective Documentation for Occupational Therapy.*

35. (D) referral. A referral is a basic request for an individual to be assessed by an occupational therapist. A referral generally includes information such as the individual's name, age, date of birth, address, physician, and diagnosis. An individual may be referred to occupational therapy for deficits in occupational performance in the areas of work, play, or leisure. A recommendation (answer A) is an advisement that an individual may benefit from a service. Plans of treatment and intervention strategies (answers B and C) are completed by the OT practitioner following the assessment. See reference: Hopkins and Smith (eds): Spencer, E: Preliminary concepts and planning. Also AOTA: Statement of occupational therapy referral.

36. (B) A mobile arm support. An individual with C5 quadriplegia typically has fair strength in shoulder flexion and abduction and at least poor– strength in the biceps, upper trapezius, and external rotators. With this level of strength, he will be able to operate a mobile arm support for self-feeding and facial hygiene activities. A wrist-driven flexor hinge splint (answer A) would be used by an individual with a lower-level spinal cord injury (C6-C8) who has functional use of the shoulder and arm muscles and has fair+ or better wrist-extension strength. This splint is indicated for individuals who lack prehension power. An electric feeder (answer C) is indicated for individuals with a higher level of involvement (C4) who demonstrate poor+ or weaker shoulder strength. Built-up utensils (answer D) may be indicated for individuals with C8 or T1 injuries who may lack the strength to tightly grasp regular utensils. See reference: Trombly (ed): Hollar, LD: Spinal cord injury.

37. (B) provide positioning and/or adaptive equipment. Positioning and adaptive equipment are necessary to maintain the integrity of the musculoskeletal system and prevent deformity. Resistive exercises (answer A) are used cautiously with individuals with RA, because of the potential for tissue damage. A newly diagnosed individual would need some emotional support (answer C), but the primary means of support is the family or a support group. Surgical intervention (answer D) would not be needed in the early stages of rheumatoid arthritis. It may be offered as a corrective measure for long-standing deformities. See reference: Melvin: Assistive devices.

38. (B) A key guard. A key guard is a device that covers the keys and provides a guide for a finger or stick without punching extra keys. A moisture guard (answer A) is a flexible plastic cover that protects the keys from drool, moisture, or dirt. An auto-repeat defeat mechanism (answer C) stops repetition of letters or numbers caused by overlong or involuntary depression of keys. One-finger-access software (answer D) allows the user to lock out keys such as the Shift or the Enter key. This enables an individual who uses only one finger or a stick to type capital letters or perform other keyboard funtions that require simultaneous depression of more than one key. See reference: Church and Glennen (eds): Church, G: Adaptive access for microcomputers.

39. (C) provide a summary of observations of the patient's behavior, including what the patient said and did during the interview. An observation summary should present a concise and accurate picture of what happened so that the OTR can understand almost as well as if she were present during the interview. It is a summary and should not include extensive descriptions (answer A) or interpretations of the interview (answer D). A treatment plan (answer B) should be developed collaboratively with the OTR. See reference: Early: Data gathering and evaluation.

40. (C) Decline the gift and explain that a COTA cannot accept gifts from patients. Accepting gifts from patients is unprofessional conduct. Fees are established based on a cost analysis of the overhead, supplies, and time required to provide a service. Therefore, answers A, B, and D are incorrect. See reference: Hopkins and Smith (eds): Hansen, RA: Ethics in occupational therapy.

41. (C) lateral trunk support. A lateral trunk support, in the frontal plane, would provide stabilization at his side to maintain correct alignment of the pelvis and trunk in the chair, counteracting asymmetrical muscle tone. A lateral trunk support would also prevent improper loading onto an unstable shoulder joint through upper extremity support. Answer A, a reclining wheelchair, would shift his weight to the posterior but not prevent the lateral shift of the trunk. An arm trough (answer B) may help maintain a more centered position of the trunk, but the weight of the affected extremity would result in instability and improper alignment of the shoulder, which could result in shoulder pain. A lateral pelvic support (answer D) would provide stabilization of the pelvis to prevent it from shifting sideways, but this support would be too low to prevent the trunk from moving laterally. See reference: Church and Glennen (eds): Harryman, S and Warren, L: Positioning and power mobility.

42. (C) extension during finger flexion and flexion during finger extension. The method used to maintain tenodesis in the hand of a person with quadriplegia is to keep the wrist extended during finger flexion and flexed during finger extension. This allows the finger flexor tendons to shorten so that tenodesis action can occur. The other methods would stretch the tendons too much, which would not allow a tenodesis grasp. See reference: Ryan (ed): Fike, ML, Weiner, M, and Darlak, S: The young adult with a spinal injury. *Practice Issues in Occupational Therapy*.

43. (D) refer him to her OTR supervisor, who has attended a workshop on sexuality and spinal cord injury. Anyone providing sexuality counseling must not only be comfortable with his or her own sexuality but must have certain competencies as well. These competencies include awareness of personal and societal attitudes concerning sexuality, knowledge of male and female reproductive systems and how different disabilities affect sexuality, and the interpersonal skills to communicate with patients about sensitive and personal issues concerned with sexuality. When an occupational therapy practitioner who has developed these skills through continuing education is available to the patient, it is not necessary to refer the patient to his physiatrist (answer C). The COTA in this situation, who is unknowledgable and embarrassed by the patient's question (answers A and B), should not be the one to counsel him on these issues. See reference: Hopkins and Smith (eds): Neistadt, ME: Human sexuality and counseling.

44. (D) no adaptive equipment. A person with a spinal-cord injury at the C8 level will have full use of his or her upper extremities and should be able to perform self-feeding independently without adaptive equipment. An injury at the C4 or C5 level would allow scapular elevation, and the individual would be able to feed himself or herself independently using a mobile arm support (answer B). An injury at the C6 level would allow enough upper-extremity function for the individual to feed himself or herself independently using a universal cuff or built-up utensils (answers C and D). See reference: Trombly (ed): Hollar, LD: Spinal cord injury.

45. (D) all individuals with open wounds. Treating blood and body substances of all individuals as though they are contaminated is the concept of universal precautions. There are several strategies to protect employees from potential exposure. Engineering controls modify the work environment to reduce risk of exposure; for example, using sharps containers, eyewash stations, and biohazard waste containers. Work practice controls are policies that require a procedure be performed a certain way so that potential for exposure is minimized. Examples of work practice controls include the technique for disposal of sharps using only one hand and frequent hand washing during and after patient contact. Personal protective equipment, another strategy, is wearing appropriate gear to prevent contact with blood or identified bodily substances. Equipment may include goggles, masks, gowns, and gloves. Answers A, B, and C are all examples of individuals with open wounds, where exposure to blood is likely. Both the healthcare provider and the patient could be placed at risk unless gloves are worn. See reference: Occupational Safety and Health Administration.

46. (C) her lower back. Touching the lower back requires shoulder abduction and internal rotation. Answers A and B are incorrect because they require external shoulder rotation. Touching the opposite shoulder (answer D) demonstrates horizontal adduction. See reference: Trombly (ed): Evaluation of biomechanical and physiological aspects of motor performance.

47. (B) combing her hair. An individual normally abducts and externally rotates the shoulder to comb his or her hair. Shoulder abduction is not required for buttoning a shirt (answer A) or tying a shoe (answer D). Tucking in her shirt in the back (answer C) requires shoulder abduction and internal rotation. Tying shoelaces (answer D) is less dependent on shoulder motion than on hip and spine flexibility. See reference: Pedretti (ed): Foti, D, Pedretti, LW, and Lillie, S: Activities of daily living.

48. (B) good (4). The individual's "available" range is the range the joint may be moved through passively. Therefore, if an individual is able to move the joint actively through the entire movement that is completed passively and then take maximum resistance, the grade is normal (5). Good (4) is the grade given when a part moves through the available range but against gravity and is able to sustain moderate resistance. Fair (3) is the grade given when an individual is able to move a part through full range against gravity but lacks strength for any resistance. Fair minus (3–) is the grade given when an individual moves a part against gravity through less than full range of motion. Fair minus is the last graded range for movement against gravity. Grades poor and trace are for gravity-eliminated movements. See reference: Trombly (ed): Evaluation of biomechanical and physiological aspects of motor performance.

49. (D) the presence of self-stimulatory behavior. Self-stimulatory behavior is often seen in autistic children and frequently interferes with function. The other answers are less relevant in terms of essential data for intervention planning; an autistic child may be normal in terms of ability to focus at close range (answer A), wrist flexibility (answer B), and hand preference (answer D) but will show poor adaptive behavior. See reference: Nelson DL: Typical strengths and weaknesses in children with pervasive disorders.

50. (A) discharge recommendations. The COTA would contribute to the process of making discharge recommendations, but this section of the discharge evaluation is to be completed by the OTR. Answers B, C, and D may be completed independently by the COTA because these areas reflect factual data at the time of discharge. This information may include discharge disposition, and data on the patient's current status. See reference: AOTA: Occupational therapy roles.

51. (C) social worker's notes. The social worker's notes will "include ... details about the patient's family and occupation, her education, cultural background, financial situation, and "habits" (p. 239). The nurse's notes (answer A) provide information about the patient's adjustment to hospitalization and ongoing functioning in the hospital. The doctor's notes (answer B) document changes in diagnosis or medication. The admitting note (answer D) includes data on circumstances of the hospital admission, tentative diagnosis and any known history. See reference: Early: Data gathering and evaluation.

52. (B) structured. "Structured interviews . . . consist of sets of questions, which are to be asked in a given order. Furthermore, the interviewer must adhere to the questions as they are written. In a semistructured interview (answer A), the questions may be rephrased and more questions added (p. 240)." Criterion-referenced tests (answer C) compare the performance of the child to a set standard or criterion. This information is usually obtained through direct observation of the child. Open-ended interviews (answer D) are designed to facilitate the expression of feelings or associations and usually have no set format aside from an opening statement. See reference: Early: Data gathering and evaluation.

53. (B) dressing habits. Certain dressing habits may be an indication of tactile defensiveness, for instance, the child may show poor tolerance of certain textures or avoid wearing turtlenecks, socks, or shoes. Conversely, some children may never take their shoes off in order to avoid tactile overstimulation. Reading skills (answer A), friendships (answer C), and the choice of hobbies (answer D) could be affected secondarily, as a result of intolerance of certain textures or human touch or the inability to concentrate. However, because of the close connection between dressing and tactile tolerance, knowledge of the child's dressing habits (answer B) will give the COTA the most reliable information. See reference: Fisher, AG, Murray, EA, and Bundy, AC (eds): Royeen, CB: Touch inventory for elementary school age children.

54. (C) following directions about objects located in front, back, and to the side. Answer C is correct because difficulty with position in space refers to difficulty perceiving the relationship of an object to the self. Answers A and B are not correct because they refer to problems of form constancy. Answer D, making judgments about moving through space, is incorrect because it refers to a problem in perceiving spatial relationships. See reference: Case-Smith, Allen, and Pratt (eds): Schneck, CM: Visual perception.

55. (C) are homebound. Homebound patients are physically unable to leave their homes with or without assistance. Homecare services are not covered if the patient merely requires a wheelchair or assistance for mobility (answers A and D). If a patient is unable to drive to an outpatient center (answer B), community transportation services can usually be arranged. See reference: Hopkins and Smith (eds): Levine, RE, Corcoran, MA, and Gitlin, L: Home care and private practice.

56. (D) joint contractures. The functional ADL problems of children with arthrogryposis multiplex congenital disorder are caused by the presence of joint contractures from birth. Independent feeding is often an initial concern. Answer A is not correct, because obstetric paralysis refers to damage of the brachial plexus occurring at birth. Answer B is incorrect, because hip dislocation is not a usual feature of this disorder; when the lower extremities are involved, the characteristic problem is also joint contracture. Answer C is not correct, because joint inflammation is characteristic of juvenile rheumatoid arthritis, not arthrogryposis. See reference: Hopkins and Smith (eds): Atkins, J: Neural tube defect.

57. (B) functional position resting splint. Bedridden individuals are often provided with splints to prevent the development of flexion contractures in the hand that can lead to problems with hygiene. A functional-position resting hand splint is most appropriate for Matthew because it will prevent flexion contractures from developing and allow the caregiver access to his hand for cleaning. Neither the dorsal or volar wrist splints (answer A and C) would keep the fingers in extension, which is necessary to prevent development of finger contractures. Dynamic finger-extension splints (answer D) are appropriate for individuals who have active finger flexion but limited active finger extension. See reference: Hopkins and Smith (eds): Fess, EE, and Kiel, JH: Upper extremity splinting.

58. (D) scoop dish. This is the best answer, because the sides of the scoop dish will aid the scooping movement. The high back of the plate provides a surface to push the food against, which makes it easier to load the food onto the spoon. Answer A is not correct, because the swivel spoon is more appropriate when supination is limited. Answer B is not correct, because the nonslip mat is designed to stabilize the plate. Answer D is incorrect, because the mobile arm support is best used to position the arm and help weak shoulder and elbow muscles position the hand. See reference: Case-Smith, Allen, and Pratt (eds): Shepherd, J, Procter, SA, and Coley, IL: Self-care and adaptations for independent living.

59. (B) dry cereals with milk. Foods selected for Julian's diet should reflect his current skill level. To increase his oral tolerance and control of food, textures are gradually modified from smooth and consistent (answer C) to smooth and slightly varied (answers A and D) to increasingly resistive foods and a combination of contrasts, for example hard and crunchy mixed with soft or liquid as given in answer B. Once he has mastered this level of control and tolerance, he can safely proceed to an even greater variety of textures, tastes, and temperatures offered at family meals. See reference: Case-Smith, Allen, and Pratt (eds): Case-Smith, J, and Humphry, R: Feeding and oral motor skills.

60. (B) the Education for all Handicapped Children Act. This bill was enacted in Congress in 1975. It requires that school systems receiving federal funds provide handicapped children with free appropriate education in the least restrictive manner. The Americans with Disabilities Act, answer A, was passed in 1990 and enacted in 1992 to provide accessibility to individuals with disabilities. Answer C, Children's Protective Services is an agency which investigates the home environment and removes children from families who neglect or abuse children. Medicare, answer D, was established in 1965 by an act of Congress as Title XVIII of the Social Security Act. The program consists of two parts. Medicare part "A" pays for inpatient hospitalization, skilled care, and hospice services. Medicare part "B" covers outpatient services, physician and other professional medical services. See reference: Bair and Gray (eds): Scott, S, and Somers, FP: Payment for occupational therapy services.

61. (C) oversized tee-shirts and elastic-top pants. For a child with difficulty in self-dressing due to incoordination (as seen in athetoid cerebral palsy), clothing should be loose fitting with simple or no fasteners. Oversized clothing is preferred to tight-fitting garments (answers A and B). Garments with elasticized waist bands are better than those using zippers (answer B) or snaps and buttons (answer D). See reference: Logigian and Ward (eds): Logigian, MK: Cerebral palsy.

62. (A) hard and firm. A firm seat or seat insert, often of a triangular shape, is best for providing a firm base of support for the child with postural difficulties. A softer, less stable surface (answers B, C, and D) adds the challenge of ongoing postural adjustments to the already difficult position of upright sitting. See reference: Logigian and Ward (eds): Logigian, MK: Cerebral palsy.

63. (B) radial-digital grasp. A radial-digital grasp is developed at 9 months and is used for precision control. A pincer grasp (answer B), or tip pinch, is characterized "by opposition of the thumb and index finger tip so that a circle is formed. This pinch pattern is used to obtain small objects." The palmar grasp (answer C) is characterized by flexing digits around an object and stabilizing it against the palm. This is used as a power grip. In a lateral pinch (answer D), the pad of the thumb is placed against the radial side of the index finger near the DIP joint. This pattern is used as a power grip on small objects. See reference: Case-Smith, Allen, and Pratt (eds): Exner, CE: Development of hand skills.

64. (B) treatment for this problem may be discontinued. The correct answer is B, because the child has developed the highest form of pencil grasp, which begins to appear at approximately 4 years of age. Answers A and C are incorrect, because these answers imply that further development of grasp can be achieved. Answer D is incorrect, because a dynamic tripod grasp of the pencil should be well-established by this age. See reference: Erhardt: Joanne.

65. (C) once a month. Levels of supervision vary depending on the expertise of the supervisee. The description of general supervision given by the AOTA includes a minimum of monthly direct contact with supervision available as needed by phone or other forms of communication. Answer A describes close supervision with direct contact occurring daily. Answer B refers to routine supervision or direct contact occurring a minimum of every 2 weeks. Answer D is minimal supervision that occurs as needed. COTAs at all levels are required to have at least general supervision from an OTR. See reference: AOTA: Occupational therapy roles.

66. (B) Head. Head control must be developed first in order to provide a stable base for oral-motor control. Answer C (trunk control) is not correct, because head control precedes trunk control in developmental progression. Although shoulder control (answer A) and hand control (answer D) both contribute to eating and feeding skills by increasing the possibility of independence in eating through improved arm and hand function, head control must be acquired first. See reference: Case-Smith, Allen, and Pratt (eds): Case-Smith, J, and Humphry, R: Feeding and oral motor skills.

67. (C) CARF. The Commission on Accreditation of Rehabilitation Facilities is the regulatory agency for the provision of rehabilitation services. AOTA (answer A) was formed in March of 1917 as the National Society for the Promotion of Occupational Therapy and does not regulate the provision of occupational therapy services. JCAHO (answer B) is the Joint Commission on Accreditation of Healthcare Organizations. The JCAHO reviews the medical care provided by healthcare organizations. The NBCOT (answer D) is the agency which develops and administers the examinations for registration as an occupational therapy practitioner. See reference: Jacobs and Logigian (eds): Cargill, L: Quality assurance.

68. (B) "Pt. will demonstrate ability to don and doff splint correctly." Correctly donning and doffing a splint is crucial for anyone using a splint. Since the patient will wear the splint to prevent further cumulative trauma to the median nerve at work, this goal is directly related to the long-term goal of returning to work. Work simplification (answer A) is modifying task performance to conserve energy, which is important for individuals with limited endurance, such as those with arthritis or COPD. Typing with wrists in flexion (answer C) is contraindicated and would aggravate the individual's symptoms. Lightweight cookware is appropriate for this individual, but it is related to a homemaking goal, not her goal of returning to work as a secretary. See reference: Reed: Carpal tunnel syndrome.

69. (B) Initiation. Inability to perform the first step of an activity without prompting indicates that the individual has initiation problems. A problem with impulsiveness (answer A) during self-care would be evidenced by the individual attempting to complete several steps of an activity rapidly, which would probably result in him cutting himself or doing a poor job of shaving. Memory or attention deficits (answers C and D) are demonstrated by the individual skipping steps of the activity, either because he does not remember the steps or is distracted by internal or external stimuli. Memory deficits could also be evidenced by the performance of task steps out of correct sequence. See reference: AOTA: Uniform terminology for occupational therapy.

70. (A) The OT department will provide inservices on relevant information on a regular basis. A policy provides information about actions that need to be taken. The steps involved in enacting a policy are the procedure. Procedures state how a policy is carried out, in what sequence, and by whom. Answers B, C, and D are all examples of procedure. See reference: Hopkins and Smith (eds): Perinchief, JM: Service management.

71. (C) discuss with her using a meals on wheels service. Interventions directed toward "improvement" are typically unrealistic in working with individuals diagnosed with organic mental disorders. These disorders are characterized by a deteriorating course. This patient would not benefit from instruction in safety or time management (answers A and B), although individuals who are cognitively impaired could. Role resumption (answer D) is more appropriate for people with mood disorders. See reference: Early: Understanding psychiatric diagnosis.

72. (D) use a tool-storage area, painted with tool shadows or outlines, that can be locked. Painting a lockable tool cabinet with shadows or outlines to indicate where tools are to be kept is a very effective method that allows easy and accurate identification of missing items. This method also makes it easy to hold clients responsible for returning tools at the end of group sessions. Keeping track of keys (answer A) is an overall safety strategy that is not specific to tools Advance preparation (answer B) is a strategy to reduce the COTA's distractions during groups. Many clients treated for psychosocial problems would be excluded from OT treatment if they had to wait until all of their behavioral risks are being managed (answer C). Clients with severe suicidal or impulsive behaviors should rarely be involved with activities requiring tools that have potential to harm. See reference: Early: Safety techniques.

73. (B) forward and side-to-side movement with the child sitting on a ball. Answer B is correct because the position of the child requires the least resistance to gravity. By tilting the child in this position, the practitioner controls how much the child will work against gravitational pull. Answers A and D are incorrect, because they would require the child to lift her head directly against gravity. Answer C is also incorrect, because the head is positioned against gravity in the quadruped position, and a child with extremely poor head control probably could not hold a quadruped position. See reference: Hopkins and Smith (eds): Erhardt, RP: Cerebral palsy.

74. (D) increased angle of flexion at the hip. The correct answer is D because increasing the angle of flexion of the hip will inhibit the extensor hypertonic pattern (or extensor reflex pattern). Answer A is not correct, because lengthening the back support will primarily aide in head and neck support and stability. Answer B is not correct, because a hip strap, although it may prevent thrusting out of the chair, primarily will stabilize the pelvis. Answer C is not correct, because a shoulder harness primarily prevents the child from falling forward. See reference: Kramer and Hinojosa: Colangelo, CA: Biomechanical frame of reference.

75. (C) Individuals presenting inservices must sign up for the conference room at least 2 weeks in advance. Procedures state how a policy is carried out, in what sequence, and by whom. A policy provides information about actions that need to be taken. Answers A, B, and D are all examples of policies. See reference: Hopkins and Smith (eds): Perinchief, JM: Service management.

76. (A) forward and backward chaining. Chaining with the child who demonstrates a cognitive disability shows the entire process of a task with all sequences. Initially, the child performs only the beginning or end of the task. Thus, the child concentrates on only a small part of the task but gradually increases participation in all sequences in their correct order. Answers B, C, and D are other methods that can be used, but forward and backward chaining are instructional methods that have been particularly successful with individuals who are mentally retarded. See reference: Hopkins and Smith (eds): Humphry, R, and Jewell, K: Mental retardation.

77. (B) yes, as long as state regulations allow autonomous practice and the COTA recognizes situa-

tions that require consultation with or referral to an OTR. Occupational therapy plays a significant role working with consumers in the independent living movement by working both with individuals and their environments. According to the AOTA position statement "The Role of Occupational Therapy in the Independent Living Movement," AOTA "supports the autonomous practice of the advanced COTA practitioner in the independent living setting." In this situation, it would be the responsibility of the COTA to recognize and seek out OTR consultation when appropriate. However, this does not supersede state regulations when they prohibit autonomous practice by the COTA. Other options for this COTA would be to find some way to fund the necessary OTR supervision (answer A), or to work as a program director, and not use the COTA credentials (answer D). See reference: AOTA: Statement: The role of occupational therapy in the independent living movement.

78. (A) Medicare. Medicare was established in 1965 by Title XVIII of the Social Security Act. The program consists of two parts. Medicare part A pays for inpatient hospitalization, skilled care, and hospice services. Medicare part B covers outpatient services along with physician and other professional medical services. Medicaid (answer B) provides health care for the poor and medically indigent. Third-party payers (answer C) are the largest source of payment for health care in the United States. These providers, which may be for-profit or nonprofit organizations, adhere to state insurance codes that require set levels of coverage. Private pay (answer D) is the term for situations in which the patient is responsible for the payment for services rendered. See reference: Bair and Gray (eds): Scott, S, and Somers, FP: Payment for occupational therapy services.

79. (D) revocation. Revocation is the permanent loss of certification from the NBCOT. A reprimand (answer A) is a formal written expression of disapproval against an OT practitioner's conduct that is retained in the NBCOT's file. This information is also communicated privately with the individual. A censure (answer B) is a formal written expression of disapproval that is made public. Probation (answer C) is the period of time a therapist is given to retain the counseling or education required to remain certified. See reference: Hopkins and Smith (eds): Hansen, RA: Ethics in occupational therapy.

80. (A) state licensure laws supersede NBCOT regulations regarding the practice of occupational therapy. AOTA and NBCOT recommend that therapists contact the state regulatory (licensure) boards since each state has legal jurisdiction over the practice of therapists within the region; therefore, answers B, C and D are incorrect. See reference: Hopkins and Smith (eds): Hopkins, HL: Scope of occupational therapy.

81. (C) prevent deformity. The most correct answer is C because a child with juvenile rheumatoid arthritis (JRA) will need splinting to prevent deformity and maintain range of motion. Answer A is not correct because hypertonus is not a characteristic of JRA. Answer B is not correct because, owing to the active nature of JRA, increasing range of motion may be contraindicated. The correction of deformity may also be contraindicated with this child because of the active nature of her disease. Therefore, answer D is not correct. See reference: Case-Smith, Allen, and Pratt (eds): Gordon, CY, Schanzenbacher, KE, Case-Smith, J, and Carrasco, R: Diagnostic problems in pediatrics.

82. (D) "Pt. has been provided with a lumbar support and a written copy of his home program." The "plan" section of a discharge summary contains the patient's discharge disposition (i.e. to a nursing home, to outpatient therapy), recommendations for additional therapy or actions on the part of the patient (e.g., outpatient therapy, home health, or performing a home program); equipment needs or equipment provided to the patient; and plans for discharge. Answer A is a subjective report. Answer B is an example of a statement that belongs in the "objective" section of a discharge summary. Answer C belongs in the assessment section. See reference: Kettenbach: Writing plans (P).

83. (A) chronic mental illness. Individuals with mild mental retardation, eating disorders and substance abuse disorders may also receive occupational therapy services, but are not the majority. See reference: Early: Treatment settings.

84. (A) learning to type. Typing is the only compensatory strategy listed. Learning to type would allow the individual to communicate legibly in writing while avoiding the need to write by hand. Answers B, C, and D are all examples of remedial strategies that do not make handwriting unnecessary. See reference: Hopkins and Smith (eds): Culler, KH: Home and family management.

85. (D) 75–84 years of age. Recent studies show that 35% of employed COTAs work primarily with patients 75–84 years of age. Only 1.5% work with infants and children up to the age of three. Eleven percent work with children aged 6–12 and 15.9% work with adults aged 19–64. See reference: AOTA: 1996 Member data survey.

86. (B) once service competency has been established. Service competency assures interrater reliability between the OTR and COTA. This concept ensures that professionals working together in a collaborative relationship for patient treatment will obtain the same or equivalent results. Techniques for assuring service competency vary between facilities. Answers A, C, and D are inappropriate, because they do not address the skill level required to administer a standardized test. See reference: Early: Data gathering and evaluation.

87. (C) assisting with stock and inventory control. Volunteer performance within an occupational therapy department should be limited so that it is in the direct line of vision of the supervisor. Transporting patients (answer A) takes them out of view of the supervisor. In addition, it is not appropriate for volunteers to treat a patient (answer B) in that they lack the skill and expertise of an occupational therapy practitioner. Answer D is incorrect because it violates the confidentiality of the patient. See reference: Ryan (ed): Jones, RA: Service operations. *Practice Issues in Occupational Therapy.*

88. (C) Both the COTA and OTR could be held accountable. If guilt or incompetence on the part of the COTA is actually established, both could ultimately be held responsible. According to the AOTA document Supervision Guidelines for Certified Occupational Therapy Assistants, the "supervising OTR is legally responsible for the outcomes of all occupational therapy services provided by the COTA." See reference: Supervision guidelines for certified occupational therapy assistants.

89. (D) may perform variable portions of the assessment process. How much a COTA contributes to the assessment process is determined by the policies of each facility and the level of competence of each COTA. The SOPs are "intended as guidelines" and "serve as a minimum standard for occupational therapy practice" (p. 1039). The SOP does not state that a COTA should or must contribute (answers A and B), and it does not limit the degree to which a COTA can contribute to the assessment process (answer C). See reference: AOTA: Standards of practice for occupational therapy.

90. (B) COTAs should read interpret and apply OT research. While there is no law or regulation requiring any OT practitioner to participate in research (answer A), graduates of OTA programs should be able to read, interpret and apply information from research in occupational therapy. Participating in data collection (answer C) and the development of a research question (answer D) are more advanced levels at which a COTA can participate. See reference: Ryan (ed): Blechert, TF and Christiansen, MF: Intraprofessional relationships and socialization. *Practice Issues in Occupational Therapy.*

91. (C) demonstrates any reliable, controlled movement. As long as Shira can produce any such movement, switches can be adapted to meet her positioning and mobility needs. Accurate reach and pointing (answer B) or isolated finger control (answer D) are not necessary to use simple pressure switches. An upright sitting position (answer A) would not be required if Shira needed to be positioned in a reclining or side-lying position. See reference: Case-Smith, Allen, and Pratt (eds): Struck, M: Augmentative communication and computer access.

92. (A) use disposable cotton swabs and have clients bring their own cosmetics. Universal precautions are related to the prevention of the spread of infection. Using disposable cotton swabs and having clients use their own cosmetics would be effective in reducing the risk of infection. Combing someone's hair (answer B) does not usually involve risks related to blood or bodily fluids. Washing equipment (answer C) that is used near eyes and mouths by several individuals is inadequate. Avoiding glass containers (answer D) is a safety precaution that is related to self-harm and not universal precautions. See reference: Early: Safety techniques.

93. (D) position the patient so she is facing a blank wall. One way to modify the environment for an individual who is easily distracted is to position him or her facing a blank wall (answer D), thereby lessening possible distracters. It may also be necessary to speak loudly in order to get the patient's attention, which is why answer A is not recommended. If the patient is unable to participate in the activity successfully, the COTA should direct her to a simpler activity. Coaxing and praising (answer B) will not increase the patient's skill level. Asking the rest of the group members to stop talking (answer C) would probably interfere with the goals of the rest of the group. See reference: Early: Responding to symptoms and behaviors.

94. (C) locate a puncture resistant container that the copper piece could be placed into before disposing of it. Answer C is the only action that is consistent with universal precautions guidelines. Answer A and D do not dispose of blood exposed items in a manner that would protect others from contact. Answer B does not include any blood exposure protection for the person applying the bandage. See reference: Occupational Safety and Health Administration.

95. (B) Photosensitivity. Photosensitivity is a side effect of neuroleptic medications that increases sensitivity to the sun, resulting in sunburn. Hypotension (answers A) and weight gain (answer D) are also known to be side effects of neuroleptics but would generally not be problematic for a community outing. Excessive perspiration (answer C) is not a side effect of these medications. See reference: Early: Psychotropic medications and somatic treatments.

96. (A) What type of chair he should sit in. Correct postural alignment and postural stability are essential to a child's self-feeding skills. Children with abnormal muscle tone often lack the stable postural base required for distal control of the arm and hand in self-feeding; therefore, seating during feeding should be addressed first. Answers A, B, and D are also important considerations but should be addressed after the seating position has been successfully solved. See reference: Case-Smith, Allen, and Pratt (eds): Case-Smith, J, and Humphry, R: Feeding and oral motor skills.

97. (A) advanced, with general supervision. Advanced is the highest level of skill, requiring only general supervision which is defined monthly contact. These individuals have refined skills in their area of expertise and may have participated in research or in providing continuing education. An intermediate therapist (answer B) will have gained skill mastery and have the ability to function as a resource person. However, they have not yet gained the refinement of special skills to be considered advanced. Entry level therapists (answer C) would be developing their skills and accepting responsibilities for relevant professional activities. Minimal supervision (answer D), with supervision on an "as needed" basis, is the level recommended for advanced-level OTRs. See reference: AOTA: Occupational therapy roles.

98. (D) Americans with Disabilities Act of 1990. Also referred to as the ADA, this act provides civil rights protection for disabled individuals in five specific areas. These areas include telecommunications, transportation, public accommodations, employment, and the activities of state and local government. The Architectural Barriers Act of 1969 (answer A) literally opened doors for changes to occur in gaining access for disabled individuals. The Federal Rehabilitation Act of 1973 (answer B) expanded service intervention for those individuals who were more severely disabled. The Fair Housing Amendment Act of 1988 (answer C) expanded the coverage of Title VIII. See reference: Hopkins and Smith (eds): Jacobs, K: Work assessments and programming.

99. (A) refuse to provide OT services to patients until an OTR has been hired to supervise her. A COTA cannot provide OT services without supervision from an OTR. Doing so could result in disciplinary action. Providing services for a limited period of time and treating only a few select patients (answers B and C) are both violations of certification, state licensure, the Code of Ethics, and the Standards of Practice. Answer D is incorrect, because the AOTA has no authority over nursing homes. In addition, no laws or regulations would be broken unless the COTA proceeded to provide OT services without supervision. See reference: Ryan (ed): Ryan, SE: COTA supervision. *Practice Issues in Occupational Therapy.*

100. (B) Begin the assessment process when individuals are admitted on the weekends. The OTR will finish the assessment on Monday. The primary role of the COTA is to implement treatment such as that described in answers A, C, and D. A COTA may not independently evaluate patients. Working on weekends, the COTA would be independently initiating evaluations. See reference: AOTA: Occupational therapy roles.

101. (B) ability to follow rules/instructions. Answer B is correct because it gives information about the student's basic ability to learn and adapt in a work situation. Answer A, leisure interests, is not correct because although important to the student's life, leisure interest knowledge is not essential to work. Answers C and D are not correct because, although they describe the student's motor control function which can affect which type of job they perform, adaptation can be made to either of these areas of need. See reference: Case-Smith, Allen, and Pratt (eds): Gordon, CY, Schanzenbacher, KE, Case-Smith, J, and Carrasco, R: Diagnostic problems in pediatrics.

102. (B) show acceptance and understanding to the individual. Paraphrasing is used to clarify and relay acceptance of what an individual has communicated. The COTA paraphrases by repeating in her or his own words what the client has said. Redirection (answer A) is used to promote healthier thoughts and behaviors. Forcing the individual to make a choice (answer C) may be accomplished by providing a question that includes two possible choices. The COTA encourages a client to provide additional information (answer D) by asking open-ended questions. See reference: Denton: Treatment planning and implementation.

103. (A) aquatic therapy program led by an OTR in a warm-water pool (bathtub temperature). Heat can contribute to symptoms of fatigue in individuals with MS. Although a water-exercise program is an excellent way for individuals with MS to maintain or promote physical fitness, they should avoid environments in which they may become overheated. All other resources mentioned are appropriate. See reference: Ryan (ed): Jensen, D, and Linroth, R: The adult with multiple sclerosis. *Practice Issues in Occupational Therapy.*

104. (C) express disagreement with her coworkers in a productive manner. Assertiveness is the ability to express feelings in an appropriate and productive manner. Answers A, B, and D are examples of other types of social interaction skills. Answers A and B are examples of good conversation. Answer D is an example of proper social conduct. See reference: Hemphill, BJ, Peterson, CQ, and Werner, PC: Social interaction skills.

105. (A) get dressed without becoming fatigued. Prevention of fatigue is the primary purpose of energy conservation. Energy conservation techniques may often result in slower, not faster (answer D) performance of activities. Using proper body mechanics may enable an individual with back pain to lift heavy cookware without pain (answer B). Using joint protection techniques may prevent further joint damage to arthritic hands when doing handicrafts (answer C). See reference: Pedretti (ed): Hittle, JM, Pedretti, LW, and Kasch, MC: Rheumatoid arthritis.

106. (B) Flex the child's hips and knees. Answer B is correct, because flexing the hips and knees prior to donning socks and shoes provides inhibition of ankle plantar flexion (which makes the task very difficult) through the key point of the hip. Answer A is not correct, because hip and knee extension is the position which already is contributing to the plantar flexion of the ankle and inhibition of plantar flexion could not occur. Answer C is not correct because the shoulder patterns may not influence the ankle patterns as significantly as hip and knee flexion and this is an extension pattern which could not be inhibitory to the abnormal ankle pattern interfering with dressing. Answer D is not correct primarily because the abnormal pattern at the ankle is usually influenced by inhibition from the key point of the hip. See reference: Case-Smith, Allen, and Pratt (eds): Hunter, JG: The neonatal intensive care unit.

107. (D) A bath using lukewarm water. A person with COPD would have difficulty breathing in hot, humid environments, such as those produced by the methods in answers A and B. Showers (answer C) result in high levels of evaporation, which also makes breathing more difficult. A lukewarm tub bath would provide the lowest humidity by using the coolest water temperature combined with the method of dispensing water that keeps evaporation at a minimum. See reference: Trombly (ed): Atchison, B: Cardiopulmonary disease.

108. (C) Mania and borderline personality disorder. Stabilizing the crisis that precipitated hospitalization is a common goal of short-term psychiatric treatment. Consistent limit setting helps stabilize individuals with mania and borderline personality, whose impaired judgment and impulsive behaviors are common admitting problems. Limit setting concerning denial is more appropriate for alcoholism and anorexia (answer B). For depression and anxiety (answer A), limit setting concerning reassurance is usually appropriate. Delirium and dementia (answer D) usually involve setting limits for decreased confusion. See reference: Hopkins and Smith (eds): Richert, GZ: Program planning, development, and implementation.

109. (A) CVA. Individuals diagnosed with a CVA represent 44 percent of the populations that COTAs treat. Individuals with fractures account for 11.6 percent, those diagnosed with developmental delay 8.6 percent, and those with cerebral palsy 3.1 percent. See reference: AOTA: 1996 Member data survey.

110. (C) notify the NBCOT of the situation and reassign the patient to a different OT practitioner. According to the Code of Ethics, OT practitioners are responsible for "maintaining a goal directed and objective relationship with all people served" as well as not engaging in behavior which may constitute a "conflict of interest that adversely reflects on the profession". The patient/therapist relationship is compromised when the OT practitioner enters into a social or intimate relationship with a patient. Every OT practitioner is responsible to report behavior that is in conflict with the Code of Ethics to the NBCOT, whether they are a supervisor or not. See reference: Hopkins and Smith (eds): Hansen, RA: Ethics in occupational therapy.

111. (D) installation of a bidet with a spray wash and air-drying mechanism. Use of a bidet for hygiene after using the toilet eliminates any upper-extremity reach requirement. Answers A, B, and C describe adaptations appropriate for a child with poor postural control in need of external stability devices; these devices would not reduce reach requirements. See reference: Case-Smith, Allen, and Pratt (eds): Dudgeon, BJ: Pediatric rehabilitation.

112. (B) do not treat the patient, because of his refusal, and document the interaction in the chart. As stated in the Code of Ethics (principle 2), "Occupational therapy personnel shall respect the individual's right to refuse professional services." Answers A and C are incorrect, because the COTA disregards the patient's refusal and proceeds to treat the patient. Answer D is incorrect, because it does not conform to Principle 4 of the Code of Ethics, "Occupational therapy personnel shall accurately record and report information related to professional activities." See reference: AOTA: Occupational Therapy Code of Ethics.

113. (A) The AOTA requires the cosignature of the supervising OTR. The AOTA does *not* require that a COTA's notes be cosigned by an OTR, unless required by the employer or legislation. It is not uncommon for insurance carriers and licensure acts to require cosignature. Cosignature indicates that an OTR has read, sanctioned, and assumed responsibility for the documentation. It is also one method of demonstrating that the OTR is supervising the COTA. See reference: Jacobs and Logigian (eds): Pagonis, J: Documentation in health care.

114. (A) Kohlman Evaluation of Living Skills (KELS). The KELS is the only item that was designed for acute care psychiatric settings. The MEDLS (answer B) is most appropriate for long term psychiatric treatment settings. The Occupational History Interview (answer C) is designed to obtain information about the patient's occupational role development. The Routine Task Inventory (answer D) is designed to assess how well an individual is able to function in the community. See reference: Early: Data gathering and evaluation.

115. (D) view of the problem and an overall goal. The interview is generally the component of the assessment process where the OT practitioner asks about the individual's goals for treatment and gains an understanding of the problems from the person's perspective. Diagnoses and medications (answers A and B) are most often found in a review of the chart. Abilities (answer C) are determined through performance measures. See reference: Denton: Assessment.

116. (C) mental imagery. Individuals with schizophrenia generally have difficulty with abstract concepts or approaches. Also, they have difficulty accurately perceiving reality. Because imagery involves abstracting and relies on the individual developing alternate perceptions, this strategy is contraindicated. All the other stress management techniques listed would be generally appropriate. See reference: Hopkins and Smith (eds): Neistadt, ME: Stress management.

117. (C) use simple, highly structured activities. Projective media, isolation, and discussing delusions are all contraindicated for people with schizophrenia. Projective activities (answer A) are most useful for encouraging expression of feelings. It may be appropriate to separate individuals (answer B) who are violent or unable to tolerate the presence of others nearby. Discussing delusions (answer D) is undesirable as it is likely to reinforce them. See reference: Early: Responding to symptoms and behaviors.

118. (C) Using a board game to introduce the concept of receiving and spending money. This activity provides an opportunity for the individual to experience the value and purpose of money. While it is important to introduce the actual value of coins and paper money, it is essential to combine this with concrete applications. Answers A, B and D are examples of graded activities to be used following the initial introduction of money concepts. See reference: Early: Daily living skills.

119. (A) wedging the clay. Individuals with tactile defensiveness often have an aversion to materials such as clay, paste and finger paints. They react most strongly to stimulation of the hands, feet, and face. Answers B, C and D involve stimuli that would not be perceived as noxious to the individual with tactile defensiveness. See reference: Reed: Developmental disorders.

120. (C) slow and predictable movement. The therapy ball provides slow, predictable, rhythmic movement for children with vestibular hypersensitivity. Answer A is not correct, because movement in any position or direction is used with children who have vestibular hyposensitivity. Answer B is not correct, because adaptation to movement will be an important goal for comfort in the child's life activities. Answer D is not correct, because it describes the type of movement most likely to be used in therapy when children are hyposensitive to movement. See reference: Hopkins and Smith: Kinnealey, M, and Miller, LJ: Sensory integration/learning disabilities.

121. (C) memory impairment. Cognitive abilities such as memory are most often initially affected in individuals with Alzheimer's Disease. Receptive and expressive aphasia, personality changes, and loss of independence in ADLs appear in the middle stage of the disease. Incontinence, inability to recognize family members and inability to walk are evident in the late stage of Alzheimer's disease. See reference Ryan (ed): Brown, I, and Epstein, CF: The Elderly with Alzheimer's disease. In Practice Issues in Occupational Therapy.

122. (D) Activity Configuration. The Activity Configuration charts how an individual spends his or her time during a typical week. Tested individuals then categorize the activity (e.g. work, recreation, rest) and indicate whether the task was required or voluntary, how adequately they believe they performed it, and whether they did it because they wanted to or because someone else wanted them to. The ACL and LCL (answers A and B) assess levels of cognitive disability. The Leisure Activity Profile (answer C) is used to distinguish between alcoholic and nonalcoholic use of leisure time. See reference: Early: Data gathering and evaluation.

123. (C) long-term memory. The ability to recall events from one's distant past is long-term memory. It is usually assessed through verbal interviews and informal testing, such as a question eliciting the individual's recall of childhood events. Comprehension (answer A) can be determined by giving the individual a command to follow. Orientation (answer B) is determined by asking about the current time and date. Short-term memory (answer D) can be determined by asking about meals eaten that day. See reference: Early: Responding to symptoms and behaviors.

124. (C) tardive dyskinesia. Long-term use of antipsychotic medications results in tardive dyskinesia in approximately 15% of individuals taking these medications. Because the side effects can seriously affect an individual's ability to perform skills of daily living as well as his or her self-concept, it is the COTA's responsibility to know about the side effects during assessment, treatment planning, and implementation. Tremors, muscular weakness, and rigid gait, signs associated with Parkinsonian syndrome (answer A), are sometimes seen as side effects of antipsychotic medications. Overdose symptoms (answer B), would vary according to the specific antipsychotic medication ingested. Lithium toxicity (answer D) is linked to antimanic medications. See reference: Early: Psychotropic medications and somatic treatments.

125. (C) the Manual Muscle Test. The manual muscle test (answer C) is an example of a nonstandardized test. Although it includes instructions for the administration and scoring of the test, it lacks validity and reliability. The interpretation of a nonstandardized test often depends on the skill, judgment, and bias of the evaluator. A standardized test has instructions for the administration and scoring as well as information regarding the validity and reliability based on established norms from a specific population. The Motor Free Visual Perception Test (answer A), the Minnesota Rate of Manipulation Test (answer B) and the Purdue Pegboard Evaluation (answer D) all have information available regarding reliability and validity based on the established norms. See reference: Pedretti (ed): Kasch, M: Hand injuries.

126. (B) mounting half-inch-diameter dowels verticaly on the markers. This adaptation will enable the client to grasp the markers with a palmar grasp. Attaching Velcro to the board and markers (answer A) is an adaptation that is more useful for a child whose precision gripping skills are limited because of a lack of stability. Placing a magnetic board upright (answer C) can help a child with visual perceptual difficulties or limitations in his or her upper-extremity range of motion. Replacing the markers with lightweight playing pieces (answer D) is an adaptation for a child with limited strength. See reference: Case-Smith, Allen, and Pratt (eds): Exner, CE: Development of hand skills.

127. (C) the cultural context and family interaction patterns. Cultural expectations may determine behavior standards and the expression of family roles. Continued feeding of a young child with a handicap may be the expression of nurturing and caring. Such an expression may be viewed as more important than the promotion of independence and self-reliance. Answers A, B, and D may be valid issues as well but should be addressed after the COTA has familiarized himself or herself with the cultural and familial context of the skill. See reference: Case-Smith, Allen, and Pratt (eds): Shepherd, J, Procter, SA, and Coley, IL: Self care and adaptations for independent living. Also: Case-Smith, J, and Humphry, R: Feeding and oral motor skills.

128. (C) Have the client use a brush with a thick handle and gradually decrease the thickness. A thick handle is easier to grasp with limited grip strength. As the client's strength increases, the COTA can gradually reduce the thickness . Using a weighted brush (answer A) helps stabilize an incoordinated limb. Using color-coding (answer B) and using a sequence of physical, gestural, and verbal cues (answer D) are methods better suited for clients with cognitive limitations. See reference: Case-Smith, Allen, and Pratt (eds): Shepherd, J, Procter, SA, and Coley, IL: Self-care and adaptations for independent living.

129. (C) National Alliance for the Mentally Ill. This is a support group that is open to clients and families and focuses on education and support related to all mental illnesses. Al-Anon (answer A) is a support group for family members of alcoholics. Family therapy (answer B) is not a support group. Recovery, Inc. (answer D) is a self-help support group for individuals with mental disorders. See reference: Hopkins and Smith (eds): Richert, GZ: Program planning, development, and implementation.

130. (B) raising the handle bars. The correct answer is B because raising the handle bars demands that the arms are raised, thus bringing the child to the upright posture. Answers A and D are not correct because the hips and lower extremities are already positioned correctly and this positioning would be disrupted. Answer D is not correct because the arms would be lowered and trunk forward flexion would be increased. See reference: Kramer and Hinojosa: Colangelo, CA: Biomechanical frame of reference.

131. (C) dynametric grip strength and the OTR to assess weight bearing status for ADLs. A dynamometer, which is a designated standardized assessment tool, is used to measure grip strength and is the only standardized assessment tool included in the choices. Upon establishing service competency, an OTR may delegate to a COTA administration of standardized assessment tools. Weight bearing status (answer A) is usually determined by the physician. Cognition (answer B) would be assessed by the psychologist on the team. Information on leisure interests (answer D) would most likely obtained by a therapeutic recreation specialist on an inpatient rehabilitation unit. See reference: AOTA: Occupational therapy roles.

132. (C) fair plus. A person with strength of fair (answer B) or fair minus (answer C) would be unable to tolerate resistance. A person with fair plus strength during manual muscle testing can tolerate minimal resistance. A person whose strength is good minus (answer D) can tolerate less than moderate resistance but more than minimal resistance. See reference: Trombly (ed): Evaluation of biomechanical and physiological aspects of motor performance.

133. (D) a raised-bed garden. The individual with back pain must avoid activities that stress the lumbar spine such as "prolonged static postures with a flexed lumbar spine, repetitive bending with a flexed spine, and lifting and carrying when the normal lumbar curve is not maintained." A raised-bed garden would allow gardening without bending. A wheelbarrow with elongated handles (answer B) would be harder to control while pushing than would a wheelbarrow with normal handles and would place undue stress on the low back. A 12-inch-high seat with tool holders could benefit an individual with low endurance, but working the ground from that position would be very difficult for an individual with back pain. See reference: Pedretti (ed): Smithline, J: Low back pain.

134. (C) baking cookies using a recipe. This is a well-delineated meal preparation activity that provides structure with a specific sequence of tasks. Setting a table or preparing a shopping list (answers A and D) do not necessarily require sequencing of tasks. Planning a meal (answer B) involves a great deal of organizational ability and would not be an appropriate choice for an initial activity to address goals relating to sequencing tasks. See reference: Early: Responding to symptoms and behaviors.

135. (C) lacing with a double cordovan stitch. The double cordovan stitch is a complex stitch requiring good fine motor coordination. The whipstitch (answer A) is simpler and does not require the same level of coordination. Punching holes with the rotary punch (answer B) requires grip strength. Measuring and cutting the leather lacing (answer D) requires range of motion and gross motor coordination. See reference: Breines: Folkcraft.

136. (B) let the boy sit at the front of the bus and use his tape player and earphones. If the boy is seated in the front of the bus, he will experience less jostling by peers, so that he will have less tactile and visual stimulation to deal with. Also, the earphones will serve to reduce auditory overload. The method described in answer A is the only one that addresses the underlying problem of the boy's low tolerance for sensory stimulation. Answers A, C, and D are behavioral management techniques that do not take his hypersensitivity into account. See reference: Case-Smith, Allen, and Pratt (eds): Cronin, AS: Psychosocial and emotional domains of behavior.

137. (D) copper tooling. The liver of sulfate used to give a copper tooling project that antiqued look has a noxious odor and can irritate the eyes. There are no odors or fumes associated with acrylic paints (Answer A), ceramic paints (answer C) or leather tooling (answer B). See reference: Drake: Copper tooling and metal craft.

138. (B) seating Mr. G. upright on a firm surface with his chin slightly tucked. The best position for feeding an individual with a swallowing disorder is upright and symmetrical, with the chin slightly tucked. "Correct positioning normalizes tone, thereby facilitating quality motor control and function of the facial musculature, jaw and tongue movement, and the swallow process, all of which minimize the potential for aspiration" (p. 180). Supine, semi-reclined and side-lying positions all place Mr. G at greater risk for choking and aspiration (entry of food material into the airway). See reference: Pedretti (ed): Nelson, KL: Dysphagia: Evaluation and treatment.

139. (C) coping strategies for continuing medication compliance. Studies designed to determine the factors related to frequent re-admission for psychiatric individuals have found medication noncompliance to be the major reason for readmission. The other strategies listed may be important issues for specific individuals however they are not the primary issue. See reference: Early: Daily living skills.

140. (D) pressure marks or redness disappear after 20 minutes. All splints made or given to a patient are checked for correct fit by adjusting any areas that still have redness or pressure marks after the splint has been removed for 20 minutes. Many types of splints may be made with the fingers not flexed or the thumb opposed and abducted (answers A and B), for example, an antispasticity ball splint or a dynamic splint for extension. Most splints are not worn at all times (answer C) but removed for activities such as self-care or exercise. A wearing schedule is issued when a splint is fitted or given to a patient. See reference: Ryan (ed): Schober-Branigan, P: Thermoplastic splinting of the hand. *The Certified Occupational Therapy Assistant.*

141. (C) pouring a glass of orange juice. Meal preparation is graded from cold to hot foods or beverages, and from simple to multiple steps. An individual beginning meal preparation training should start with a cold item involving the least number of steps possible, such as pouring a glass of juice or other cold beverage. Cold sandwich preparation (answer A) adds another step as each topping to the bread is added and as the use of utensils is introduced. After preparation of cold items has been mastered, training in hot food or beverage preparation (answers B and D) may be initiated. See reference: Kovich and Bermann (eds): Van Dam-Burke, A, and Kovich, K: Self-care and homemaking.

142. (B) flaccidity. Flaccidity, or hypotonicity, is often present initially following a stroke, and may later change to spasticity (answer D), or increased muscle tone. The flaccid extremity feels heavy and hangs limply at the individual's side. The weight of the arm may eventually pull the humerus out of the glenohumeral joint, resulting in subluxation (answer C). Paralysis (answer A) may be accompanied by either flaccidity or spasticity, and is not an adequate answer. See reference: Pedretti (ed): Undzis, MF, Zoltan, B and Pedretti, LW: Evaluation of motor control.

143. (A) project group. Project groups should focus on short-term tasks in which the group participants are expected to demonstrate some interaction and sharing. Groups in answers B, C, and D involve more interaction among the members and longer-term tasks and feature less involvement by the COTA. See reference: Ryan (ed): Blechert, TF, and Kari, N: Interpersonal communication skills and applied group dynamics. *The Certified Occupational Therapy Assistant.*

144. (D) Present only a few blocks at a time. Like other children with his diagnosis, Cesar has poor impulse control and has great difficulty completing a task. By presenting a few blocks at a time, the COTA can help Cesar focus on a few relevant stimuli and make it possible for him to complete a short-term task successfully. This experience will then help him increase his attention span. The use of soft foam blocks (answer A) can help prevent injury if thrown, but is not essential in increasing his attention span. Providing blocks of only one color (answer B) may reduce visual stimulation somewhat and using interlocking blocks (answer C) may make manipulation of the pieces easier, but the presentation of the full amount of blocks all at once would still be perceived as overwhelming to Cesar. See reference: Case-Smith, Allen, and Pratt (eds): Cronin, AS: Psychosocial and emotional domains of behavior.

145. (A) index and middle fingers; place your thumb on the child's cheek." The correct position of the adult's hand for jaw control when feeding the child from the side is as described in answer A. Answers B and D are incorrect, because the thumb should be placed on the cheek to provide jaw stability. Answer C is incorrect, because controlling the child's jaw movement with the adult's whole hand provides less control of the child's jaw than the recommended method. Placing the adult's thumb on the ear (answer D) is also incorrect, because it would create discomfort for the child; in addition, thumb placement should be near the fulcrum of jaw movement (temporomandibular joint). When the child is fed from the front, the adult's thumb should be placed on the chin and the middle finger should be placed under the chin to control opening and closing of the jaw. The index finger then rests on the side of the child's face to provide stability. See reference: Case-Smith, Allen, and Pratt (eds): Parham, LD, and Mailloux, Z: Sensory integration.

146. (C) Pencil gripper. These are all adaptive devices that can be used with a child who has juvenile rheumatoid arthritis for various reasons. However, the correct answer is C, because the pencil gripper will probably make grasping the pencil easier and reduce hand grasp fatigue. Because of weak hands, and because printing and handwriting is a common task for children this age, it is important that fatigue be reduced. The reacher (answer A) is not correct because it frequently requires grip strength, although it is an important piece of equipment for children who have problems with extended reach. The jar opener (answer B) is not incorrect in terms of its adaptation for hand-strength problems, but jar opening is not a task frequently performed by a school-aged child (as is handwriting). The plate guard (answer C) will provide adaptation for incoordination, one-handedness, and limitations in hand/arm function but is not particularly necessary when hand strength is decreased (adapting the utensil would be more reasonable). See reference: Case-Smith, Allen, and Pratt (eds): Gordon, CY, Schanzenbacher, KE, Case-Smith, J, and Carrasco, R: Diagnostic problems in pediatrics.

147. (B) The COTA asks members of a small group to draw pictures of themselves on a piece of paper. The COTA then leads a discussion about body-image concerns and links the discussion to the group members' drawings. Adapting the activity procedures allows the COTA to use one activity to address different treatment goals. Selecting an activity appropriate for eating disorders is based on a primary problem focus for this population—body image distortions. Only answer B focuses on this problem area. Answer A focuses on cognitive deficits; answer C focuses on family dynamics; and answer D is an assessment task from the BAFPE. See reference: Denton: Treatment planning and implementation.

148. (B) examining an analysis of the individual's job. The job analysis is a detailed description of the physical, sensory, and psychological demands of a job. Examples of performance requirements include tasks such as lifting, walking, sitting, standing, and reaching, as well as seeing and hearing and interpersonal skills. Interviewing the individual (answer B) is useful to obtain information about his or her perception of the injury, motivation for returning to work, and sense of responsibility for rehabilitation. However, the worker may not be able to give an objective, detailed, and concise analysis of the job. The Dictionary of Occupational Titles (answer C) provides generic job descriptions but does not contain as much specific information as a job analysis. A physician (answer D) is unlikely to have the depth of information necessary or the time available to provide the necessary information. See reference: Pedretti (ed): Burt, CM, and Smith, P: Work evaluation and work hardening.

149. (A) ease the patient onto the floor, cushioning his fall. Proper body mechanics must be used when transferring patients. No one should "attempt a transfer that seems unmanageable because of the discrepancy between the patient's size and her own or because of the patient's level of dependency (p. 294)." Attempting to continue or reverse the transfer of an obese patient who has already begun to slip (answers B and C) is likely to result in injury to the COTA and perhaps to the patient as well. Once the patient has started to slip, the COTA should begin easing him to the floor immediately. Although calling for assistance is an appropriate action, the higher-priority action is to begin easing the patient to the floor to prevent injury to the individuals involved. See reference: Trombly (ed): Retraining basic and instrumental activities of daily living.

150. (B) allow the chin to remain tucked when drinking. Tucking the chin toward the chest maximizes airway protection for individuals with dysphagia. Methods the caregiver can use to control or slow the rate of liquid intake for individuals who demonstrate poor judgment or impulsivity (answers A and C) include using a drinking spout with a small opening, pinching a straw, or using a vacuum feeding cup with a control button. Plastic cups and plastic coated utensils are best for individual's with a bite reflex (answer D) to prevent damage to their oral structures. See reference: Trombly (ed): Konosky, KA: Dysphagia.

151. (A) remove all throw or scatter rugs. Whether an individual with instability during walking uses a walker, cane, or no equipment, the floor should be cleared of any obstacles that may cause slipping or tripping. Scatter or throw rugs may catch on a person's foot or the tip of an assistive device, resulting in a fall. Alternatively, rugs can be firmly taped down or secured with nonskid backing. Installing lever handles, a ramp, or a handheld shower (answers B, C, and D) would make certain tasks easier for this individual but would not be necessary for safety. See reference: Ryan (ed): Gower, D, and Bowker, M: The elderly with a hip arthroplasty. *Practice Issues in Occupational Therapy.*

152. (A) consistently obtain the same results as a competent practitioner performing the same procedure. The term "service competency" indicates an interrater reliability between two OT practitioners. Service competency is achieved or demonstrated through passing the certification examination (answer B). Continuing education and experience (answers C and D) may contribute to the development of service competency but do not guarantee competence. See reference: Early: Data gathering and evaluation.

153. (B) a class about job seeking strategies. The purpose of applying remedial strategies is to enhance underlying abilities. Teaching and training methods are commonly used techniques. Answer A, the NPI Interest Checklist, is a tool used to identify the degree of an individual's interest in a variety of leisure areas. Answer C is an example of a compensatory strategy. Answer D provides opportunities for exploration and expression. See reference: Early: Cognitive and sensorimotor activities.

154. (B) provision of foot support. This is probably the first concern of the therapist, in order for the child to feel secure on the toilet and to be positioned for bowel control. Answer A is not correct since management of fasteners can be developed later, after positioning for stability has been achieved. Answer C is not correct because provision of a seat belt may not be necessary if foot support (or back support) is provided. Answer D is not correct because climbing onto the toilet independently may be developed later (as it occurs with normal developmental progression). See reference: Case-Smith, Allen, and Pratt (eds): Shepherd, J, Procter, SA, and Coley, IL: Self care and adaptations for independent living.

155. (A) a canister vacuum cleaner. A canister vacuum cleaner may be managed by someone with weakness and impaired balance while sitting down. The hose is light enough to be easily pushed, and the canister is on wheels and may be moved by a seated person by pushing it with the foot or having someone else move it. An upright vacuum cleaner (answer B) is too heavy for repetitive pushing and pulling and can cause exhaustion or pull the individual off balance. A self-propelled vacuum cleaner (answer C) could also pull the individual off balance by moving too fast for the individual to respond with appropriate postural adjustments. A hand-held vacuum cleaner (answer D) requires too much stooping to do anything but a very small area of the floor. Repetitive bending can cause fatigue quickly and challenges impaired balance. See reference: Trombly (ed): Stewart, C: Retraining housekeeping and child care skills.

156. (C) stand at a high table while working on a puzzle for increasing amounts of time each day. To increase standing tolerance, or endurance, the cashier needs to stand for progressively longer periods of time each day. Answer A would be appropriate for an individual with a back injury who needs to improve his ability to lift. Answer B would be appropriate for an individual who needs to increase the distance he is able to walk. Answer D would be appropriate for an individual who needs to increase lower extremity strength. See reference: Pedretti (ed): Pedretti, LW and Wade, IE: Therapeutic modalities.

157. (D) quotes from the individual. SOAP is an acronym for Subjective, Objective, Assessment, and Plan. The SOAP format is a common format in the medical fields for documentation. The subjective portion of the SOAP note contains information found in the chart provided by the patient or family. Measurement results (answer A) are based on a patient's performance during the evaluation and are included in the objective section. Answer B, analysis of the measurements, is recorded in the assessment area of the SOAP note. Speculative information (answer C) should not be included in documentation. See reference: Hopkins and Smith (eds): Perinchief, JM: Service management.

158. (C) skilled nursing facilities. The largest number of certified occupational therapy assistants (42.2%) work in skilled nursing facilities. School systems are next with 14%. Rehabilitation hospitals employ 9.3% and psychiatric hospitals 1.8%. See reference: AOTA: 1996 Member data survey.

159. (A) partial hospitalization. Partial hospitalization is appropriate for individuals who are experiencing acute psychiatric symptoms and who have a place or family to stay with at night. Partial hospitalization offers most of the structure, staffing, and services available on an inpatient unit except for overnight provisions. Day treatment (answer C) focuses on assisting individuals to adapt to their illness and develop daily living skills at the program site. Day treatment services are typically verbal activities and group therapy within a 3- to 6-month period. Day care (answer B) is long term care that provides structured daily activities and medications to maintain current levels of functioning. Community mental health centers (answer D) provide a wide range of individual and outpatient services that address a variety of individual goals. See reference: Hopkins and Smith (eds): Richert, GZ, and Gibson, D: Practice settings.

160. (C) CVA/hemiplegia. A 1996 study completed by the American Occupational Therapy Association revealed that the diagnosis most frequently being treated by COTAs was CVA/hemiplegia. The second most commonly seen diagnosis was fractures (11.6%). This was followed by developmental delay (8.6%) and learning disabilities at (4.7%). See reference: AOTA: 1996 Member data survey.

161. (C) IEP. The individual education plan is a form that must be completed for children receiving services in the school system. This documentation standard was defined in the Education of the Handicapped Act (1975 and 1986). The UB-82 form (answer A), is used to process insurance claims. FIM (answer B), which stands for "functional independence measure" is a method used on rehabilitation units to measure an individual's level of independence. The HCFA-1500 form (answer D) is used to bill Medicare and other insurance carriers for health care services. See reference: Hopkins and Smith (eds): Perinchief, JM: Service management.

162. (C) lordosis. Lordosis, a concave posterior curvature of the spine, is a result of excessive anterior pelvic tilt. Scoliosis (answer B) is a result of a lateral curve of the vertebral column and is unaffected by anterior pelvic tilt. Kyphosis (answer D), a concave anterior curvature of the spine, may develop in response to exaggerated lordosis. Stenosis (answer A) is a disease of the spine resulting in narrowing of the spinal column. See reference: Norkin and Levangie: The vertebral column.

163. (A) remotivation. Remotivation approaches are used to encourage the expression of thoughts and feelings related to intact long-term memories. The topic should be linked to past experiences that are easy to understand. Reality orientation (answer B) is designed to maintain or improve awareness of time, situation, and place. Compensatory strategies (answer C) are appropriate when cognitive impairment is not expected to improve. Environmental modification (answer D) is a type of compensatory strategy. See reference: Early: Cognitive and sensorimotor activities.

164. (C) Doffing socks. Answer C is correct because, according to most developmental scales, children first learn to remove garments, especially socks. Answer A is not correct, because the ability to don garments with the front and back correctly placed is a skill that is developed later. Buttoning and tying bows (answer D) is incorrect for the same reason. Answer B is incorrect, because children are able to remove garments before they are able to put them on. See reference: Case-Smith, Allen, and Pratt (eds): Shepherd, J, Procter, SA, and Coley, IL: Self-care and adaptations for independent living.

165. (B) federal and state governmental agencies and third-party payers. AOTA (included in answers A, C, and D) does not require physician referral for the provision of OT services. Federal, state, and local governmental agencies, third-party payers, regulatory and state agencies, and individual facilities may require physician referral. See reference: AOTA: Statement of occupational therapy referral.

166. (A) playing "Whisper Down the Lane." When working with the individual with paranoid ideation, it is important to select structured activities that use "controllable" materials. Answers B, C, and D all meet this criterion. The game "Whisper Down the Lane" involves whispering, and the paranoid individual is likely to believe the other players are talking, or whispering, about her. See reference: Early: Responding to symptoms and behaviors.

167. (D) swivel spoon. A swivel spoon allows the head of the spoon to rotate as the individual moves the handle into varying positions, thus compensating for poor supination. An individual who is unable to reach her mouth because of limitations in shoulder or elbow flexion would benefit from a spoon with an elongated handle (answer A). An individual who is unable to hold a spoon because of difficulty with grasp would benefit from a spoon with a built-up handle (answer C). A spork (answer B) is helpful for those who need to use one utensil as both fork and spoon. See reference: Hopkins and Smith (eds): Kohlmeyer, KM: Assistive and adaptive equipment.

168. (D) use dust mitt to keep fingers fully extended. Using dust mitts "keeps fingers straight and prevents the static contraction and potentially deforming forces of holding a dust cloth." Pushing the vacuum (answer A) forward by straightening the elbow completely, then pulling it back close to the body uses *long* strokes and promotes good elbow and shoulder range of motion. When ironing (answer B), trying to get the elbow into full *extension* helps to maintain elbow range of motion. Keeping lightweight objects (answer C) on *high* shelves encourages reaching, which helps maintain shoulder range of motion. See reference: Pedretti (ed): Hittle, JM, Pedretti, LW, and Kasch, MC: Rheumatoid arthritis.

169. (A) her goals have been met and she can no longer benefit from OT services. Discontinuation of occupational therapy should occur when an individual has met her goals, and/or further progress is not anticipated within the therapeutic environment. Frequently, the individual's goals have been met but the individual could benefit from continued services (answer C). In this situation, new goals are established and intervention continues since further progress is anticipated. If the individual's goals have not been met and she could benefit from continued services (answer B), therapy would continue until goals are achieved. Depending on an individuals status at discharge, recommendations may be made for community services, outpatient care, day care, or home health services. A vital role of the occupational therapy practitioner is to provide appropriate linkages to the community for those individuals served. The preparation for discharge planning should include the patient's support system, discharge environment, and possible need for continued health care services. Discharge of an individual should be made based on objective information. If an individual does not "feel" that they are making progress (answer D), the COTA needs to clarify with the individual her status based on objective measurements and observations. See reference: Reed and Sanderson: Direct service functions.

170. (B) universal precautions. Health care personnel are to follow universal precautions when blood or certain body fluids are present. OSHA has identified materials that require universal precautions to be blood, semen, vaginal secretions, cerebrospinal fluid, synovial fluid, pleural fluid, pericaridal fluid, pertoneal fluid, amniotic fluid, any body fluid with visible blood, any unidentifiable body fluid and saliva from dental procedures. Suicidal, escape and medical precautions are guidelines developed for individuals identified with those risks which are not noted in this question. See reference: Occupational Safety and Health Administration.

171. (B) confront the individual's behavior: "Are you aware that your frequent interruptions prevent others from having a chance to contribute?" In general, the group leader should try A, C, or D before confronting the individual who is monopolizing. Confrontation within a group setting is difficult for many individuals to accept. See reference: Posthuma: What to do if....

172. (C) Acute care hospitalization. The emphasis of acute care hospitalization is on symptom reduction, medications, and discharge planning. The club house format (answer A) emphasizes belonging and security. Community mental health centers (answer B) focus on medication management, crisis intervention and outpatient therapy. Quarterway houses (answer D) emphasize increasing autonomy and decreasing supervision. See reference: Hopkins and Smith (eds): Richert, GZ, and Gibson, D: Practice settings.

173. (B) activity adaptation. Modifying how directions are provided is one way to adapt activities. Activity analysis (answer A) is the process of identifying the aspects, steps, and materials used in performing the activity. Grading activities (answer C) is a gradual progression of steps toward a goal. Clinical reasoning (answer D) is the problem-solving process that practitioners use in thinking about a client's treatment. See reference: Early: Analyzing, adapting, and grading activities.

174. (C) wheeling efficiency. Answer C is correct because the light weight of this type of wheelchair allows the child with weakness to be independent for longer periods of time. This type of chair is also easier for parents to handle when lifting it in and out of a car. Answer A is not correct because the removable armrest wheelchair feature is helpful in sliding transfers. Answer B is not correct because the desk arm feature allows children to sit closer to tables for school work and other table-top activities.

Answer D is not correct because it is the adjustable arm rest feature that allows adjustment for varying heights of lap trays or work surfaces. See reference: Case-Smith, Allen, and Pratt (eds): Wright-Ott, C, and Egilson, S: Mobility.

175. (B) bingo. Luck is the key element in games of chance. Bingo is a game that uses chance in calling out numbers randomly. Baseball card collecting (answer A) is considered to be a hobby versus a game. Charades and balloon volleyball (answers C and D) are strategy and skill-based games. See reference: Early: Leisure skills.

176. (B) capitation. Capitation is a uniform payment or fee per diagnosis. This form of reimbursement has evolved with healthcare reform. Fee for service (answer A) is an outdated model, in which health care providers were paid what they billed. This type of system allowed for various forms of abuse in the healthcare system. Cost shifting (answer C) occurs when a facility increases prices for all individuals who need service to cover the shortfalls in reimbursement by some of the carriers. Cost control (answer D) is the strategy that focuses on keeping the expenses below the revenue generated. See reference: Bair and Gray (eds): Scott, SJ and Somers, FP: Payment for occupational therapy services.

177. (A) prepare a tossed salad, make garlic bread, make spaghetti sauce and meatballs. Grading should progress from simple to complex. Using the oven is more complex than using the stove, which is more complex than preparing cold food. Making spaghetti sauce is a complex task which involves making meatballs, frying them, cutting and sautéing vegetables, opening cans and jars, and combining ingredients in a large pot. Making garlic bread requires fewer steps and could be done with a toaster oven. Preparing a tossed salad involves no cooking at all, and is the most simple task in the sequence. In answer B, making a grilled cheese sandwich is more complex than making instant pudding and should be last in the sequence. In answer C, broiling a steak is the most complex of the three tasks and should be last in the sequence. In answer D, scrambling eggs is the most complex task, and should be last. See reference: Boserup (ed): A kitchen training program as an occupational therapy activity.

178. (A) Complete independence with self-care and transfers. An individual with T3 (or lower) paraplegia will have the trunk balance and upper extremity strength and coordination to complete self-care and work activities independently. See reference: Trombly (ed): Hollar, LD: Spinal cord injury.

179. (D) clinical reasoning. Clinical reasoning is the problem solving process that OT practitioners use in thinking about an individual's treatment. Modifying how directions are provided, such as using demonstration rather than verbal instruction, is an example of activity adaptation (answer B). Activity analysis (answer A) is the process of identifying the aspects, steps and the materials used in performing the activity. Grading activities (answer C) is a gradual progression of steps toward a goal. See reference: Early: Analyzing, adapting, and grading activities.

180. (B) whether the program allows the "teacher," i.e., the COTA, to adjust the number, type, and frequency of attempts the individual can make to use the program. The use of computer applications within psychosocial settings should be linked to the overall goals of treatment. In the treatment of behavioral disorders, behavior management and reinforcement are overall goals. Answer B includes the software features that best enable the COTA to grade and adapt reinforcement. Answers A and C are criteria that are important for individuals with social-skill deficits. Noncompetitive games (answer D) are appropriate for individuals with paranoia. See reference: Hopkins and Smith (eds): Simon, CJ: Use of activity and activity analysis.

181. (B) wearing permanent press clothing. Using a wrinkle-resistant fabric eliminates or decreases the amount of ironing needed. The side-loading washer (answer A) is an example of household equipment adapted to eliminate excessive reaching from a wheelchair. An extended-handle dustpan (answer C) eliminates bending or stooping from a standing or sitting position. Neither the dustpan nor the washer, however, eliminates or reduces the amount of work needed for the tasks. Good body mechanics (answer D) are necessary to protect or maintain physical health, but they do not eliminate or reduce the amount of work either. See reference: Trombly (ed): Retraining basic and instrumental activities of daily living.

182. (D) adapted teaching techniques. Answer D is correct, because a child with this type of disability will characteristically have learning problems that require such teaching methods as "chaining" or behavior modification. Answers A, B, and C are of secondary importance, because physical coordination may be impaired, or other physical limitations such as abnormal muscle tone or significant problems with balance could also be present. These additional problems may require adaptive equipment, clothing, or techniques. However, all aspects of dressing are dependent on the child's ability to learn procedures of dressing, and therefore it is necessary to consider task analysis and teaching approach first. See reference: Case-Smith, Allen, and Pratt (eds): Wright-Ott, C, and Egilson, S: Mobility.

183. (D) a weighted pen and weighted wrists. Weighting body parts and utensils (or writing tools) is effective with individuals with ataxia in improving control during performance of a task. Hitting the keys on a keyboard (answer A) would be difficult for Carolyn, although weighting her wrists could make performance of the activity possible. A keyboard is a good alternative for individuals with difficulty writing due to weakness, limited ROM, or incoordination. A universal cuff with a pencil-holder attachment (answer B) would be appropriate for an individual with hand weakness who uses a universal cuff for other tasks. A balanced forearm orthosis (answer C) is appropriate for individuals with severe muscle weakness. In addition, individuals with muscle weakness find felt-tip pens easier to write with than ballpoint pens. See reference: Pedretti (ed): Schlageter, K, and Zoltan, B: Traumatic brain injury.

184. (C) to both sides of the body. Answer C is correct because the individual will need to be able to transfer to both sides of her body at home. Layouts of many home fixtures do not lend themselves to transferring the individual only from one side. If the transfers are not practiced to both sides, the individual may find it easy to transfer to the commode, but not from the commode. The family also needs to know the differences in the way the individual is handled, with more or less support. Thus, answers (A) to the unaffected side, (B) to the affected side and (D) to the side the commode will be approached, are all incorrect because they all involve transfer to only one side. See reference: Trombly (ed): Retraining basic and instrumental activities of daily living.

185. (A) baking brownies. Progressive levels of meal preparation include: access a prepared meal; prepare a cold meal; prepare a hot beverage, soup, or prepared dish; prepare a hot one-dish meal; and prepare a hot multi-dish meal. Making a fresh fruit salad (answer D) is a less challenging activity because no cooking is involved. While both involve heating an item, preparing toast (answer C) is more simple than heating soup because opening a plastic bag is a less complex task than opening a can. Baking brownies (answer A) is slightly more complex because of the progression from stove top to oven and the addition of several ingredients that need to be mixed. Therefore, this would be the appropriate upgrade. Making an apple pie (answer B) involves a higher level of task performance and complexity than brownies, and would be an appropriate task after the individual demonstrates competence in the less complex task of baking brownies. See reference: Hopkins and Smith (eds): Culler, KH: Home and family management.

186. (A) apply the stimuli beginning at an area distal to the lesion progressing proximally. The general guidelines for sensation testing are that the person's vision should be occluded, the stimuli should be randomly applied with false stimuli intermingled (opposite of answer C), a practice trial should be performed before the test, and the unaffected side or area should be tested before the affected side or area (opposite of answer B). Also, the tested individual should be given a specified amount of time in which to respond; therefore, answer D is incorrect. See reference: Trombly (ed): Bentzel, K: Evaluation of sensation.

187. (D) unclamp the individual's catheter and tap over the bladder. The individual is suffering from a condition called autonomic dysreflexia. If not promptly addressed, death may result. This condition may be caused by a bowel impaction, plugged catheter, or suppository insertion. Do not recline the individual in that this may result in a higher cerebral blood pressure. The condition must be treated promptly so taking a heart rate and blood pressure postpone action on the condition. A drop in blood sugar is usually associated with diabetes which is counteracted by having the individual consume fruit juice to raise the blood sugar level. Autonomic dysreflexia causes the blood pressure to increase to dangerous levels, so no actions should be performed to the individual which would cause the blood pressure to rise. See reference: Trombly (ed): Hollar, LD: Spinal cord injury.

188. (D) attached to a cuff that fits around his palm. Individuals with C6 quadriplegia may have a tenodesis grasp or no grasp at all available to them. Therefore, a buttonhook that fits onto the palm or a buttonhook with a built-up handle are the only appropriate choices. A buttonhook with a knob handle (answer B) or on a 1/2-inch dowel (answer C) is appropriate for an individual with a functional grasp but limited dexterity. A buttonhook with an extra-long, flexible handle benefits an individual with limited range of motion. See reference: Trombly (ed): Retraining basic and instrumental activities of daily living.

189. (D) discuss her concerns with an OTR who is present. Although her own supervisor is absent, an OTR present would become the acting supervisor for the COTA for the day. The COTA should always discuss concerns with the supervisor first. Going to the administration (answer C) would not only disregard the chain of command, but could escalate a problem that should be handled internally. ADL training is a skilled service beyond the scope of what an aide can do. The COTA should not allow the aide to finish the treatment session (answer A). It may not be feasible in a busy department for the COTA to complete the session herself (answer B). See reference: Early: Supervision.

190. (A) setting up or cleaning up treatment activities. Aides are noncredentialed personnel who are delegated routine nonskilled tasks. Answers B, C, and D require skill and judgment to complete the task. See reference: Ryan (ed): Ryan, SE: COTA supervision. *Practice Issues in Occupational Therapy.*

191. (C) "You sound like things are looking pretty bad to you right now." This is an example of paraphrasing the patient's comment. This type of response conveys to the patient that you understood what he says and that you are listening to him. Answers A, B, and D are examples of well-meaning but poorly designed responses. Answer A may give him false hope. Answer B may imply his concerns are trivial and can be soothed away with idle chit-chat. Answer D may imply that the COTA knows more than the patient does about the types of things that will make his life meaningful. See reference: Denton, PL: Effective communication.

192. (B) flexed at all joints. When weight bearing, the fingers should be flexed at all joints (the fisted position). This preserves the tenodesis function by protecting the finger flexors from over-stretching, which could result if fingers are positioned as described in answers A, C, and D. Another reason for this position is to prevent claw-hand deformity by protecting the intrinsic hand muscles from over-stretching. See reference: Hill (ed): Farmer, A: Setting goals.

193. (C) swing away leg rests, removable arm rests. After swinging away the leg rests and removing the armrests, the individual can move across the sliding board without being blocked by the wheelchair. Answers A and B are incorrect because they would not facilitate a sliding board transfer. Answer D is incorrect because a removable arm rest may make transfers easier, but elevating leg rest would not. A leg rest would need to be detachable or swing away in order for it to be moved out of the way. See reference: Pedretti (ed): Adler, C and Tipton-Burton, M: Wheelchair assessment and transfers.

194. (B) high contrast and defined borders. Answer B is correct because it provides the only combination of features when adapting visual material which will assist the child with visual discrimination problems. High contrast of the stimuli (shape, letter, numbers, etc.) in relation to the background, and defining important areas of the stimuli with a border will attract the eye and provide clear input. Answer A is incorrect because low contrast of the stimuli, such as blue ditto lettering, is difficult to discriminate. Answer D is incorrect because undefined borders around the important stimuli makes for less clear input. Answer D is incorrect because both features of the visual stimulus would make it difficulty to discriminate. See reference: Kramer and Hinojosa (eds): Todd, VR: Visual perceptual frame of reference: An information processing approach.

195. (C) applying grout to a tile trivet and waiting for it to dry. Activities provide a variety of opportunities for therapeutic gains. The process of grouting a tile trivet involves covering the individual's tile design with the grout mixture, which is a messy step. The individual then sees that the tile pattern is emphasized with the addition of the grout. Waiting for the grout to dry requires an individual to delay gratification. Working in a group (answer A) promotes cooperation. Selecting a tile design (answer B) involves decision making. Cleaning off the table (answer D) may promote the experience of success after a mess but does not involve delayed gratification. See reference: Hopkins and Smith (eds): Simon, CJ: Use of activity and activity analysis.

196. (A) slip a piece of cylindrical foam onto the fork handle. The criteria for selecting adaptive equipment include effectiveness, affordability, operability, and dependability. For this assessment, the COTA needs something fast and inexpensive; durability is not an issue because this is not a permanent piece of equipment. A cylindrical foam handle meets these criteria. Thermoplastic material (answer B) is easy to clean and durable, but it is expensive and takes more time to fabricate. Adhesive-backed foam (answer C) is expensive and difficult to clean, and once it is attached to a fork it is difficult to remove. It is not a good idea to use plastic forks (answer D) for feeding evaluations because they are easily broken, although wrapping a washcloth around a fork handle is quick and inexpensive, easily washable, and appropriate for a temporary need. See reference: Hopkins and Smith (eds): Kohlmeyer, KM: Assistive and adaptive equipment.

197. (C) frequent handwashing. Hands should be washed at specified times during the day, including before and after patient treatment, before and after removing gloves, and before eating or preparing food, to name a few. Specific handwashing procedures have been developed and should be followed. Gloves (answer A), masks, and gowns (answers B and D) are examples of protective barriers to be worn when encountering bodily fluids, but handwashing is the primary and most effective method used. See reference: Early: Safety techniques.

198. (C) Requiring moderate assistance. Requiring moderate assistance is defined as having the ability to complete the task with supervision and cueing while requiring physical assistance for 20 to 50 percent of the task. The individual who requires minimal assistance (answer A) is able to complete a task with supervision and cueing while requiring physical assistance for less than 20 percent of the task. An individual who needs supervision, cueing, and physical assistance for from 50 to 80 percent of the task is performing at the maximal assistance level (answer D). An individual is rated dependent (answer A) when he or she is able to perform less than 20 percent, or a few steps, of the activity independently. This individual may require elaborate equipment, may perform the activity extremely slowly, and may fatigue easily. See reference: Pedretti (ed): Foti, D, Pedretti, LW, and Lillie, S: Activities of daily living.

199. (B) NPI Interest Checklist. This tool is frequently used to initiate discussion of how a patient usually spends his leisure time and to identify areas of specific interest. While the KELS and the Scorable Self-Care Evaluation (answers A and D) address the use of leisure time, they are used primarily to assess skills in personal care, safety and health, money management, transportation, use of the telephone, and work. The Activity Configuration (answer C) is used to assess the patient's use of time and his feelings about all of the activities he performs in a typical day or week. See reference: Early: Data gathering and evaluation.

200. (C) provide enjoyable activities in a safe and accepting environment. Answer C is correct because children who learn to enjoy activities alone will be more likely to cooperate with peers in a group activity. Answer A is not correct because the child will not initiate and develop social interaction in an environment that inhibits independence (such as an authoritarian environment). Answer B is not correct because children with peer interaction problems will need to be taught some basic social skills in order to increase peer interaction. Answer D is not correct because the children will more likely learn and accept rules and limits established by their group. See reference: Kramer and Hinojosa (eds): Olson, L: Psychosocial frame of reference.

BIBLIOGRAPHY

American Occupational Therapy Association, Inc: 1996 Member Data Survey. American Occupational Therapy Association, Rockville, MD.

American Occupational Therapy Association, Inc: Commission on Standards and Ethics: Enforcement procedure for the occupational therapy code of ethics. Am J Occup Ther 50:848-852, 1996.

American Occupational Therapy Association, Inc: Essentials and guidelines for an accredited educational program for the occupational therapy assistant. Am J Occup Ther 45:1085-1092, 1991.

American Occupational Therapy Association, Inc: Guide To Fieldwork Education. American Occupational Therapy Association, Rockville, MD, 1991.

American Occupational Therapy Association, Inc: Commission on Standards and Ethics: Occupational therapy code of ethics. Am J Occup Ther 48:1037-1038, 1994.

American Occupational Therapy Association, Inc: Intercommission Council: Occupational Therapy Roles. Am J Occup Ther 47:1087-1099, 1993.

American Occupational Therapy Association, Inc: Policy: Registered Occupational therapists and certified occupational therapy assistants and modalities. Am J Occup Ther 45:1112-1113, 1991.

American Occupational Therapy Association, Inc: Position Paper: Use of occupational therapy aides in occupational therapy practice. Am J Occup Ther 49:1023-1025, 1995.

American Occupational Therapy Association, Inc: Commission on Practice: Standards of practice for occupational therapy: Am J Occup Ther 48:1039-1043, 1994.

American Occupational Therapy Association, Inc: Statement Of Occupational Therapy Referral. Am J Occup Ther 48:1034-1035, 1994.

American Occupational Therapy Association, Inc: Statement: The role of occupational therapy in the independent living movement. Am J Occup Ther 47:1079-1080, 1993.

American Occupational Therapy Association, Inc: Commission on Practice: Guide for supervision of occupational therapy personnel. Am J Occup Ther 48:1045-1046, 1994.

American Occupational Therapy Association, Inc: Terminology Task Force: Uniform terminology for occupational therapy - third edition. Am J Occup Ther 48:1047-1054, 1994.

American Occupational Therapy Association, Inc: Effective Documentation For Occupational Therapy. American Occupational Therapy Association, Rockville, MD, 1991.

Ayres, AJ: Sensory Integration and the Child. Western Psychological Services, Los Angeles, 1983.

Bailey, DM: Research and the Health Professional, ed 2. FA Davis, Philadelphia, 1997.

Bair, J and Gray, M (eds): The Occupational Therapy Manager. American Occupational Therapy Association, Rockville, MD, 1992.

Bonder, BR and Wagner, MB: Functional Performance in Older Adults. FA Davis, Philadelphia, 1994.

Boserup, E (ed): A Kitchen Training Program as an Occupational Therapy Activity. American Occupational Therapy Association, Rockville, MD, 1985.

Breines, EB: Occupational Therapy Activities From Clay to Computers. FA Davis, Philadelphia, 1995.

Case-Smith, J, Allen, AS, and Pratt, PN (eds): Occupational Therapy for Children, ed 3. CV Mosby, St. Louis, 1996.

Christiansen, C and Baum, C: Occupational Therapy: Overcoming Human Performance Deficits. Slack, Thorofare, NJ, 1991.

Church, G. and S. Glennen, The Handbook of Assistive Technology. Singular Publishing Group, San Diego, 1992.

Denton, PL: Psychiatric Occupational Therapy: A Workbook of Practical Skills. Little Brown, Boston, 1987.

Drake, MD: Crafts in Therapy and Rehabilitation. Slack, Thorofare, NJ, 1992.

Dunn, W: Pediatric Occupational Therapy. Slack, Thorofare, NJ, 1991.

Early, MB: Mental Heath Concepts and Techniques for the Occupational Therapy Assistant, ed 2. Raven Press, NY, 1993.

Erhardt:, RP: Developmental Hand Dysfunction: Theory, Assessment, Treatment. Tucson Therapy Builders, Tucson, 1989.

Finnie, NR: Handling the Young Cerebral Palsied Child at Home. JB Lippincott, NY, 1993.

Fisher, AG, Murray, EA, and Bundy, AC (eds): Sensory Integration: Theory and Practice, FA Davis, Philadelphia, 1991.

Gilfoyle, EM, Grady, AP and Moore, JC: Children Adapt. Slack, Thorofare, NJ, 1990.

Glickstein, JK: Therapeutic Interventions in Alzheimer's Disease: A Program of Functional Communication Skills for Daily Living. Aspen Publishers, Rockville, MD, 1988.

Hansen, RA and Atchison, B (eds): Conditions in Occupational Therapy. Williams and Wilkins, Baltimore, 1993.

Hemphill, BJ (ed): Mental Health Assessment in Occupational Therapy. Slack, Thorofare, NJ, 1988.

Hemphill, BJ, Peterson, CQ, and Werner, PC: Rehabilitation in Mental Health. Slack, Thorofare, NJ, 1991.

Hill, JP (ed): Spinal Cord Injury: A Guide to Functional Outcomes in Occupational Therapy. A Rehabilitation Institute of Chicago procedure manual. Aspen Publishers, Rockville, MD, 1988.

Hopkins, HL and Smith, HD (eds): Willard and Spackman's Occupational Therapy, ed 8, JB Lippincott, Philadelphia, 1993.

Howe, MC and Schwartzberg, SL: A Functional Approach to Group Work in Occupational Therapy., ed 2. JB Lippincott, Philadelphia, 1995.

Jacobs, K and Logigian, M: Functions of a Manager in Occupational Therapy, revised edition. Slack Incorporated, Thorfare, NJ, 1994.

Johnson, C, Lobdell, K, Nesbitt, J and Clare, M: Therapeutic rafts. Slack, Thorofare, NJ, 1996.

Kettenbach, G: Writing SOAP Notes, ed 2. FA Davis, Philadelphia, 1995.

Kovich, KM and Bermann, DE (eds): Head Injury: A Guide to Functional Outcomes in Occupational Therapy. A Rehabilitation Institute of Chicago procedure manual. Aspen Publishers, Rockville, MD, 1988.

Kramer, P and Hinojosa, J (eds): Frames of Reference for Pediatric Occupational Therapy. Williams and Wilkins, Baltimore, 1993.

Logigian, MK and Ward, JD, (eds): A Team approach for Therapists: Pediatric Rehabilitation. Little Brown, Boston, 1989.

National Board for Certification in Occupational Therapy: NBCOT 1997 Candidate Handbook. NBCOT, Gaithersburg, MD, 1996

Nelson, DL: Children with Autism. Slack, Thorofare, NJ, 1984.

Norkin, CC and Levangie, PK: Joint Structure and Function: A Comprehensive Analysis, ed 2. FA Davis, Philadelphia, 1992.

Norkin, CC and White, DJ: Measurement of Motion: A Guide to Goniometry, ed 2. FA Davis, Philadelphia, 1995.

Occupational Safety and Health Administration: Standard #1910. 1030, 61 FR 5507, February 13, 1996.

O'Sullivan, SB and Schmitz, TJ (eds): Physical Rehabilitation: Assessment and Treatment, ed 3. FA Davis, Philadelphia, 1994.

Palmer, ML and Toms, JE: Manual for Functional Training, ed 3. FA Davis, Philadelphia, 1992.

Pedretti, L (ed): Occupational Therapy: Practice Skills for Physical Dysfunction, ed 4. Mosby-Yearbook, St. Louis, 1996.

Posthuma, BW: Small Groups in Counseling Therapy: Process and Leadership, ed 2. Allyn and Bacon, Needham Heights, MA, 1996.

Punwar, AJ., Occupational Therapy Principles and Practice, ed 2. Williams and Wilkins, Baltimore, 1994.

Reed, KL and Sanderson, SN: Concepts of Occupational Therapy, ed 3. Williams and Wilkins, Baltimore, 1992.

Rothstein, JM, Roy, SH, and Wolf, SL: The Rehabilitation Specialist's Handbook. FA Davis, Philadelphia, 1991.

Ryan, SE (ed): Practice Issues in Occupational Therapy: Intraprofessional Team Building. Slack, Thorofare, NJ, 1993.

Ryan (ed): The Certified Occupational Therapy Assistant: Principles, Concepts and Techniques, ed 2. Slack, Thorofare, NJ, 1993.

Trombly, CA (ed): Occupational Therapy for Physical Dysfunction, ed 4. Williams and Wilkins, Baltimore, 1995.

Zoltan, B: Vision, Perception and Cognition: A Manual for the Evaluation and Treatment of the Neurologically Impaired Adult, ed 3. Slack Incorporated, Thorofare, NJ, 1996.